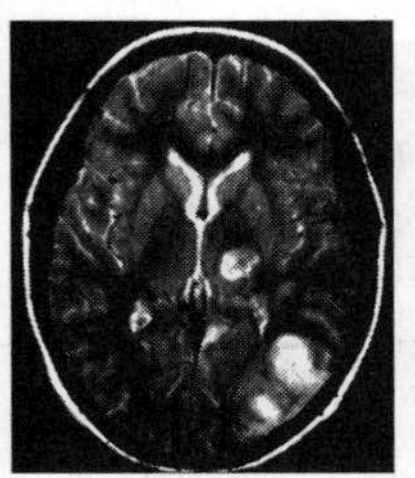

Vascular Neurology

Questions and Answers

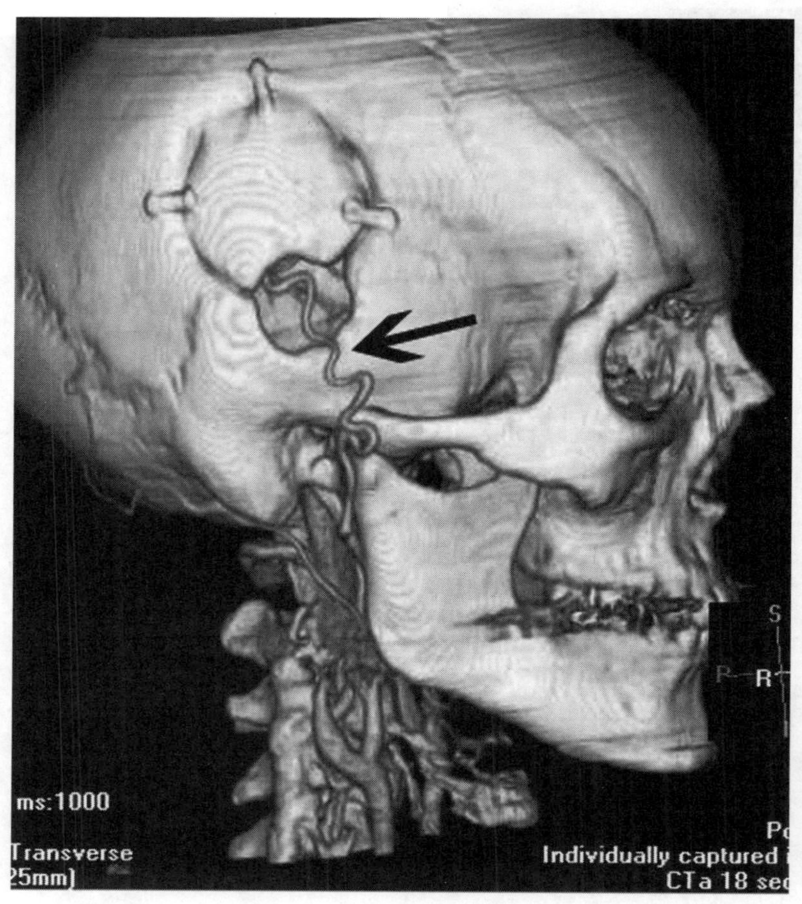

S
R
ms:1000
Transverse
25mm]
Individually captured i
CTa 18 sec

VASCULAR NEUROLOGY
QUESTIONS AND ANSWERS

Nancy Futrell, MD

Director
Intermountain Stroke Center
Salt Lake City, Utah

Dara G. Jamieson, MD

Associate Professor of Clinical Neurology
New York Presbyterian Hospital
Weill Medical College of Cornell University
New York, New York

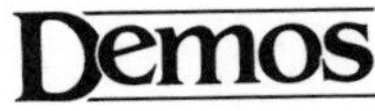

ACQUISITIONS EDITOR: R. Craig Percy
COVER DESIGN: A Good Thing
COPYEDITOR: Joann Woy
COMPOSITOR: Patricia Wallenburg
PRINTER: Transcontinental Printing

Visit our website at www.demosmedpub.com

LIBRARY OF CONGRESS CATALOGING-IN-PUBLICATION DATA
Futrell, Nancy.
Vascular neurology : questions and answers / Nancy Futrell, Dara G. Jamieson.
p. ; cm.
Includes bibliographical references and index.
ISBN-13: 978-1-933864-24-2 (pbk. : alk. paper)
ISBN-10: 1-933864-24-9 (pbk. : alk. paper)
1. Cerebrovascular disease—Examinations, questions, etc. 2. Neurology—Examinations, questions, etc. I. Jamieson, Dara G. II. Title.
[DNLM: 1. Cerebrovascular Accident—Examination Questions. 2. Neurology—Examination Questions. WL 18.2 F996v 2008]
RC388.5.F88 2008
616.8'10076—dc22

2007046823

MADE IN CANADA

08 09 10 5 4 3 2 1

CONTENTS

PREFACE

STROKE IS THE THIRD MOST COMMON CAUSE of death and disability in the US. It is a complex disease, with many causes, many presentations, and many levels of severity. Despite recent medical advances, stroke remains a difficult disease to diagnose and treat. In recognition of the importance of this common disorder, the American Board of Psychiatry and Neurology (ABPN) instituted a new subspecialty examination in 2005. According to the ABPN's website, this exam is intended "to officially establish the field of vascular neurology as a definite area of subspecialization in neurology and child neurology and to provide a means of identifying properly trained and experienced vascular neurologists."

Vascular Neurology: Questions and Answers, is intended to be a comprehensive study guide for the ABPN's vascular neurology subspecialty exam. In addition, this book can be used by any physician who wants to thoroughly and systematically review the topic of vascular neurology, self-assess his or her skills, or prepare for another examination that contains questions on this important topic.

While the ABPN's exam consists of 200 multiple-choice questions administered during a 4-hour period, *Vascular Neurology: Questions and Answers* contains over 500 multiple-choice questions, each with an answer, detailed explanation, and one or more references for further study and review as desired. We have included almost 100 illustrations (some in full color) keyed to many of the questions. The book is divided into chapters with questions providing detailed coverage of basic science, pharmacology, clinical stroke, hematology, cardiology, pediatrics, neuroimaging, neuropathology, and rehabilitation. All of these topics are important components to an in-depth understanding of the field, and all are important components of the ABPN's vascular neurology subspecialty examination.

Those readers who are preparing for the ABPN's exam are strongly encouraged to visit the ABPN website for information about, and requirements for, the exam: www.abpn.org. It is important to note that there will be a "grandfathering period" through 2009. During this time, Board-certified neurologists may apply to take the exam if they can provide documentation that they have "a minimum of 25% of practice time devoted to vascular neurology." After 2009, all applicants will need to have successfully completed a 1-year vascular neurology fellowship program.

Stroke is a topic of critical relevance to neurologists, cardiologists, emergency room physicians, internists, vascular and neurosurgeons, and physiatrists worldwide. While not intended to be an authoritative reference source, *Vascular Neurology: Questions and Answers* will provide these professionals with an excellent (and fun) resource that will enable them to test their knowledge, clinical skills, and exam-readiness in a relatively short period of time.

As with any book, the authors may learn the most. Developing questions in areas outside of neurology required gaining a higher level of understanding in some areas, such as fetal development of the heart and perinatal changes in circulation. The questions and answers contained in this book are designed to synthesize complex information into an easily understood format. As we wrote this book, each of us developed half of the questions and the other did a self-test with these questions. We found approaching the questions as a test, while comparing our answers with the correct answer, was fun and informative. We hope our readers will have the same experience.

For those using this book to prepare for the ABPN's vascular neurology subspecialty exam, we wish you luck. For those using this book as a means of better understanding this important topic, we wish you happy reading and learning.

Nancy Futrell, MD
Salt Lake City, Utah

Dara G. Jamieson, MD
New York, New York

ACKNOWLEDGMENTS

THE AUTHORS WISH TO THANK:

Ehud Lavi, MD, my husband, who encouraged me in the writing of this book and provided the neuropathology pictures.

— DJ

Clark Millikan, MD, my spouse and mentor in vascular neurology. The recognition of vascular neurology as a board certified specialty is the culmination of his lifetime work in establishing this field.

— NF

We would also like to thank NeuroLogica Corporation, Danvers, Massachusetts, for their generosity in making the color prints possible.

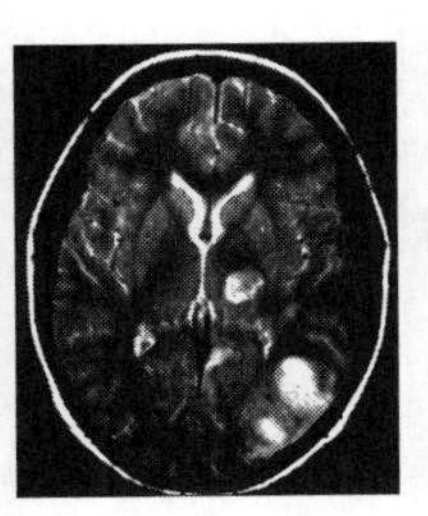

Vascular Neurology
Questions and Answers

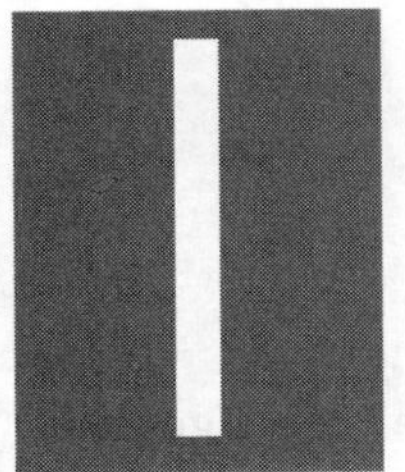

Basic Science Questions

1. The atherogenicity of lipoproteins is related to size. Which of the following statements is true?

A. The largest lipoproteins are the most atherogenic.
B. The smallest lipoproteins are the most atherogenic.
C. The intermediate sized lipoproteins are the most atherogenic.
D. The large- and intermediate-sized lipoproteins are most atherogenic.
E. The intermediate- and small-sized lipoproteins are most atherogenic.

2. The intimal layer of arteries is lined with endothelial cells and also contains:

A. Smooth muscle cells in humans and rodents.
B. Smooth muscle cells in humans, but not in rodents.
C. Extracellular matrix, but no smooth muscle cells in humans or animals.
D. Adipose cells.
E. T cells.

3. Which of the following substances is atherogenic?

A. Tissue factor.
B. Interferon-γ.
C. $CD4^+$ T cells.
D. Heat shock proteins.
E. All of the above.

4. Intimal thickening at arterial bifurcations:

A. Is present at birth.
B. Is present in infancy and childhood only in individuals at high risk for the development of diffuse atherosclerosis during adulthood.
C. Develops shortly after puberty.
D. Develops in early adulthood.
E. Develops in middle adulthood.

5. Fatty streaks in arteries:

A. Do not develop in the fetus.
B. Can be seen in the aorta in children.
C. Are composed of extracellular lipids.
D. Form most often in individuals who will eventually develop significant atherosclerosis.

6. The main regulator of blood pressure is:

A. The sympathetic nervous system.
B. The parasympathetic nervous system.
C. The kidneys.
D. The adrenal gland.

7. Which of the following contributes to elevated blood pressure?

A. Vasopressin.
B. Renal sympathectomy.
C. Atrial natriuretic peptide.
D. The parasympathetic nervous system.

8. The artery of Percheron:

A. Arises from the distal basilar artery.
B. Supplies the cerebellar peduncle.
C. When occluded, results in bilateral thalamic/midbrain infarcts.
D. Is a vestigial remnant seen in 1% of cerebral arteriograms.

9. Nitric oxide (NO):

A. Raises blood pressure.
B. Lowers blood pressure.
C. Has variable effects on blood pressure.
D. Has no effect on blood pressure.

10. Shear stress causes:

A. Stretching injury of the vessel.
B. Alignment of endothelial cells along the linear axis of the laminar flow.
C. Decreased release of NO.
D. Increased superoxide levels.

11. Vascular smooth muscle hypertrophy is stimulated by:

A. Mechanical vascular injury.
B. Platelet-derived growth factor.
C. Angiotensin II.
D. Fibroblast-derived growth factor (FDGF).

12. Vascular smooth muscle hyperplasia is stimulated by:

A. Hypertension.
B. Thrombin.
C. Angiotensin II.
D. Inflammatory cytokines.

13. Which statement best describes apolipoprotein A-1 (apoA-1)?

A. Elevated levels of apoA-1 may indicate vascular risk in women.
B. ApoA-1 comprises about 70% of the total protein mass of high-density lipoprotein (HDL).
C. ApoA-1 plays a minimal role in reverse cholesterol transport.
D. ApoA-1 is a less accurate predictor of vascular risk than is HDL.
E. ApoA-1 levels must be measured after fasting leading to variable and poorly standardized results.

14. When decreased cerebral perfusion causes autoregulatory failure, what happens to each of the following parameters? Each response may be used more than once.

A. Cerebral blood flow (CBF).
B. Cerebral blood volume (CBV).
C. Mean transit time (MTT).
D. Oxygen extraction fraction (OEF).
E. Cerebral metabolic rate of O_2 ($CMRO_2$).

1. Increased.
2. Decreased.
3. Unchanged.

15. Lipoprotein-associated phospholipase A2 (Lp-PL A2):

A. Is an enzyme that is secreted by macrophages, T lymphocytes, and mast cells.
B. Is primarily bound to HDL and very low-density lipoprotein (VLDL).
C. Should be assayed routinely to dictate patient management and vascular risk reduction.
D. Is a risk factor for cardiovascular disease that is dependent on diabetes.
E. All of the above.

16. Which of the following usually mediates neuronal apoptosis (programmed cell death) in brain ischemia?

A. Cysteine-requiring aspartate-directed proteases (caspases).
B. Apoptosis-inducing factor (AIF).
C. Endonucleases.
D. Matrix metalloproteinases (MMPs).
E. Bradykinin.

17. Vascular endothelial growth factor (VEGF):

A. Affects blood vessels but not neurons or glial cells and plays no role in neurogenesis.
B. Has no role in diseases of the peripheral nervous system.
C. Is induced by hypoxia through hypoxia-inducible factor (HIF-1) transcription factor.
D. Promotes angiogenesis, the differentiation of angioblasts into endothelial cells to form de novo blood vessels.
E. Has a deleterious effect on recovery from cerebral ischemia.

18. Match the level of cerebral blood flow to the cellular events:

A. 35–25 mL/100 g/min.	1. Electrical failure.
B. 18–25 mL/100 g/min.	2. Deterioration of transmembrane ionic gradients.
C. 50–55 mL/100 g/min.	3. Homeostasis.
D. < 10–12 mL/100 g/min.	4. Increased glycolysis.

19. Which of the following statements best describes the role of glutamate in cerebral ischemia?

A. Glutamate is released into the extracellular space with an rCBF of 10% of normal (<5 mL/100 g/min).
B. Antagonism of glutamate receptors in animal models of ischemia has translated into efficacy in human neuroprotection.
C. Glutamate may mediate anoxic and hypoglycemic hippocampal and cortical neuronal injury.
D. Ischemia results in the release of glutamate, which activates ligand-gated calcium (Ca^{2+}) channels in presynaptic neurons.

20. Endothelial cells produce:

A. Anticoagulant and thrombolytic substances, but no prothrombotic substances.
B. Anticoagulant, thrombolytic, and prothrombotic substances.
C. Only thrombolytic substances, with no anticoagulant or prothrombotic substances.
D. Anticoagulant substances, with no thrombolytic or prothrombotic substances.

21. Nitric oxide:

A. Is a byproduct of L-arginine.
B. Release is decreased by shear stress.
C. Production is decreased by exercise.
D. Produces vasoconstriction.

22. The posterior spinal artery generally branches from which artery?

A. Vertebral artery.
B. Basilar artery.
C. Posterior inferior cerebellar artery.
D. Anterior inferior cerebellar artery.

23. Which cranial nerve exits the brainstem between the posterior cerebral artery and the superior cerebellar artery?

A. Nerve III.
B. Nerve IV.
C. Nerve V.
D. Nerve VI.

24. Lipoprotein(a):

A. Consists of apolipoprotein(a) covalently linked to apolipoprotein B-100.
B. May be involved in thrombolysis based on the apoB-100 moiety.
C. Differs from low-density lipoprotein (LDL) cholesterol LDL-C by the apoB-100 component.
D. Has little role in the pathogenesis of cerebrovascular disease.

25. The labyrinthine artery most frequently originates from which artery?

A. Basilar artery.
B. Anterior inferior cerebellar artery.
C. Superior cerebellar artery.
D. Posterior inferior cerebellar artery.
E. Posterior cerebral artery.

26. Which infectious agent is most closely associated with atherosclerosis?

A. Chlamydia pneumoniae.
B. Helicobacter pylori.
C. Cytomegalovirus (CMV).
D. Mycoplasma pneumoniae.
E. Human immunodeficiency virus (HIV).

27. Which one of the following decreases blood pressure?

A. Aldosterone.
B. Endothelin.
C. Angiotensin II.
D. Atrial natriuretic peptide.

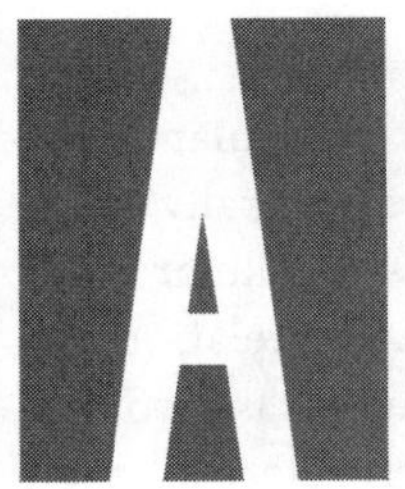

Basic Science Answers

1. The answer is C. Very low-density lipoprotein (VLDL) and chylomicrons are the largest lipoproteins. These are too large to enter the vessel wall, so they are not atherogenic. High-density lipoprotein (HDL) are small lipoproteins that can both enter and leave the blood vessel wall. Thus, HDL does not accumulate in the vessel wall. They may also serve a role in transporting cholesterol out of the vessel wall, although the exact mechanism of protection by HDL is not known. Low-density lipoprotein (LDL) is the major cholesterol-containing lipoprotein. It can enter the vessel wall, but high LDL levels reduce the efflux of cholesterol from the vessel wall. (Strandness, Chapter 9)

2. The answer is B. Smooth muscle cells proliferate in the formation of atherosclerosis. In humans, smooth muscle cells are present in the intima (although most are in the media), but smooth muscle cells are not found in the intima in rodents and many other animals. This is one of several differences in the vessel wall that have added to the difficulty in developing animal models of human atherosclerosis. Neither adipose cells nor T cells are normally found in the intimal layer of arteries. (Fuster, Chapter 44)

3. The answer is E. Heat shock proteins induce cytotoxicity in T cells, which in turn induces tissue factor production in macrophages. T cells also produce the inflammatory cytokine interferon-γ. This is part of the cascade that induces atherosclerosis. (Stoll et al., *Stroke* 2006)

4. The answer is A. Intimal thickening is present at birth in atherosclerosis-prone locations, such as bifurcations. Atherosclerosis will form first in such areas, but atherosclerotic plaque formation is not limited to these areas. (Fuster, Chapter 44)

5. The answer is B. Fatty streaks can develop in the fetus, particular if the mother has hypercholesterolemia. The lipids in fatty streaks are generally intracellular, found mainly in lipid-filled macrophages (foam cells). Extracellular lipids are present in atherosclerotic plaques but not in the fatty streaks. The relationship between fatty streaks and the eventual development of atherosclerosis is inconsistent. Although fatty streaks form in areas that are prone to atherosclerosis, their development in various patient populations does not necessarily correlate with the risk of atherosclerosis. For example, fatty streaks occur in women at younger ages than in men, even though men develop atherosclerosis earlier than women. Early in life, fatty streaks are more common in the thoracic aorta but, later in life, atherosclerosis is more prominent in the abdominal aorta. (Fuster, Chapter 44)

6. The answer is C. The sympathetic nervous system elevates blood pressure, particularly in situations of stress. The parasympathetic system responds to elevated blood pressure and mediates the production of substances to lower blood pressure. In the long run, however, the kidneys have the main responsibility of controlling blood pressure and blood volume. (Fuster, Chapter 61)

7. The answer is A. Vasopressin does not cause essential hypertension, but it does contribute to the maintenance of elevated blood pressure in hypertensive patients, particularly African Americans. In this population, the inhibition of vasopressin receptors decreases blood pressure. Renal sympathectomy lowers blood pressure in experimental models of hypertension. Atrial natriuretic peptide is a vasodilator that lowers blood pressure. The parasympathetic nervous system acts to lower blood pressure. (Fuster, Chapter 61)

8. The answer is C. The central artery of Percheron arises from the first segment of one of the posterior cerebral arteries, giving rise to bilateral medial thalamic perforators. When occlusion produces bilateral paramedian thalamic infarcts, the patient may present with alteration in consciousness and eye-movement abnormalities. This artery is one of the few examples of a cerebral artery that supplies a bilateral structure. (Raphaeli, et al. *Neurology* 2006)

9. The answer is C. Nitric oxide (NO) plays an important role in maintaining appropriate blood pressure. It is a vasodilator and is produced by the endothelium in response to vasoconstricting substances. In this setting, it counterbalances forces that would produce hypertension. In individuals with insulin resistance, however, NO plays a major role in the production of hypertension. (Fuster, Chapter 61)

10. The answer is B. Shear stress is protective against atherosclerosis, and stretching injury is detrimental. The major cause of stretching injury is hypertension. Shear stress, associated with laminar flow, is particularly low at branch points and vascular curvatures. Bifurcations, tortuous vessels, and kinks in vessels are associated with turbulent flow, rather than laminar flow, and are at higher risk for the formation of atherosclerotic plaques. Laminar flow causes an alignment of cells along the linear axis of blood flow. It increases the release of NO and prostacyclin, which are protective against atherosclerosis. Stretching injury causes increased superoxide levels, which increase the formation of atherosclerotic plaques. (Fuster, Chapter 7)

11. The answer is C. Smooth muscle in vessels has two mechanisms of growth—hypertrophy and hyperplasia. Hypertrophy refers to an increase in the size of the smooth muscle cells. Angiotensin II promotes hypertrophy. The other answers refer to factors that promote hyperplasia of vascular smooth muscle. (Fuster, Chapter 7; Geisterfer et al., *Circulation Res* 1988)

12. The answer is D. Smooth muscle cells can undergo hypertrophy (enlargement of individual cells) or hyperplasia (cellular proliferation). Growth factors produced following vascular injury are strong stimulants of smooth muscle hyperplasia, an important mechanism of restenosis following endarterectomy or angioplasty. Inflammatory cytokines contribute to smooth muscle hyperplasia. The role of inflammation is a major topic of investigation in the pathogenesis of atherosclerosis. The other three answers refer to stimuli for smooth muscle hypertrophy. (Fuster, Chapter 7; Dussailant, et al., *J Am Coll Cardiol* 1995)

13. The answer is B. ApoA-1 comprises about 70% of the total protein mass of HDL. It is involved in the transport of phospholipids and unesterified cholesterol from peripheral cells to be converted to HDL, thus providing HDL with a core of cholesterol esters and facilitating cholesterol excretion into bile. Lower levels of apoA-1 appear to be more predictive of vascular risk than low HDL levels. Automated measurement of ApoA-1 can be carried out on nonfasting blood samples with reproducible and standardized results. (Khuseyinova & Keonig, *Curr Atherosclerosis* Rep 2006)

14. The answers are A 2, B 1, C 1, D 1, E 3. With decreased cerebral perfusion pressure, cerebral blood flow (CBF) is stable over a wide range of pressure owing to vascular autoregulation. Increases in mean arterial pressure (MAP)—an estimate of cerebral perfusion pressure—produce vasoconstriction and increased vascular resistance, thus maintaining CBF in a normal range. With decreased MAP, CBF will be maintained through vasodilation. However, with autoregulatory failure, as perfusion pressure continues to drop, CBF falls linearly as a function of pressure. CBV generally increases with increase in MTT (CBV/CBF). To maintain $CMRO_2$ unchanged, the oxygen ejection fraction (OEF) increases. (Derdeyn, *Neuroimag Clin N Am* 2005)

15. The answer is A. Lipoprotein-associated phospholipase A2 (Lp-PL A2) is produced by macrophages, T lymphocytes, and mast cells. It is mainly bound to LDL, with only 20% bound to HDL and VLDL. The role of Lp-PL A2 is not clear, because it may have both prothrombotic and antithrombotic mechanisms. Lp-PL A2, as a specific marker of vascular inflammation, may be an independent risk factor for cardiovascular disease, which is relatively unaffected by conventional vascular risk factors. However the clinical utility of the Lp-PL A2 assay needs further investigation, and routine screening is not indicated. (Garza et al., *Mayo Clin Proc* 2007)

16. The answer is A. Neuronal loss after cerebral ischemia involves energy-dependent programmed cell death (apoptosis). Caspases are a family of proteases that are upregulated and activated in animal models of focal and global ischemia. Caspases are activated by the release of mitochondrial cytochrome c, along with other pathways and effectors. Apoptosis-inducing factor (AIF) and endonucleases are less commonly involved mediators of apoptosis, and their role in cerebral ischemia appears limited. Matrix metalloproteinases and bradykinin are involved in the loss of the blood–brain barrier and the microvascular extracellular matrix after cerebral ischemia. (Love, *Prog Neuro-Psychopharmacol Biol Psychiatry* 2003)

17. The answer is C. Angiogenesis is the sprouting of new capillaries from pre-existing vessels, as opposed to vasculogenesis, which is the differentiation of angioblasts into endothelial cells for the production of de novo blood vessels. Vascular endothelial growth factor (VEGF) is an important signaling molecule in the central and peripheral nervous system, which is involved in both angiogenesis and neurogenesis. It is induced by hypoxia, in which case it may have a neuroprotective role as a promoter of cerebral angiogenesis. Infarct volume is increased and neurological function is more impaired with cerebral ischemia in VEGF-knockout than in wild-type mice. VEGF modifies acute and chronic central and peripheral neurodegenerative processes through effects on blood vessels, neurons, and perhaps glia. (Greenberg & Jin, *Nature* 2005)

18. The answers are A 4, B 1, C 3, D 2. The normal range of CBF (50–55 mL/100 g/min) is maintained by cerebral autoregulation. With a decrease in CBF, oxygen extraction increases to maintain the normal cerebral metabolic rate of oxygen consumption. As CBF declines further, to 35 to 25 mL/100 g/min, protein synthesis decreases and energy demands are met by glycolysis. With CBF at 18 to 25 mL/100 g/min, there occurs slowing of the electroencephalogram, attenuation of evoked potentials, and decline in synaptic potentials. With further decline of CBF, to less than 10 to 12 mL/100 g/min, normal ionic gradients are reversed, with influx of calcium and sodium and efflux of potassium. (Chaturvedi & Levine, Chapter 2)

19. The answer is C. Glutamate is an excitatory amino acid, released during ischemia, that plays a role in the initiation and elaboration of ischemic injury. Exposure to glutamate produces swelling of cortical neurons and intracellular accumulation of calcium. Glutamate is released into the extracellular space when rCBF is at 40% of normal (< 20 mL/100 g/min). Release of glutamate activates ligand-gated Ca^{2+} channels in postsynaptic neurons. The beneficial effects of glutamate antagonism in animal ischemia models have not been replicated in human trials. (Chaturvedi & Levine, Chapter 2)

20. The answer is B. Anticoagulant and thrombolytic substances are produced by the endothelium, along with prothrombotic substances. The generation of prothrombotic substances is enhanced by injury, inflammation, or the metabolic syndrome. Anticoagulant substances include prostacyclin, NO, antithrombin III, and heparin-like molecules. The endothelium produces endogenous tissue plasminogen (t-PA), a potent thrombolytic. Prothrombotic molecules produced by the endothelium include tissue factor, factor VIII, plasminogen activation inhibitor, and factor Va. (Fuster, Chapter 7)

21. The answer is A. L-arginine contains guanidine nitrogens that are oxidized to citrulline and NO by nitric oxide synthetase (NOS). NO was initially described as endothelium-derived relaxing factor. The release of NO is increased by shear stress, and it is protective against the formation of atherosclerotic plaques in areas of high shear stress. NOS expression is increased in endothelial cells by exercise, thus increasing the production of NO. (Fuster, Chapter 7)

22. The answer is C. The paired posterior spinal arteries usually branch from the posterior inferior cerebellar arteries, although they may occasionally come off the vertebral arteries. The single anterior spinal artery branches from the vertebral arteries. (Haines, 2004)

23. The answer is A. The oculomotor nerve exits the dorsal surface of the brainstem between the quadrigeminal branch of the posterior cerebellar artery and the superior cerebellar artery. (Haines, 2004)

24. The answer is A. Lp(a) is a LDL-like plasma lipoprotein that consists of apolipoprotein(a) covalently linked to apolipoprotein B-100. The unique glycoprotein apo(a) component, which has a marked size heterogeneity, distinguishes it from LDL-C. It is measurable in human plasma, and its role in the promotion of vascular disease, including ischemic stroke, has been investigated based on several putative mechanisms. Gene expression of apo(a) has been found in atherosclerotic intracerebral and carotid vessels and may presage the development of atherosclerotic plaque in cerebral vessels. Lp(a) may have a role in the inhibition of t-PA, based on the structural homology between apo(a) and plasminogen. Thus, it may interfere with intrinsic fibrinolysis. Lp(a) is involved in endothelial dysfunction and in the induction of inflammation. (Ariyo et al., *N Engl J Med* 2003; Danik et al., *JAMA* 2006; Jamieson, *Exp Mol Pathol* 2001; Ohira et al., Stroke 2006)

25. The answer is B. Although the labyrinthine artery may occasionally arise from the basilar artery, it most frequently branches from the anterior inferior cerebellar artery. (Haines, 2004)

26. The answer is A. Multiple organisms have been associated with atherosclerosis and risk of stroke. Helicobacter pylori, cytomegalovirus (CMV), and human immunodeficiency virus (HIV) have been implicated in atherosclerosis, but the evidence is strongest for Chlamydia pneumoniae, an obligate intracellular organism with respiratory transmission. C. pneumoniae has been identified in atheroma, and repeated infection with the organism may trigger or accelerate development of cerebral and coronary atherosclerosis. Antibody titers, especially IgA, appear to be associated with stroke risk, although some data do not show a link. Stroke in HIV infection may be due to a prothrombotic state, vasculitis, or noninflammatory vasculopathy. H. pylori, CMV, and M. pneumoniae are not clearly associated with atherosclerotic stroke. (Elkind & Cole, *Sem Neurol* 2006)

27. The answer is D. Atrial natriuretic peptide is produced when receptors in the atria detect overfilling of the atria. It is a vasodilator that lowers blood pressure. Aldosterone, a product of the adrenal gland, elevates blood pressure. Aldosterone-producing adrenal adenomas and adrenal hyperplasia are causes of hypertension. Endothelin is a vasoconstrictor that can contribute to hypertension. Endothelin antagonism can lower blood pressure. Angiotensin II also produces hypertension. (Rosenthal, Chapter 61)

2 Pharmacology Questions

28. Sodium nitroprusside (Nipride, Nitropress):

A. Dilates arterioles but not venules.
B. Impairs renal perfusion.
C. Has a therapeutic effect that lasts only 12 minutes after cessation of infusion.
D. Has toxicity that can be reduced by the simultaneous administration of sodium thiosulfate.
E. Has no effect on intracranial pressure.

29. In patients with diabetes mellitus, the treatment of chronic hypertension should be initiated with:

A. Calcium channel blockers.
B. β-Blockers.
C. Angiotensin-converting enzyme (ACE) inhibitors.
D. Thiazide diuretics.

30. Thiazide diuretics:

A. Are rarely used in the management of hypertension, with the advent of newer agents.
B. Do not cross the placental barrier so may be used safely during pregnancy.
C. Do not cause impotence.
D. Elevate low-density lipoprotein (LDL) levels.
E. Elevate high-density lipoprotein (HDL) levels.

31. Calcium-channel blockers:

A. Should be avoided in patients with diastolic dysfunction.
B. Should be avoided in the elderly and in African Americans.
C. Are indicated in patients with congestive heart failure.
D. Lower exercise tolerance.

32. Angiotensin-converting enzyme (ACE) inhibitors:

A. Are safe during pregnancy.
B. May lower blood pressure excessively when combined with diuretics.
C. Do not alter sodium homeostasis.
D. Do not alter potassium homeostasis.

33. Digitalis:

A. Is effective in decreasing the ventricular response in patients with atrial fibrillation and in preventing recurrent atrial fibrillation following cardioversion.
B. Has negative inotropic effects.
C. Is effective in heart rate reduction in patients with thyrotoxicosis.
D. Is excreted unchanged by the kidney.

34. Methyldopa (Aldomet):

A. Is a relatively safe drug for use during pregnancy.
B. Is a peripherally active antihypertensive.
C. Does not produce sedation or depression.
D. Does not produce symptomatic orthostatic hypotension.

35. Variant angina (Prinzmetal angina):

A. Is best treated by sublingual nitroglycerin.
B. Is best treated by aspirin.
C. Is best treated with β-blockers.
D. Is best treated by calcium-channel blockade.

36. Calcium-channel blockers:

A. Increase coronary vascular resistance.
B. Increase coronary blood flow.
C. Are useful in variant (Prinzmetal) angina, but not in exertional angina.
D. Are of no utility in unstable angina.

37. Which statement about hyperlipidemia in children is true?

A. The treatment of choice is niacin.
B. Children with LDL levels of over 130 mg/dL and a family history of atherosclerotic vascular disease should be treated pharmacologically.
C. Statins are contraindicated in children.
D. Bile-acid sequestrants can be used safely in children.

38. Which of the following statements best describes blood pressure treatment in patients with diabetes?

A. Calcium-channel blockers are used because of their renal protective effect.
B. More rigorous control of blood pressure has not been shown to decrease ischemic stroke risk.
C. Blood pressure management does not impact the development of microalbuminuria.
D. Therapy using multiple antihypertensive agents should be avoided.
E. The first choice of agent for treatment should be an ACE inhibitor or an angiotensin receptor blocker (ARB).

39. Which statement is true about total cholesterol?

A. Cholesterol control reduces the risk of heart disease more in men than in women.
B. Reduction of total cholesterol below 150 mL/dL results in an elevated noncardiac mortality.
C. Excess alcohol intake elevates both triglycerides and total cholesterol.
D. Diet is more effective in reducing total cholesterol than in reducing triglycerides.

40. Statins lower cholesterol by:

A. Decreasing dietary absorption of cholesterol and triglycerides.
B. Increasing the numbers of LDL receptors on hepatocytes.
C. Decreasing levels of hydroxy-3-methylglutaryl coenzyme A (HMG-CoA) reductase.
D. Increasing the synthesis of apolipoprotein B-100 in the liver.

41. The most common side effect of statins is:

A. Cough.
B. Elevation of liver enzymes.
C. Myopathy.
D. Rhabdomyolysis.

42. The bile-acid sequestrants cholestyramine (Questran) and colestipol:

A. Have an outstanding safety record.
B. Are contraindicated in children.
C. Are useful in patients with severe hypertriglyceride levels.
D. Enhance the absorption of warfarin.

43. Which statement is true about vascular endothelium and endogenous antithrombotic substances in humans?

A. Platelet aggregation and thrombus formation generally do not occur on the surface of an intact blood vessel.
B. Tissue factor is an endogenous anticoagulant.
C. Heparan sulfate is a plasma protein that exerts an anticoagulant effect near the endothelial cell.
D. Prostacyclin is an anticoagulant synthesized by endothelial cells.

44. Of the following choices which is the most common source of commercial heparin?

A. Rabbit lung.
B. Porcine intestinal mucosa.
C. Human endothelial cells.
D. Human mast cells.

45. The anticoagulant effect of heparin requires:

A. Fibroblast growth factors.
B. Heparan sulfate.
C. Antithrombin III.
D. Endothelial cells.

46. Which statement is true about unfractionated heparin?

A. High doses of heparin produce platelet activation.
B. Heparin crosses the placenta.
C. Heparin produces thrombocytopenia via direct destruction of platelets.
D. Osteoporosis is a potential complication of heparin.

47. The most accurate measure of the therapeutic effect of heparin is:

A. Activated partial thromboplastin time (aPTT).
B. Plasma heparin level.
C. Bleeding time.
D. D-dimer levels.
E. High-sensitivity C-reactive protein.

48. After an initial IV bolus of 5,000 units of unfractionated heparin in a 70-kg-man, the plasma half-life ($t_{1/2}$) of heparin is:

A. 1 hour.
B. 2 hours.
C. 4 hours.
D. 8 hours.

49. The standard subcutaneous dose of enoxaparin (Lovenox) is:

A. 1 mg/kg/day.
B. 2 mg/kg/day.
C. 100 mg/day.
D. Must be adjusted according to laboratory measures of therapeutic anticoagulation.

50. Which statement is true about danaparoid (Orgaran)?

A. It is a hirudin derivative.
B. It prolongs the PTT in standard recommended doses.
C. It is an inhibitor of factor Xa.
D. Its therapeutic effect is measured by direct blood levels of the agent.

51. Lepirudin (Refludan).

A. Is administered subcutaneously.
B. Can be reversed by protamine sulfate.
C. Is monitored using aPTT.
D. Is not associated with antibody production.

52. Of the coagulation factors affected by Coumadin (warfarin), the one with the shortest $t_{1/2}$ is:

A. Coagulation factor II.
B. Coagulation factor VII.
C. Coagulation factor IX.
D. Coagulation factor X.

53. A 56-year-old man who was taking warfarin because of atrial fibrillation was seen in a Coumadin clinic and found to have an international normalized ratio (INR) of 4.3, using finger-stick testing. The most appropriate immediate measure is:

A. Oral vitamin K as an outpatient.
B. Hospital admission for IV vitamin K.
C. Hold warfarin for 1 week.
D. Hold warfarin for 1 day.

54. A 75-year-old man in atrial fibrillation who was on Coumadin (warfarin) was admitted to a subacute rehabilitation facility after a hip replacement. On discharge, he was given a prescription for warfarin 5 mg daily. At home, he had an old bottle of Coumadin 5-mg tablets. He was not aware that Coumadin and warfarin were the same medication, so he took one pill from each bottle on a daily basis. He went out to dinner with his family and became nauseated. When he began vomiting blood, his family rushed him to the emergency department where his finger-stick INR was too high to be recorded. The patient was in a small rural hospital, and only the agents listed here were available. Which of the following is the most appropriate treatment for this man?

A. Vitamin K orally, 3 mg hourly for 4 hours.
B. Vitamin K IV, 10 mg by slow infusion.
C. Fresh frozen plasma.
D. Fresh frozen plasma and vitamin K 10 mg IV.
E. Subcutaneous vitamin K.

55. The action of warfarin is caused by:

A. Decreased production of clotting factors by the liver.
B. Decreased carboxylation of clotting factors, resulting in clotting factors that are less active.
C. Both decreased production and decreased carboxylation of clotting factors.
D. Decreased production and carboxylation of clotting factors, along with interference with the activity of circulating clotting factors.

56. A patient with atrial fibrillation presents to the Coumadin clinic for a routine INR. He has a recent episode of bronchitis that was treated with antibiotics. During this illness, he had 2 days when he could not remember if he had taken his warfarin, so he took a pill "just in case." He was sure he had not missed any doses, but he was concerned he might have taken a couple of extra doses. His INR by finger stick was 7.0. Blood was obtained for blood counts and a repeat INR from the clinical lab. His hematocrit and hemoglobin were normal. According to the laboratory, his INR was 8.6. The appropriate measures include:

A. Immediate hospitalization for reversal of the excess level of anticoagulation using fresh frozen plasma.
B. Administration of 2.5 mg of vitamin K orally, hold warfarin, and perform daily INR measurements on an outpatient basis.
C. Administer 1.0 mg of vitamin K orally, hold warfarin, and perform daily INR measurements on an outpatient basis.
D. Stop warfarin and restart when the INR is 2.0.
E. Administer 5 mg of oral vitamin K and continue warfarin at a reduced dosage.

57. Tissue plasminogen activator (t-PA):

A. Is a strong activator of plasminogen.
B. Is a poor activator of plasminogen unless exposed to fibrin.
C. Is cleared mainly by the kidney.
D. Is less expensive than streptokinase.

58. Aminocaproic acid (Amicar):

A. Is a procoagulant substance.
B. Is an inhibitor of fibrinolysis.
C. Is a useful therapy to prevent rebleeding in patients with subarachnoid hemorrhage.
D. Is proven to be an effective treatment to reduce bleeding during surgery.

59. Which statement about aspirin is true?

A. The degree of stroke risk reduction with aspirin increases with increasing dose up to 650 mg daily.
B. Aspirin enhances the activity of cyclooxygenase.
C. Aspirin blocks the production of thromboxane A2, a platelet activator and vasoconstrictor.
D. Aspirin toxicity is not clearly dose-dependent.

60. Dipyridamole (Persantine):

A. Has mild vasoconstrictor effect in high doses.
B. Inhibits platelets by inhibiting cyclooxygenase.
C. Decreases the intracellular concentration of cyclic adenosine monophosphate (cAMP).
D. Blocks the uptake of adenosine.

61. Ticlopidine (Ticlid) and clopidogrel (Plavix) are:

A. Similar in toxicity profiles.
B. Rapidly absorbed, resulting in rapid therapeutic effect.
C. Thienopyridine agents closely related in chemical structure.
D. Platelet inhibitors and vasodilators.

62. Abciximab (ReoPro):

A. Inhibits platelet activation induced by thrombin, collagen, or thromboxane A2.
B. Inhibits platelet activation by promoting the action of von Willebrand factor.
C. Can be administered orally or parenterally.
D. Has a $t_{1/2}$ of 2 hours following IV administration.
E. Is extracted from porcine intestine.

63. Eptifibatide (Integrilin) is:

A. A monoclonal antibody that is directed toward the platelet glycoprotein IIb/IIIa receptor.
B. A peptide that inhibits platelet activation by interaction with the vitronectin receptor on platelets.
C. An antibody that inhibits platelets by binding the collagen receptor.
D. A peptide that inhibits the platelet glycoprotein IIb/IIIa receptor.
E. Administered orally.

64. A 48-year-old man presented with amaurosis fugax in the right eye lasting 5 minutes. His evaluation revealed right carotid atherosclerosis with less than 40% stenosis. His LDL was 135. He was placed on a platelet inhibitor and a statin for his elevated cholesterol. Three weeks later, his LDL was 86 but he complained of muscle cramps. What is the next appropriate intervention?

A. Check creatine kinase (CK) levels and then obtain a thyroid-stimulating hormone (TSH) level if the CK is elevated to five times the normal upper limit.
B. Check CK and discontinue the statin immediately if the CK is elevated to three times the upper limit of normal.
C. Discontinue statin treatment immediately.
D. Use quinine to control the muscle cramps, because the statin has adequately controlled the LDL.
E. Order an electromyogram (EMG).

65. The most common side effect of Aggrenox (extended-release dipyridamole and aspirin) is:

A. Gastric irritation.
B. Headache.
C. Leukopenia.
D. Insomnia.
E. Hematuria.

66. The therapeutic effect of low-molecular-weight heparin therapy can be monitored in the laboratory by checking the blood for:

A. Partial thromboplastin time (PTT).
B. Factor Xa levels.
C. Factor Xa inhibition.
D. D-Dimer.

67. A 26-year-old woman, who is 10 weeks pregnant, presents with headache along with right hemiparesis and aphasia. Cerebral venous thrombosis was diagnosed. Her mother had a spontaneous deep vein thrombosis (DVT) and a pulmonary embolus 3 years earlier, and she is on chronic warfarin therapy. What is the main contraindication to warfarin in this patient?

A. Hemorrhagic risk of pregnancy and delivery.
B. Gastric irritation.
C. Predisposition to preeclampsia.
D. Teratogenicity.

68. Which of the anticonvulsants listed here is the safest to give to an anticoagulated patient, specifically to avoid interaction with warfarin?

A. Keppra (levetiracetam).
B. Dilantin (phenytoin).
C. Depakote (valproic acid).
D. Phenobarbital.

69. Which of the following statements about amiodarone is correct?

A. Amiodarone is contraindicated in patients with atrial fibrillation.
B. Amiodarone increases the refractory period of the left atrium.
C. Amiodarone increases ventricular response in patients with atrial fibrillation.
D. Amiodarone is effective in preventing recurrence of atrial fibrillation after cardioversion only when administered in very high doses.

70. The most common side effect of clopidogrel (Plavix) is:

A. Thrombocytopenia.
B. Headache.
C. Gastrointestinal (GI) distress.
D. Rash.
E. Intraocular bleeding with vision loss.

71. Cilostazol (Pletal):

A. Is an effective agent in the secondary prevention of stroke.
B. Produces vasoconstriction in therapeutic doses.
C. Is not used in stroke prevention because of frequent, serious side effects.
D. Is administered parenterally.

72. Ezetimibe (Zetia):

A. Inhibits cholesterol synthesis in the liver.
B. Decreases cholesterol levels by decreasing bile acid availability.
C. Decreases absorption of cholesterol in the intestine.
D. Produces higher blood levels in men than in women.

73. Of the agents listed, which one produces the greatest elevation of HDL?

A. Ezetimibe (Zetia).
B. Rosuvastatin (Crestor).
C. Niacin.
D. Fenofibrate (Tricor).
E. Red wine.

74. Side effects from high-dose niacin:

A. Are ameliorated by aspirin and, in many patients, by taking the medication with food.
B. Are not dose-dependent.
C. Are infrequent.
D. Are not influenced by alcohol intake.
E. Include dangerous lowering of blood glucose in patients with diabetes.

75. Which statement is true about niacin?

A. As a natural product, niacin has less toxicity than any of the "standard medications" for lowering lipids.
B. Over-the-counter sustained-release niacin is preferred to crystalline (immediate-release) niacin, because less liver toxicity is associated with the sustained release preparation.
C. Niacin lowers LDL and triglycerides, along with raising HDL. It is particularly useful in patients with the combination of elevated triglycerides and low HDL.
D. Elevation of liver transaminases is most common during the first 6 months of treatment with niacin.

76. Fibric-acid derivatives (clofibrate, gemfibrozil, fenofibrate, ciprofibrate, bezafibrate):

A. Have no effect on the coagulation and fibrinolytic systems.
B. Increase the risk of cholelithiasis.
C. Are the second-line treatment for severe hypertriglyceridemia in patients at risk for pancreatitis, with ω-3-acid esters (Omacor) being the first-line agent.
D. Are safe in patients with renal failure.

77. Which of the following agents can be given in combination with a statin without increasing the risk of muscle toxicity?

A. Fibric-acid derivatives (e.g., gemfibrozil).
B. Niacin.
C. Bile-acid sequestrants (e.g., cholestyramine, colestipol).
D. Fenofibrate (Tricor).

78. Omega-3-acid esters (Omacor):

A. Lowers triglycerides and LDL.
B. Lowers triglycerides and raises HDL.
C. Lowers triglycerides and raises VLDL.
D. Has no effect on triglycerides, but lowers LDL and raises HDL.

79. Which statement is true regarding chronic hypertension in pregnancy?

A. Hydralazine is contraindicated during pregnancy.
B. Calcium-channel blockers may be used during pregnancy.
C. Maternal, but not fetal, outcome is worsened by mild to moderate maternal hypertension.
D. Magnesium sulfate is the treatment of choice for chronic hypertension during pregnancy.
E. Beta blockers are absolutely contraindicated during pregnancy.

80. Patient self-testing and self-management of warfarin:

A. Is less effective in maintaining a therapeutic INR than a well-run "Coumadin clinic."
B. Is effective only when managed by telephone or telemedicine by an appropriate provider.
C. Is limited more by insurance issues than by quality issues.
D. Has not been studied.

81. Which of the following intravenous treatments for an intractable migraine headache is contraindicated in patients with vascular disease?

A. Magnesium.
B. Dihydroergotamine (DHE).
C. Steroids.
D. Sodium valproate.
E. Metoclopramide.

82. A patient with transient ischemic attacks (TIAs) and hypertension is on multiple medications, including a platelet inhibitor, a statin, and an ACE inhibitor for stroke prevention. He has had a myocardial infarction in the past and is on a β-blocker. He is on levodopa-carbidopa (Sinemet) for Parkinson disease. He presents to the clinic with near-syncope when he gets out of bed or stands up from a chair. Which of his medicines are likely contributors to this problem?

A. Statin, ACE inhibitor, β-blocker, and Sinemet.
B. ACE inhibitor, β-blocker, and Sinemet.
C. ACE inhibitor and β-blocker.
D. Only the β-blocker.

83. Which of the following statements best describes lipid management in patients with cerebrovascular disease?

A. Elevated lipids are strong risk factors for cerebrovascular disease, similar to cardiovascular disease.
B. Statin therapy is of no benefit to patients with ischemic stroke or TIA of presumed atherosclerotic origin who have normal cholesterol levels.
C. Patients with ischemic stroke or TIA with low HDL cholesterol may be considered for treatment with niacin or gemfibrozil.
D. The recommendation in very-high-risk patients is to aim for an LDL cholesterol level of less than 100 mg/dL.
E. The risk reduction with statin therapy in cerebrovascular disease is solely due to cholesterol reduction.

84. A 27-year-old man has a strong family history of coronary artery disease and stroke. His LDL was 184 mg/dL. Three months after starting a statin, his liver enzymes were elevated, at two times the upper limit of normal. Based on his liver tests:

A. The statin should be stopped.
B. Liver function tests should be followed until they normalize.
C. The statin should be stopped if there is a single result of transaminases elevated above three times normal.
D. The statin should be stopped if there is a persistent elevation of transaminases about three times normal.

85. Prothrombin complex concentrates (PCCs):

A. Are inexpensive, easily available products that prevent bleeding in patients with factor IX deficiency.
B. Are safe to give to patients with severe liver disease.
C. Contain varying amounts of factors II, VII, IX, and X.
D. Treat warfarin induced intracerebral hemorrhage through normalization of the INR more slowly than does fresh frozen plasma (FFP) infusion.
E. Should not be combined with intravenous vitamin K.

86. Which parenteral agent used for treatment of hypertension may cause cerebral vasodilation, elevated intracranial pressure, and impaired cerebral autoregulation?

A. Labetalol (Normodyne, Trandate).
B. Esmolol (Brevibloc).
C. Sodium nitroprusside (Nipride, Nitropress).
D. Nicardipine (Cardene).
E. Enalaprilat (Vasotec).

87. Match the parenteral antihypertensive agent used in neurologic emergencies with its mechanism of action. Use each answer only once.

A. Labetalol (Normodyne, Trandate).	1. α_1-, β_1-, β_2-antagonist.
B. Esmolol (Brevibloc).	2 DA_1 agonist.
C. Nicardipine (Cardene).	3. β_1-antagonist.
D. Enalaprilat (Vasotec).	4. ACE inhibitor.
E. Fenoldopam (Corlopam).	5. L-Type calcium-channel blocker.

88. Which antihypertensive agent used in neurologic emergencies is favored in patients with acute renal insufficiency?

A. Labetalol (Normodyne, Trandate).
B. Esmolol (Brevibloc).
C. Fenoldopam (Corlopam).
D. Nicardipine (Cardene).
E. Enalaprilat (Vasotec).

89. Which of these antihypertensive medications is most appropriate as initial therapy for patients with chronic renal disease?

A. Ramipril (Altace).
B. Metoprolol (Lopressor).
C. Amlodipine (Norvasc).
D. Verapamil (Calan).
E. Doxazosin (Cardura).

90. Which of the following statements about ticlopidine is true?

A. Because of serious side effects, this agent is no longer available.
B. Thrombocytopenia is the most frequent serious side effect.
C. This agent has been approved for primary prevention of stroke.
D. Digestive and skin disturbances are the major limitations to compliance.

91. Which of the following supplements could be taken by a patient on long-term anticoagulation or antiplatelet therapy, without bleeding concerns?

A. Fish oil.
B. Garlic.
C. L-Arginine.
D. Ginkgo.
E. Ginseng.

92. Which of the following produces the greatest increase in HDL levels?

A. Alcohol.
B. Statins.
C. Fibrates.
D. Nicotinic acid.
E. Thiazolidinediones.

93. Which of the following puts a patient starting a statin medication at increased risk for the development of myopathy?

A. Taking amiodarone for atrial fibrillation.
B. Drinking a 6-oz glass of grapefruit juice daily.
C. Obesity.
D. Male gender.

94. Which statement is true about monitoring blood work in patients taking statins?

A. The CK level should be monitored in 12 weeks and then yearly, unless patients develop symptoms.
B. The hepatic enzymes should be monitored before treatment, 12 weeks following treatment, and then yearly unless otherwise indicated.
C. The CK level is of no utility in patients taking statin, because symptoms of muscle soreness necessitate cessation of the agent regardless of the CK level.
D. Complete blood counts should be monitored yearly.

95. Statin-induced myopathy:

A. Is rare at low doses.
B. Is idiosyncratic rather than dose-dependent.
C. Is increased in patients with familial hyperlipidemia.
D. Is increased in patients taking warfarin.

96. An 82-year-old man with multiple vascular risk factors complained that his medications are too expensive. You look at all his medications and suggest one that he can stop without increasing his vascular risk. Which medication did you suggest that he should discontinue?

A. Atorvastatin (Lipitor).
B. Ramipril (Altace).
C. Clopidogrel (Plavix).
D. Vitamin E supplements.
E. Glipizide (Glucotrol).

97. Which statement is true about the treatment of hypertension in patients with heart failure?

A. Calcium-channel blockers have positive inotropic effects and are useful in patients with heart failure.
B. β-Blockers are contraindicated in patients with heart failure because of negative inotropic effects.
C. Angiotensin-converting enzyme (ACE) inhibitors are the treatment of choice in patients with left ventricular dysfunction and hypertension.
D. Digitalis glycosides can reduce left ventricular hypertrophy in patients with chronic hypertension.

98. Corticosteroids are the initial treatment of choice to prevent stroke in patients with:

A. Hypereosinophilic syndrome.
B. Wegener granulomatosis.
C. Systemic lupus erythematosus (SLE).
D. Granulomatous angiitis of central nervous system.
E. Periarteritis nodosa.

99. The CT scan of a 71-year-old man with the sudden onset of a headache, nausea, vomiting, and ataxia shows a large cerebellar hemorrhage. He is taking warfarin for a DVT, and his INR is 3.2. The neurosurgeon asks you what to do about the elevated INR and how long it will take to normalize the value, because she wants to decompress the posterior fossa. Match the management option with the time for anticoagulant reversal. Use each answer only once.

A. Just stop warfarin.
B. Intravenous vitamin K.
C. Fresh frozen plasma (FFP).
D. Prothrombin complex concentrate (PCC).
E. Factor VIIa concentrate.

1. Twelve to 32 hours.
2. Fifteen minutes after a 1-hour infusion.
3. Five to 14 days.
4. Six to 24 hours.
5. Fifteen minutes after a bolus.

100. A 53-year-old woman with hypertension and elevated total cholesterol has had a long history of episodic migraine. Her blood pressure is still elevated, and she only complies intermittently with antihypertensive therapy. She had a small-vessel infarct 3 years ago, from which she had excellent recovery. She asked you for injectable sumatriptan for her severe migraines, which occur about 15 days a month. What do you do?

A. You suggest that she try a long-acting triptan because of the frequency of her headaches.
B. You discuss the use of a daily preventative medication to decrease her need for acute therapy.
C. You suggest that she try a short-acting triptan, warning her not to use more than two or three doses a week.
D. You tell her that her headaches will go away eventually and that she can use over-the-counter (OTC) medications, up to four to five doses daily.
E. You give her a butalbital/acetaminophen/caffeine preparation to take whenever she has a headache, up to 10 doses a week.

101. Contraindications in intravenous immunoglobulin (IVIG) treatment in a patient with myasthenia gravis include:

A. Past history of stroke.
B. Past history of renal disease.
C. Decreased IgA levels.
D. Age over 65.

102. Which statement is true about glycerol for treatment of cerebral edema?

A. Glycerol does not cross the blood–brain barrier.
B. Glycerol decreases serum osmolarity.
C. Glycerol reduces intracranial pressure (ICP) quickly, with this effect lasting for up to 60 minutes.
D. Glycerol reduces ICP, with the effect starting 30 to 60 minutes after administration and lasting for 6 to 8 hours.

103. Which of the following agents has been shown to reduce mortality from malignant cerebral edema following a large middle cerebral artery stroke?

A. Mannitol.
B. Glycerol.
C. Corticosteroids.
D. Furosemide (Lasix).
E. None of the above.

104. Ancrod, when administered to patients within 3 hours of an acute ischemic stroke:

A. Has a greater symptomatic intracranial hemorrhage rate than does tissue t-PA.
B. Decreases mortality.
C. Decreases the proportion of severely disabled patients.
D. Decreases fibrinogen levels maximally within 60 minutes of the IV bolus.
E. All of the above.

105. Which statement is true regarding vitamin (B_6, B_{12}, folic acid) treatment for stroke prevention?

A. The Vitamin Intervention for Stroke Prevention (VISP) trial showed a benefit for vitamin therapy in secondary stroke prevention.
B. The VISP trial failed to show a benefit for primary stroke prevention in patients with elevated homocysteine levels, but a secondary prevention trial is needed.
C. The VISP trial failed because the vitamin therapy prescribed failed to lower homocysteine levels.
D. Although the VISP trial failed to show a clinical benefit for stroke prevention, the data are conflicting about vitamin treatment in prevention of myocardial infarction (MI).

106. Which of the following is a contraindication to metformin (Glucophage)?

A. Congestive heart failure requiring pharmacologic treatment.
B. Administration of cationic contrast agents.
C. Elevated serum creatinine.
D. Metabolic acidosis.
E. All of the above.

107. Match each medication used for stroke prevention with its main mechanism of action. Each answer may be used only once.

A. Aspirin.
B. Clopidogrel (Plavix).
C. Argatroban.
D. Dipyridamole.
E. Enoxaparin (Lovenox).

1. Inhibition of thromboxane A_2.
2. Inhibition of thrombin-catalyzed or thrombin-induced reactions.
3. Inhibition of adenosine diphosphate (ADP)-dependent activation of the glycoprotein IIb/IIIa receptor.
4. Antithrombin III-mediated inhibition of factor Xa.
5. Inhibition of platelet phosphodiesterase.

108. Match each medication used for stroke prevention with its main mechanism of action. Each answer may be used more than once.

A. Eptifibatide (Integrilin).
B. Danaparoid (Orgaran).
C. Abciximab (ReoPro).
D. Hirudin.
E. Dalteparin (Fragmin).
F. Fondaparinux (Arixtra).

1. Inhibition of platelet phosphodiesterase.
2. Antithrombin III-mediated inhibition of factor Xa.
3. Direct inhibition of the platelet glyco protein IIb/IIIa receptor.
4. Inhibition of thrombin-catalyzed or thrombin-induced reactions.
5. Increased platelet adenosine.

109. Appropriate anticoagulation treatment for patients with a history of heparin-induced thrombocytopenia (HIT) is:

A. Intravenous unfractionated heparin.
B. Intravenous low-molecular-weight heparin.
C. Subcutaneous enoxaparin (Lovenox).
D. Intravenous argatroban (Novastatin).
E. Oral anticoagulation with dabigatran.

110. Which of the following antiepileptic drugs (AEDs) has been associated with potential harmful effects on functional recovery after a stroke?

A. Phenytoin (Dilantin).
B. Gabapentin (Neurontin).
C. Lamotrigine (Lamictal).
D. Carbamazepine (Tegretol).
E. Levetiracetam (Keppra).

111. Which AED would be most appropriate for use in a patient with seizures after a stroke due to atrial fibrillation?

A. Phenytoin (Dilantin).
B. Gabapentin (Neurontin).
C. Phenobarbital.
D. Carbamazepine (Tegretol).
E. Levetiracetam (Keppra).

112. What is the time window for treatment of intracerebral hemorrhage (ICH) using recombinant factor VIIa?

A. One hour.
B. Four hours.
C. Six hours.
D. Twelve hours.
E. Twenty-four hours.

113. The recommended prevention of clinical worsening due to vasospasm in subarachnoid hemorrhage is:

A. Nimodipine 60 mg orally every 4 hours for 21 days.
B. Nicardipine.
C. Nimodipine 40 mg orally every 6 hours for 21 days.
D. Aminocaproic acid 5 g IV.
E. Intra-arterial verapamil.

114. Which of the following agents used for stroke prevention has the lowest risk of symptomatic hemorrhage?

A. Clopidogrel (Plavix) and aspirin combination.
B. Warfarin (Coumadin).
C. Dipyridamole and aspirin combination (Aggrenox).
D. Intravenous unfractionated heparin.

115. Which of the following have been shown to lower homocysteine levels and decrease the incidence of ischemic stroke?

A. Folic acid 0.8 mg, vitamin B_{12} 0.4 mg, vitamin B_6 40 mg.
B. Fish oil.
C. Folic acid 2.5 mg, vitamin B_{12} 1 mg, vitamin B_6 50 mg.
D. Vitamin E.
E. None of the above.

116. Digoxin is:

A. No longer used in patients with atrial fibrillation.
B. Useful in preventing recurrent atrial fibrillation.
C. Useful in decreasing ventricular response in patients with atrial fibrillation.
D. Derived from the delphinium flower.

117. In which of the following has hormone replacement therapy (HRT) been shown to be of benefit?

A. Prevention of ischemic stroke in healthy women.
B. Prevention of ischemic stroke in women with coronary artery disease.
C. Prevention of ischemic stroke in women with a prior ischemic stroke.
D. Prevention of hemorrhagic stroke in healthy women.
E. None of the above.

118. The Stroke Prevention by Aggressive Reduction in Cholesterol Levels (SPARCL) Study:

A. Examined the role of cholesterol-lowering in primary risk reduction of ischemic stroke.
B. Showed that simvastatin (Zocor) 80 mg daily lowered risk of recurrent ischemic stroke.
C. Found that cholesterol lowering decreased overall mortality.
D. Found that cholesterol lowering was associated with an increased risk of hemorrhagic stroke.
E. Examined the role of cholesterol lowering in patients with known coronary artery disease.

119. Which of the following is most appropriate to treat cigarette abuse in patients who have had a stroke?

A. Bupropion (Zyban).
B. Varenicline (Chantix).
C. Nicotine gum or patches.
D. Hypnosis.
E. Telephone "quit line."

120. Which of the following chemotherapeutic agents is most associated with ischemic stroke?

A. Tamoxifen.
B. Anthracycline.
C. Trastuzumab.
D. Doxorubicin.
E. Cyclophosphamide.

121. Angiotensin-converting enzyme (ACE) inhibitors:

A. Reduce the risk of stroke in patients without hypertension.
B. Have frequent serious side effects.
C. Are approved for use during pregnancy.
D. Are contraindicated in patients with diabetes and renal dysfunction.

122. Angiotensin receptor blockers (ARBs) were compared with calcium-channel blockers in the Morbidity and Mortality after Stroke, Eprosartan (MOSES) trial. Patients were known hypertensives with stroke within 24 months. The end-point was a combination of stroke and vascular death. Which statement is correct about the results?

A. ARBs lowered blood pressure more rapidly and more effectively than did calcium-channel blockers.
B. ARBs decreased the occurrence of primary end-points more so than calcium-channel blockers, although the rapidity and efficacy of blood pressure lowering was identical between the two agents.
C. ARBs had more side effect than did calcium-channel blockers.
D. ARBs are more effective than ACE inhibitors in lowering blood pressure.

123. Which statement is true when comparing ARBs to ACE inhibitors?

A. Both agents cause cough, a nonserious side effect that leads to the discontinuation of the agents by some patients.
B. ACE inhibitors are favored over ARBs in patients with renal failure.
C. Unlike ACE inhibitors, ARBs can be used safely during pregnancy.
D. ACE inhibitors are more expensive than ARBs.

124. Which of the following statements best describes the use of anticoagulants in acute stroke patients not eligible for thrombolysis?

A. Intravenous unfractionated heparin has been shown by meta-analysis to result in a significant reduction in death or dependency.
B. Bolus infusion of intravenous unfractionated heparin should be given prior to a continuous infusion.
C. Intravenous heparin has been shown to halt progression of "stroke in evolution."
D. The use of low-dose subcutaneous heparin is appropriate to reduce the risk of DVT.
E. High-dose subcutaneous heparin decreases the risk of early stroke recurrence without risk of hemorrhagic stroke.

125. Decrease in risk of recurrent ischemic stroke through treatment with a HMG-CoA reductase inhibitor was found in which clinical trial?

A. The Stroke Prevention by Aggressive Reduction in Cholesterol Levels (SPARCL) Study.
B. The British Heart Protection Study (HPS).
C. The Cholesterol And Recurrent Events (CARE) Study.
D. The Scandinavian Simvastatin Survival Study (4S).
E. The Long-Term Intervention with Pravastatin in Ischemic Disease (LIPID) Study.

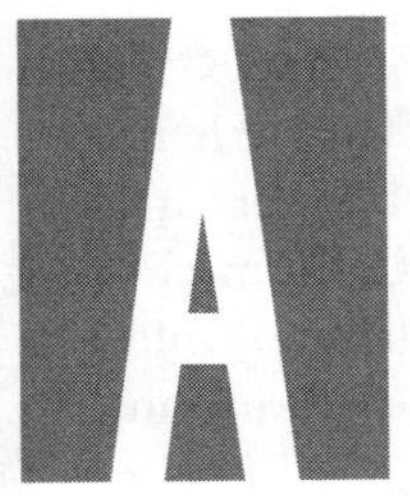

PHARMACOLOGY ANSWERS

28. The answer is D. Cyanide can accumulate and cause severe lactic acidosis in patients treated with sodium nitroprusside. This usually occurs in patients receiving high doses of nitroprusside, but it can also occur after treatment with moderate doses. Sodium thiosulfate enhances the metabolism of nitroprusside but can itself be toxic if administered for more than 24 to 48 hours. Nitroprusside dilates arterioles and venules, leading to a more profound hypotensive effect when the patient is upright. It does not impair renal perfusion but it increases intracranial pressure (ICP). The therapeutic effect of nitroprusside lasts less than 3 minutes after cessation, making it an ideal hypotensive agent, because it is immediately reversible. This has led to its use in the acute stroke patient, although its toxicity and the availability of alternate agents in recent years has decreased its role in the acute stroke patient. (Brunton, Chapter 32)

29. The answer is C. Angiotensin converting enzyme (ACE) inhibitors are preferred, because they delay the development of renal dysfunction in patients with diabetes. Calcium-channel blockers are recommended as the second agent if monotherapy is inadequate. β-Blockers may mask symptoms of hypoglycemia. Thiazide diuretics may raise glycosylated hemoglobin in diabetic patients. (Brunton, Chapter 32)

30. The answer is D. Thiazides elevate low-density lipoprotein (LDL) levels and increase the ratio of LDL to high-density lipoprotein (HDL). However this has not been shown to increase coronary artery disease. Thiazides remain the most frequently used class of agents for the treatment of hypertension in the United States. Thiazides do cross the placental barrier but have no direct teratogenic effects. They can cause volume depletion, resulting in placental hypoperfusion. They also appear in breast milk, so they should not be used by nursing mothers. Thiazides can cause impotence. (Brunton, Chapter 32)

31. The answer is A. Calcium-channel blockers can worsen cardiac hemodynamics in patients with diastolic dysfunction. Calcium-channel blockers are particularly effective in elderly patients and in African Americans. Calcium-channel blockers should not be used in patients with congestive heart failure. Unlike β-blockers, calcium-channel blockers generally do not exacerbate asthma and do not interfere with exercise tolerance. (Brunton, Chapter 32)

32. The answer is B. ACE inhibitors potentiate the effect of diuretics. They decrease the aldosterone response to sodium loss, so they can lower sodium when used in combination with diuretics. They generally have only small, clinically insignificant effects on potassium. However, because of the interaction with aldosterone, clinically significant elevations of potassium may occur in patients on potassium-sparing agents or in patients with renal failure. ACE inhibitors are contraindicated during pregnancy; therefore, they should be used with caution in women of childbearing age. (Brunton, Chapter 32)

33. The answer is D. Eighty percent of digitalis is excreted by the kidney. Dosages, or dosage intervals, must be modified in patients with renal failure. Digitalis has positive inotropic effects, making it a useful agent in heart failure. It is effective in decreasing the ventricular response in patients with atrial fibrillation, but it does not prevent recurrence of atrial fibrillation. Patients with thyrotoxicosis should be treated with β-blockers rather than digitalis, which does not decrease the heart rate in these patients. (Brunton, Chapter 34)

34. The answer is A. Methyldopa is an adrenergic agent used infrequently in the treatment of hypertension, because of side effects, which include immunologic abnormalities and headache. It can be used during pregnancy because it is relatively effective and safe for both mother and fetus. This drug is centrally active. Because it does not inhibit the baroreceptors as peripherally active agents do, it rarely produces symptomatic orthostatic hypotension. It can produce transient sedation and depression. (Brunton, Chapter 34)

35. The answer is D. The exact cause of variant angina has not been completely explained, and the standard treatments for angina have not been effective. Nitrates do not favorably alter mortality in this group of patients, but calcium-channel blockers are effective. Abnormal coronary anatomy has been found in autopsied cases of variant angina, but the lack of effect of aspirin suggests that platelet aggregation is not a precipitating factor of acute symptoms. β-Blockade is deleterious in this type of angina. (Brunton, Chapter 31)

36. The answer is B. Calcium-channel blockers decrease coronary vascular resistance and increase coronary blood flow. They are useful in variant angina but are also useful in the treatment of exertional angina. Calcium-channel blockers also have some utility in unstable angina, although alternate therapies including platelet inhibition, thrombolysis, and β-blockade are clearly more effective. (Brunton, Chapter 31)

37. The answer is D. Current guidelines suggest that children with LDL levels over 160 mL/dL and a family history of atherosclerosis should be treated pharmacologically. Statins have been used successfully and safely in children, as have bile-acid sequestrants. Either of these are reasonable choices as lipid-lowering agents in children. (Holmes, *Curr Cardiol Rep* 2005; Wiegman, *JAMA* 2004)

38. The answer is E. Primary prevention studies have shown marked benefit to blood-pressure lowering in patients with diabetes, with the Joint National Committee-7 guidelines suggesting a reduction target in diabetic patients of 115/75. Blood pressure management using thiazide diuretics, β-blockers, angiotensin receptor blockers (ARBs), and ACE inhibitors is of benefit in reducing cardiovascular and cerebrovascular events in patients with diabetes. Angiotensin receptor blockers and ACE inhibitors should be used as first-line agents in diabetic patients because of the reduction of progression to nephropathy and albuminuria. Calcium-channel blockers should be considered add-on agents, because they do not appear to reduce the progression of renal disease in diabetic patients. Most diabetic patients need multiple agents for the optimum control of blood pressure. (Sacco et al., *Stroke* 2006)

39. The answer is C. Several secondary causes of hyperlipidemia exist, including diabetes, excess alcohol, estrogen therapies, nephrotic syndrome, glucocorticoid excess (both endogenous and iatrogenic), obstructive liver disease, and hypothyroidism. The last two elevate total cholesterol more than triglycerides, and the others elevate triglycerides more than total cholesterol. Clinical trials have shown a benefit of total cholesterol-lowering therapy in both men and women, but women benefit more than do men. Populations with low total cholesterol, such as the Chinese and patients with congenital disorders associated with very low cholesterol, do not have higher cardiac or noncardiac mortality. The consequence of lowering cholesterol to below 150 mL/dL has not been systematically tested. Diet is effective in reducing lipids, with more dramatic effect on triglycerides than cholesterol. Dietary cholesterols are a major constituent of chylomicrons, and the only method for reducing chylomicron levels is reducing dietary fats. (Brunton, Chapter 35)

40. The answer is B. Statins enhance the synthesis and decrease the degradation of LDL receptors on hepatocytes, resulting in enhanced removal of LDL from the blood. Statins do not alter the absorption of dietary fats. Statins competitively inhibit hydroxy-3-methylglutaryl coenzyme A (HMG-CoA) reductase activity (without changing levels), decrease hepatic synthesis of apolipoprotein B-100 and decrease the synthesis of triglyceride-rich lipoproteins. (Maron, *Circulation* 2001)

41. The answer is B. The incidence of elevation of liver enzymes with statin use is about 1%. Liver function tests should be done before starting a statin, and then should be checked in 3 months and in 6 months after starting the drug. Because this side effect is dose-dependent, liver functions tests should also be checked 3 and 6 months after increasing the dose. Once the dosage is stable, liver functions can be checked every 6 to 12 months. Statins do not produce cough, which is the most common side effect of ACE inhibitors. Myopathy is a rare side effect of statins, although combination therapy with some other cholesterol-lowering drugs, particularly fibric-acid derivatives, increases the risk. Rhabdomyolysis can occur in patients with statin-induced myopathy and can produce renal failure. Cerivastatin (Baychol), the statin most highly associated with myopathy and rhabdomyolysis, was taken off the market in 2001. (Brunton, Chapter 32)

42. The answer is A. These agents are among the oldest and safest cholesterol-lowering agents. Because of their safety, they were previously the only agents recommended in children. Trials of statins in children with familial hypercholesterolemia who had LDL levels of at least 155 mL/dL found that statins were safe and effective. Bile-acid sequestrants are contraindicated in patients with very high triglycerides, because they can further elevate triglycerides. These agents interfere with the absorption of numerous drugs, including warfarin. (Brunton, Chapter 35; Wiegman, *JAMA* 2004)

43. The answer is A. Normal vascular endothelium produces substances that generally prevent platelet aggregation and thrombus formation. In situations in which the endothelium is disrupted or there are deficiencies of endogenous protective mechanisms, platelet aggregation and thrombus formation may occur. Tissue factor is an endogenous procoagulant substance. Heparan sulfate is an endogenous anticoagulant, but it is not a plasma protein. Heparan sulfate is synthesized in the endothelial cells. Prostacyclin is also synthesized by endothelial cells, but it inhibits platelet aggregation and does not directly affect the coagulation cascade. (Brunton, Chapter 54)

44. The answer is B. The first source of heparin available for study was extracted from dog liver and had major toxicity in humans. Beef liver proved to be less toxic, but when the price of beef liver increased (because of a growing demand for pet food), investigators discovered that beef lung and intestine were also good sources of heparin. The most common sources of heparin today are porcine intestinal mucosa and bovine lung. Bioavailability of heparin from various sources is very similar. Rabbit is a common source of thromboplastin used in the prothrombin time (PT) analysis, but is not a standard source of heparin. Human cells are not a commercial source of heparin. (Brunton, Chapter 54)

45. The answer is C. Antithrombin is a critical heparin cofactor. Heparin is a strong catalyst for the thrombin-antithrombin reaction. Fibroblast growth factors do bind to heparin, but this interaction produces endothelial proliferation and angiogenesis rather than anticoagulation. Heparan sulfate is an anticoagulant substance produced by the endothelial cells, but neither it nor any other endothelial product is necessary for the action of heparin. (Brunton, Chapter 54)

46. The answer is D. Osteoporosis is a potential, but not a common, complication of heparin and is generally associated with extended administration (3–6 months) of full-dose heparin. High doses of heparin have an antiplatelet effect. Heparin does not cross the placenta. Heparin can produce thrombocytopenia, but this is through an antibody-mediated effect on platelets. (Brunton, Chapter 54)

47. The answer is B. The therapeutic range for heparin is 0.3 to 0.7 U/mL, depending on the intensity of anticoagulation desired. The partial thromboplastin time (aPTT) that corresponds to this range is variable, depending on the equipment and the reagents used to perform the test. Some aPTT tests will overestimate the level of anticoagulation of heparin. Bleeding time is a measurement of platelet inhibition. Although it will be extended by high doses of heparin, the bleeding time is not an accurate measurement of heparin anticoagulant activity. D-Dimer is a measure of fibrin split products. C-reactive protein is an inflammatory marker that is directly proportional to the risk of vascular disease. (Brunton, Chapter 54)

48. The answer is B. The plasma half-life ($t_{1/2}$) of heparin is dose-dependent. At a dose of 100 U/kg of heparin administered intravenously, which is in the range of the standard 5,000-unit initial bolus frequently used clinically, the $t_{1/2}$ is very short. Because of this phenomenon, immediate administration of an IV drip is necessary if continued anticoagulation is desired. Higher doses of heparin result in a longer $t_{1/2}$. Subcutaneous administration results in a prolonged absorption, with a long $t_{1/2}$, but a lower peak level. It should be noted that, before the advent of automated infusion pumps, heparin was frequently administered by hourly IV infusions of maintenance doses. This is a technique that is still useful in situations where patients need to be removed from infusion pumps to obtain diagnostic studies or for rehabilitation activities. (Brunton, Chapter 54)

49. The answer is B. The dose is 1 mg/kg b.i.d., for a total of 2 mg/kg/day in two equally divided doses. The 100-mg daily dose is appropriate only for patients weighing approximately 110 pounds. The standard dose for Lovenox is based on weight and was determined in trials of deep venous thrombosis (DVT) prevention. At this dose, monitoring is not necessary. Higher doses can be used, but require monitoring with factor Xa inhibition levels. This assay is not always available in many areas of the country, and it may require 2 to 3 days to obtain the results. In those situations where more aggressive anticoagulation is needed (e.g., patients with DVT that progresses on standard-dose Lovenox), IV unfractionated heparin may be necessary if factor Xa inhibition levels are not readily available. (Brunton, Chapter 54)

50. The answer is C. Danaparoid is a mixture of heparin sulfate, dermatan sulfate, and chondroitin sulfate that is derived from porcine intestine. It is not related to hirudin and does not prolong standard clotting assays (PT, aPTT) at recommended doses. It does inhibit factor Xa. Although factor Xa levels are not required for monitoring in most patients, monitoring may be required in the setting of renal failure. This drug is approved for the prevention of DVT in patients who cannot be given heparin because of heparin antibody–induced thrombocytopenia. (Frangos, *J Am Coll Surg* 2000)

51. The answer is C. Lepirudin is a recombinant derivative of hirudin and is approved for anticoagulation in patients with heparin-induced thrombocytopenia. It is monitored using the aPTT, but is not reversible with any agent. It can produce antihirudin antibodies, which can cause a paradoxical increase in the aPTT. A daily aPTT should be obtained during therapy. It is administered IV. (Brunton, Chapter 54)

52. The answer is B. The $t_{1/2}$ of factor VII is only 6 hours. Factor II has the longest $t_{1/2}$ of 50 hours. Because of the long $t_{1/2}$ of factor II, the full anticoagulant effect of warfarin is not achieved for several days, despite possible early elevations of the PT and international normalized ratio (INR) when the factors with shorter half times are reduced. (Brunton, Chapter 54)

53. The answer is D. In the absence of bleeding complications, oral vitamin K is not recommended for an INR of 4.3. Vitamin K given intravenously should be reserved for a seriously elevated INR with active bleeding. Even in this setting, fresh frozen plasma is considered safer than intravenous vitamin K and will more quickly reverse the coagulopathy. The exception to this might be in a patient with congestive heart failure, a setting in which volume overload from fresh frozen plasma could worsen the heart failure. Warfarin should be held 1 or 2 days, but 1 week without warfarin is excessive and will result in complete loss of effective anticoagulation in most patients. (Ansell, *Chest* 2001; Sachdev, et al. *Am J Health Syst Pharm* 1999)

54. The answer is D. This is a massive overdose, with active bleeding, so immediate reversal is necessary. Vitamin K's effect requires several hours, because the synthesis of fully active coagulation factors is required for its effect. Fresh frozen plasma is the fastest way to provide active coagulation factors, but the infused coagulation factors with short t½ (namely factor VII) will be cleared from the system faster than the residual blood levels of the warfarin. Thus, IV vitamin K is necessary to stimulate liver production of active coagulation factors and to maintain the reversal of the excess anticoagulation. There is a risk of anaphylaxis with IV vitamin K, so it should be used with caution and only in situations of massive anticoagulation overdose or active bleeding with warfarin overdose. The action of oral vitamin K takes 24 to 48 hours and is not fast enough to be useful in this situation. Intravenous vitamin K acts in 6 to 24 hours. Subcutaneous vitamin K takes longer for its action and is less reliably absorbed. (Aguilar, *Mayo Clin Proc* 2007)

55. The answer is C. Therapeutic warfarin decreases the production of coagulation factors by the liver by 30% to 50%. Full carboxylation of the factors is necessary for maximum activity, and warfarin decreases the carboxylation, resulting in a 10% to 40% decrease in the bioactivity of the clotting factors. Warfarin does not interfere with the activity of fully carboxylated clotting factors. Heparin is the agent that interferes with the activity of circulating clotting factors. (Brunton, Chapter 54)

56. The answer is B. In the absence of bleeding, a patient with an INR 7 to 9 can be managed as an outpatient. The administration of fresh frozen plasma is not necessary, and oral vitamin K is sufficient. The dose of oral vitamin K varies from 1 to 2.5 mg for an INR from 5.0 to 9.0, and 3 to 5 mg for an INR above 9. Higher doses of vitamin K will overcorrect the anticoagulation. Warfarin should be discontinued until the INR is clearly moving lower, although the delayed action of warfarin requires it be restarted at a slightly lower dose before the INR reaches the standard therapeutic range, in order to avoid a subtherapeutic INR 3 to 5 days later. (Brunton, Chapter 54)

57. The answer is B. In the absence of fibrin, tissue plasminogen (t-PA) is a poor fibrinolytic agent. The initial hope when this agent was developed was that the fibrin specificity would prevent significant hemorrhagic complications of the drug. Even though hemorrhage is a significant side effect, the fibrin specificity prevents diffuse plasminogen activation and a systemic lytic state. Clearance of t-PA occurs mainly through the liver. Streptokinase is much less expensive than t-PA, but is not used in cerebrovascular disease because of excess hemorrhage. (Brunton, Chapter 54)

58. The answer is B. Aminocaproic acid is a lysine analog that blocks the binding of lysine to plasminogen and plasmin, thus inhibiting fibrinolysis. It has no procoagulant activity. Aminocaproic acid has been tried for various bleeding conditions and, in the past, was given to prevent rebleeding in subarachnoid hemorrhage, but the thrombotic complications outweigh its potential therapeutic benefit. This agent has been studied to prevent bleeding during surgery, but benefit has not been established. (Brunton, Chapter 54)

59. The answer is C. Aspirin decreases the activity of cyclooxygenase, blocking the production of thromboxane A2, a compound with both antiplatelet and vasoconstrictor effect. The antiplatelet activity of aspirin is present at low dose, with the clinical recommendation that it be dosed from 50 to 325 mg daily for secondary stroke prevention. Gastrointestinal toxicity and bleeding risk increase at higher doses. (Brunton, Chapter 54)

60. The answer is D. Dipyridamole produces its antiplatelet effect by increasing the intracellular concentration of cyclic adenosine monophosphate (cAMP). It blocks the uptake of adenosine, which is a stimulator for platelet adenyl cyclase. It also inhibits cyclic nucleotide phosphodiesterase. Dipyridamole has a vasodilatory effect, which is the major contributor to the transient headaches sometimes seen when initiating this agent at high doses. It does not interfere with cyclooxygenase, the method of platelet inhibition of aspirin. (Brunton, Chapter 54)

61. The answer is C. Clopidogrel has a much more favorable toxicity profile than does ticlopidine. Although ticlopidine is still available, it is rarely used because of the hematologic side effects, mainly neutropenia and thrombotic thrombocytopenia purpura. Nausea and vomiting, which are common with ticlopidine, are infrequent with clopidogrel. Both agents are rapidly absorbed, but maximal inhibition of platelets takes 8 to 11 days. It is thought that these agents are probably prodrugs, requiring metabolism to the active (as-yet unknown) ingredients. Loading doses do result in a more rapid onset of action. Loading doses of ticlopidine 500 mg and of clopidogrel 300 mg are commonly used. Both agents inhibit platelets, but neither has a vasodilatory effect. They are both thienopyridines and are closely related chemically. The only platelet inhibitor in common usage that has vasodilatory effect is dipyridamole, most commonly used in combination with low-dose aspirin and marketed as Aggrenox. (Brunton, Chapter 54)

Ticlopidine

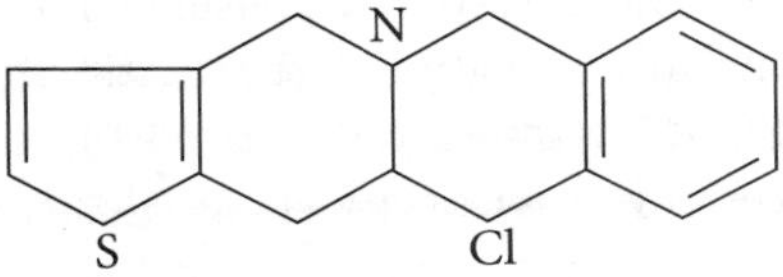

Clopidogrel

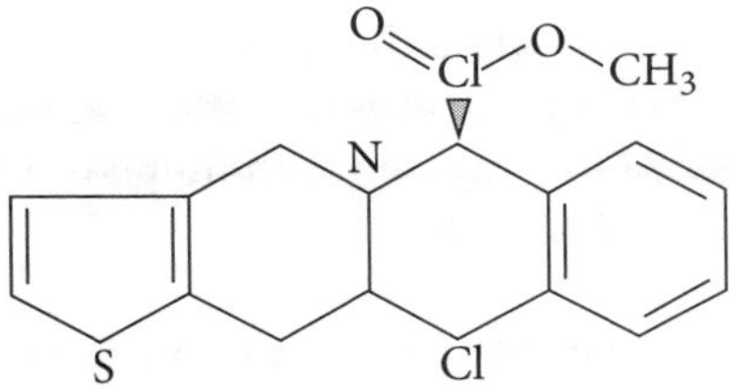

62. The answer is A. Abciximab is the Fab fragment from a humanized monoclonal antibody that is directed toward the platelet glycoprotein IIb/IIIa receptor. It interacts with this dimeric receptor, inhibiting the receptor for fibrinogen and for the procoagulant substance von Willebrand factor. The unbound antibody has a short half-life of only 30 minutes, but the bound antibody remains on the receptor and exhibits platelet inhibitory effects for 18 to 24 hours. It is administered IV with a 0.25 mg/kg bolus followed by a 0.125 mg/kg/min IV infusion. This agent has been demonstrated to prevent restenosis following coronary angioplasty. Its role in stroke is not yet established. (Brunton, Chapter 54)

63. The answer is D. Eptifibatide is a peptide, not an antibody. It inhibits platelets via interaction with the platelet glycoprotein IIb/IIIa receptor, but does not interact with the vitronectin receptor. Thus, its antiplatelet effect should be less than that of abciximab (ReoPro), which interacts both with the platelet glycoprotein IIb/IIIa receptor and the vitronectin receptor. Eptifibatide has a short $t_{1/2}$ of 6 to 12 hours following IV infusion. This agent is presently used in the setting of unstable angina or following coronary angioplasty. Tirofiban (Aggrastat) has a similar method of action to eptifibatide, but is a small nonpeptide molecule that is also administered intravenously. The development of oral agents to inhibit the platelet glycoprotein IIb/IIIa receptor has been thwarted by serious side effects. (Brunton, Chapter 54)

64. The answer is A. Muscle weakness, pain, or cramps is a symptom of a potentially serious complication of statin therapy. Muscle breakdown (rhabdomyolysis) can lead to myoglobinuria and renal failure. Rhabdomyolysis occurs at creatine kinase (CK) levels greater than 10 times the upper limit of normal. Elevations of CK are relatively common, so it is recommended by many experts that a CK be obtained before starting statin therapy, so that a baseline for the individual patient is available for comparison during treatment. The statin guidelines state that a statin should be discontinued if the CK elevation is greater than *ten* times the normal range or if progressive elevations occur on serial testing in a given patient. Elevations of three to ten times the upper limit of normal should prompt an evaluation for common causes of elevated CK, such as trauma or exercise. Thyroid function tests should be checked, because hypothyroidism predisposes to myopathy. The symptoms should not be masked with quinine, and an EMG is of no value. (Pasternak, *J Am Coll Cardiol* 2002)

65. The answer is B. In the European Stroke Prevention Study 2 (ESPS-2), headache was more frequent in patients on Aggrenox compared to aspirin. This is thought to be due to the vasodilatory effect of the dipyridamole. This side effect generally resolves within 1 to 2 weeks, but headache is the most common reason for discontinuation of this medication. The dose of aspirin is small, 25 mg b.i.d., so gastric irritation is unlikely. In patients with true aspirin allergy, however, this medication should not be administered. Leukopenia and insomnia are not side effects of this medication. Hematuria would be an occasional side effect with any platelet inhibitor. (Diener, *J Neuro Sci* 1996)

66. The answer is C. Low-molecular-weight heparin decreases the inhibition of factor Xa and does not affect the level of Xa. D-Dimer measures fibrin breakdown products and is a measure of active thrombus formation. The PTT measures the therapeutic effect of unfractionated heparin. (Brunton, Chapter 54)

67. The answer is D. Warfarin is teratogenic and should not be administered during pregnancy, although use of this agent may be considered after the first trimester of pregnancy. Subcutaneous low-molecular-weight heparin may be given to women at risk of thrombosis during pregnancy. Although obvious hemorrhagic risks are related to pregnancy and delivery, which will be increased by anticoagulation therapy of any type, this is a relatively minor problem in clinical practice. Answers B and C are distractors, because warfarin does not irritate the gastric mucosa, nor does it cause preeclampsia. If a patient were to develop preeclampsia, hypertension would increase the hemorrhagic risk of anticoagulation. (Greer, *J Thromb Thrombolysis* 2006)

68. The answer is A. The interaction between levetiracetam and warfarin has been specifically studied, and warfarin kinetics and INR levels were not influenced by the addition of levetiracetam (Keppra). In general, the anticonvulsant agents developed in the last two decades have fewer drug interactions that do older agents. They are not metabolized by the cytochrome P system, making interactions with warfarin much less likely, although this has not been formally studied with all these agents. The other three agents listed all interact with the cytochrome P system and will alter warfarin metabolism and INR levels. (Patsolos, *Epilepsia* 2002)

69. The answer is B. Amiodarone, which increases the refractory period of the left atrium, is now frequently used in the treatment of atrial fibrillation. It *decreases* the ventricular response in patients with atrial fibrillation. Both of these effects are useful in decreasing heart rate in patients with atrial fibrillation. After cardioversion, amiodarone dosage may be reduced. (Tieleman, *Am J Cardiol* 1997)

70. The answer is D. Rash occurs in about 4.2% of patients taking Plavix. There were no reports of thrombocytopenia in the initial trial of Plavix, but postmarketing reports include an incidence of thrombotic thrombocytopenia purpura of about 4 in 1million users of the agent. Headache is not a side effect of Plavix. Intraocular bleeding with visual loss is very rare with Plavix. (*Physician's Desk Reference*)

71. The answer is A. Cilostazol (Pletal) is a quinolinone derivative approved in the United States for treatment of claudication. It is an oral agent that inhibits phosphodiesterase, producing platelet inhibition, and it also has vasodilatory effects. Side effects are relatively minor and include headache, diarrhea, and dizziness. It was studied in Japan in 1,000 patients in a randomized, double-blind trial, and was found effective in reducing stroke ($p = 0.015$). Unfortunately, because patients were randomized to Pletal versus placebo, we do not know whether it is any better than aspirin alone. Pletal is not approved in the United States for secondary stroke prevention. (Matsumoto, *Atheroscler Suppl* 2005)

72. The answer is C. Suppression of production of cholesterol by the liver is the mechanism of action of statins. Bile acid sequestrants (cholestyramine [Questran], colestipol [Colestid], and colesevelam [Welchol]) cause bile acids to be excreted in the stool. Blood levels of Zetia are slightly higher (<20%) in women than in men, but can be twice as high in the elderly. There were no differences based on ethnic origin. (*Physician's Desk Reference*)

73. The answer is C. Niacin in high doses raises HDL by 30% to 40%. Zetia alone has little or no effect on HDL, with reports of both increases and decreases of 1% to 2%. With the use of Zetia in combination with atorvastatin (Zocor), HDL was elevated by 3% to 9%. Rosuvastatin (Crestor) increased HDL by 3% to 22%, depending on the dose and the patient population being studied. Tricor and red wine increase HDL by 19% and 15%, respectively. (Brunton, Chapter 35; *Physician's Desk Reference*)

74. The answer is A. The major side effects of niacin are flushing and dyspepsia. A daily dose of 325 mg of aspirin will reduce the problem with flushing in many patients. Taking the medication with food may decrease the dyspepsia. The side effects worsen with increasing dosage. They occur frequently, and lead to patient noncompliance. They are worsened by taking the medication with hot drinks or with alcohol. In patients with diabetes, niacin can cause insulin resistance, which can elevate blood glucose. Niacin should be used with caution (if at all) in patients with diabetes. Niacin can also elevate uric acid, so it should be used with caution in patients with gout. (Brunton, Chapter 35)

75. The answer is C. Niacin is an extremely effective treatment for dyslipidemia. It is the oldest agent used for this purpose and has an advantage of positive effects on essentially all lipid parameters. Many patients prefer "natural" treatments to "medications," and niacin appeals to such individuals. Unfortunately, both the major and minor side effects are significant. The discontinuation rate of niacin is high because of flushing and dyspepsia. More serious is the liver toxicity, which can occur at any time during therapy. Liver function tests should be ordered every 3 to 6 months. Sustained-release niacin has a much higher level of liver toxicity than does crystalline niacin. Because both these preparations are available over-the-counter, it is important that physicians counsel patients against the sustained-release niacin. (Brunton, Chapter 35)

76. The answer is B. Omacor does decrease triglyceride levels, but it has not been studied for the prevention of pancreatitis in patients with very high triglycerides. Fibric-acid derivatives have both anticoagulant and fibrinolytic effects. They are the treatment of choice in patients with triglyceride levels above 1,000 mg/dL who are at risk for pancreatitis. They are relatively contraindicated in patients with either liver or kidney disease. (Brunton, Chapter 35; *Physician's Desk Reference*)

77. The answer is C. Many patients do not achieve adequate treatment of dyslipidemia on a statin alone. Combining statins with other agents carries an increased risk of muscle toxicity in many cases. The combination of statins with bile-acid sequestrants is particularly effective when large reductions of LDL are needed. The risk of myopathy is not increased by this combination. The effect of statins is also enhanced by niacin, but the risk of myopathy increases. This combination can only be used with low-dose (less than 25% of the maximum dose) statins. Fibric-acid derivatives are very useful in combination with statins in patients with both high triglycerides and high LDL. Because of the increased risk of myopathy, the statin dose should again be limited to 25% of the maximum. Tricor is also used in combination with statins, but again with an increased risk of rhabdomyolosis. (Brunton, Chapter 35)

78. The answer is B. Omacor lowers triglycerides, raises LDL, raises HDL, and lowers very-low-density lipoprotein (VLDL). No safety studies have been done on its use in pregnant women, and toxicity during pregnancy in animals have been at doses many times the standard dose in humans. Omacor is given a category C classification for pregnancy. The side effects of Omacor are relatively mild. The major serious side effect with Omacor is elevation of LDL. (*Physician's Desk Reference*)

79. The answer is B. Hydralazine, methyldopa, β-Blockers and calcium-channel blockers are reasonable choices to treat chronic hypertension in pregnancy. Hydralazine is used in pregnancy with only rare reports of fetal thrombocytopenia. Methyldopa has a well-documented safety record for chronic use in pregnancy. β-Blockers, especially atenolol, may be associated with intrauterine growth retardation. Calcium-channel blockers at high doses should be avoided in the first trimester. No randomized trials have evaluated the treatment of chronic hypertension in pregnancy. Both maternal and fetal outcomes are worsened by hypertension. Magnesium sulfate is the treatment of choice for preeclampsia, but it is not used for treatment of chronic hypertension during pregnancy. Intravenous hydralazine or labetolol may also be used to treat acutely elevated blood pressure in pregnancy. (Subai, *Obstet Gynecol* 2005)

80. The answer is C. Studies have shown that patients who are taught to self-test and manage their own warfarin maintain a therapeutic INR range longer than do patients managed by a clinic using traditional measures. The major drawback is cost, because most insurance companies are not paying for the testing devices and reagents. Of note, Medicare has recently approved payment of point-of-care warfarin monitoring equipment for patients with mechanical heart valves. (Gardiner, *Br J Haematol* 2006)

81. The answer is B. All of these agents can be used in patients with a severe migraine headache lasting longer than 72 hours and refractory to usual oral migraine therapies. Dihydroergotamine (DHE) is a vasoconstrictor that has an effect on arteries, including in the carotid and coronary beds, and on veins. Ergot alkaloids, including DHE and ergotamine, should not be used in patients with known or symptomatic vascular disease. (Oleson J, et al., 2006)

82. The answer is B. Statins do not produce orthostatic hypotension. Many antihypertensives and diuretics contribute to orthostatic hypotension, along with phenothiazines, antidepressants, antiparkinsonian agents, and central nervous system depressants. A thorough review of the patient's medications is necessary in the evaluation of orthostatic hypotension. (Fuster, Chapter 40)

83. The answer is C. Elevated lipids are not as well established as risk factors for cerebrovascular disease as they are for cardiovascular disease. The stroke risk reduction seen in patients with cerebrovascular disease who are treated with statins extends beyond the effects of cholesterol reduction, so statin treatment reduces stroke risk even in patients with normal cholesterol levels. Nonstatin medications to treat dyslipidemias (e.g., niacin, fibrates, cholesterol absorption inhibitors) can be used in cerebrovascular patients who cannot tolerate statins, but evidence of their efficacy in prevention of secondary stroke is scant. Some data indicate the benefit of niacin and gemfibrozil in stroke risk reduction in persons with low HDL levels. The recommendation in patients with symptomatic atherosclerotic is to aim for an LDL level of less than 100 mg/dL. The recommendation in very-high-risk patients with multiple risk factors is to aim for an LDL level of less than 70 mg/dL. (Sacco et al., *Stroke* 2006)

84. The answer is D. Statins frequently produce transient elevation in liver enzymes and a single elevation of liver enzymes does not dictate discontinuation. But if there is a persistent elevation above three times normal, the statin should be discontinued. (*Physician's Desk Reference*)

85. The answer is C. Prothrombin complex concentrates (PCCs) contain varying amounts of Factors II, VII, IX, and X, and are used to prevent bleeding in patients with factor IX deficiency. The concentrates are expensive and not readily available. They can be used to treat warfarin-induced intracerebral hemorrhage through normalization of the INR much more rapidly than does fresh frozen plasma (FFP) infusion. The PCC infusion should be combined with vitamin K when reversing an elevated INR. They are generally not used in patients with severe liver disease. (Aguilar, *Mayo Clin Proc* 2007)

86. The answer is C. Nitroprusside, a nitrovasodilator, lacks a smooth dose response and can cause excess hypotension in the elderly and rebound hypertension with withdrawal. There is a potential for cyanide and thiocyanate toxicity with prolonged use. It may also elevate intracranial pressure through its vasodilatory effect. For these reasons, it is now rarely used in neurologic emergencies. (Rose & Mayer, *Neuro Crit Care* 2004)

87. The answers are A 1, B 3, C 5, D 4, E 2. Labetalol is an adrenergic receptor-blocking agent with greater blockade of the $\beta_1$and β_2 receptors than of the α_1 receptors. Esmolol is a cardioselective β_1 receptor antagonist that rapidly lowers blood pressure with a short duration of action. Nicardipine is a dihydropyridine calcium channel blocker that lowers blood pressure acutely without increasing intracranial pressure. Enalaprilat is an ACE inhibitor for intravenous injection. It is the active metabolite of the orally administered pro-drug enalapril maleate. Enalaprilat is poorly absorbed orally. Fenoldopam (Corlopam) is a selective, dopamine (DA_1) receptor agonist that causes both systemic and renal arteriolar vasodilation. (Rose & Mayer, *Neuro Crit Care* 2004)

88. The answer is C. Fenoldopam (Corlopam) is a selective, dopamine (DA_1) receptor agonist that causes both systemic and renal arteriolar vasodilation. In hypertensive patients, fenoldopam decreases blood pressure, increases renal blood flow, and maintains or improves the glomerular filtration rate. Selective DA_1 agonists that decrease renal vascular resistance, increase renal blood flow, and increase sodium excretion and urine volume may be useful in acute renal failure. (Rose & Mayer, *Neuro Crit Care* 2004)

89. The answer is A. In patients with chronic renal disease, the goals of lowering blood pressure are to slow the deterioration of renal function and to prevent vascular disease. The ACE inhibitors and ARBs can decrease the progression of diabetic and nondiabetic renal disease. With advanced renal disease, loop diuretics may be combined with other drug classes. Ramipril (Altace) is an ACE inhibitor and would be indicated for initial therapy. Metoprolol (β-blocker), amlodipine and verapamil (calcium-channel blockers), and doxazosin (α-blocker) are not recommended initial drugs in renal patients. (Chobanian et al., *JAMA* 2003)

90. The answer is D. Although the reported digestive upset is on the order of 6%, in clinical practice discontinuation for digestive problems is more likely two to three times higher than that number. Allergic reactions with rash or urticaria occur early in 10% to 15% of patients. The drug is still available. Thrombocytopenia can occur from ticlopidine, but the most serious blood dyscrasia is leukopenia. Blood counts should be monitored every 2 weeks in patients for the first 3 months. Ticlopidine has been studied and approved for secondary stroke prevention, not for primary prevention. (*Physician's Desk Reference*)

91. The answer is C. Alternative pharmacotherapy, including fish oils, garlic supplements, ginkgo biloba, and ginseng, used in the management of cardiovascular disease may have bleeding effects in combination with antiplatelet or anticoagulant medications. L-Arginine's most common side effects are gastrointestinal. (Chagan et al., *Am J Manag Care* 2002)

92. The answer is D. Elevating low HDL levels has cardiovascular benefit. Mild to moderate alcohol consumption may be associated with raising HDL levels but treatment of low levels is generally achieved by medication. Statins and fibric-acid derivatives result in a 5% to 10% and 10% to 20% increase in HDL levels, respectively. Thiazolidinediones result in around a 15% increase in patients with diabetes and other metabolic disorders. Nicotinic acid inhibits the hepatic uptake of apo A-1 and decreases hepatic lipase activity, leading to an increased level up to 30% to 35%. (Khuseyinova & Keonig, *Curr Athero Rep* 2006)

93. The answer is A. Multiple medications in general, and multiple organ disease, all predispose to the development of statin-induced myopathy. Medications that are particularly risky include amiodarone, other cholesterol-lowering agents (particularly fibrates, but sometimes also nicotinic acid), cyclosporine, "azole" antifungals (e.g., ketoconazole), erythromycin, macrolide antibiotics, verapamil, and HIV protease inhibitors. Large quantities of grapefruit juice, in excess of a quart a day, also pose a risk. The impression that grapefruit juice is "contraindicated" is incorrect. (Unfortunately, this is something often promulgated by pharmacies, and appropriate patient education is important.) Small body frame increases the risk, as does age (over 80), particularly in females. (Pasternak, *J Am Coll Cardiol* 2002)

94. The answer is B. Creatine kinase levels should also be checked prior to treatment to obtain a baseline. There is no role for checking CK levels unless the patient is symptomatic (muscle pain or severe weakness). Because the potentially dangerous side effect of statins is rhabdomyolysis leading to renal failure, muscle weakness or pain alone without an elevation of CK is *not* a dangerous problem. Most patients will stop the drug with weakness, but in the absence of an elevated CK this is not an emergency. Blood count measurements are not a routine part of the monitoring of statins. (Pasternak, *J Am Coll Cardiol* 2002)

95. The answer is A. Statin-associated myopathy is clearly dose-dependent, occurring more often at higher doses. It is a relatively rare problem that occurs almost always in patients with other risks. The nature of the lipid problem being treated does not predispose to myopathy. Warfarin is not a drug than increases the incidence of statin-induced myopathy. (Pasternak, *J Am Coll Cardiol* 2002)

96. The answer is D. At one time, high-dose vitamin E was thought to have vascular risk-reduction properties, but the negative results of multiple recent clinical trials of vitamin E indicate that it may be at best ineffective and, at worst, harmful. The recently published Women's Health Study and the Heart Outcome Prevention Evaluation—The Ongoing Outcomes both found lack of vascular benefit. Recent studies of vitamin E in patients with Alzheimer disease and amyotrophic lateral sclerosis have also shown no benefit in treating those diseases. There is no reason why this elderly man needs to take high-dose vitamin E supplements. (Guallar et al., *Ann Int Med* 2005)

97. The answer is C. Angiotensin II has a major role in the development of cardiac fibrosis and hypertrophy. Long-term ACE inhibition is recommended in patients with cardiac failure and hypertension. Calcium-channel blockers have negative inotropic effects and are not recommended for treatment of cardiac failure. The benefits of β-blockers in patients with heart failure are now well defined. The combination of β-blockers and ACE inhibitors should be used in patients with heart failure, unless contraindications are present. Digitalis glycosides are the only oral inotropic agents available for the treatment of heart failure. They increase cardiac contractility. The usefulness of digitalis glycosides in right-sided heart failure and in ischemia-induced heart failure is limited, and side effects are numerous. (Fuster, Chapter 25)

98. The answer is A. Patients with hypereosinophilic syndrome are initially treated with prednisone. For the unusual cases that do not respond interferon-α or cytotoxic chemotherapy are options. Wegener's granulomatosis, granulomatous angiitis CNS, and periarteritis nodosum are all vasculidities that may not be controlled by corticosteroids alone, and that almost invariably require immunosuppressive agents. It should be noted that there is a benign form of CNS vasculitis that occurs most often in young women. It generally responds to corticosteroids, and does not require the same aggressive therapy as that required by the classic granulomatous angiitis of the CNS. Stroke in SLE is often related to a hypercoagulable state or to cardiogenic emboli, in which case anticoagulation may be the preferred treatment. Patients with SLE rarely have underlying vasculitis as a cause of stroke. (Futrell & Millikan, *Stroke* 1989; Rich, Chapter 56)

99. The answers are A 3, B 4, C 1, D 2, E 5. Both intravenous vitamin K (10 mg) and FFP take many hours to reduce the INR. The volume of FFP needed to reverse the anticoagulant effect completely (up to 2–4L) may be risky. A rapid infusion of FFP is necessary to increase the plasma protein levels significantly, but a risk of volume overload exists. The use of PCC, which is made up of multiple coagulation factors including factor IX, normalizes the INR more quickly than FFP infusion, but it is expensive and not readily available. Recombinant factor VIIa has been used to reverse anticoagulation in patients with intracerebral hemorrhage. Although it reverses the factor VII deficiency, it does not replace the other factors, and it may need to be repeated frequently or combined with vitamin K and FFP. The short half-life of factor VIIa concentrate makes induction of a prothrombotic state unlikely. (Aguilar et al., *Mayo Clin Proc* 2007)

100. The answer is B. Triptans, 5HT1B/1D agonists, are effective medications to abort acute episodic migraines. However, they should not be used in migraine sufferers who have untreated or symptomatic vascular disease, including uncontrolled hypertension and ischemic cerebrovascular or cardiovascular disease. She should not be put on either a short- or a long-acting triptan for her migraines. Given the frequency of her headaches, she will not be comforted by lack of treatment and is at risk of medication-overuse headaches should you start frequent use of over-the-counter (OTC) medications or a butalbital/acetaminophen/caffeine combination. She should be offered a daily preventative medication to decrease the frequency and severity of her migraines. (Olesen, et al., Chapter 51)

101. The answer is C. IgA deficiency–related anaphylactic response can be prevented by checking levels prior to the initial treatment. Ischemic stroke is a rare complication of intravenous immunoglobulin (IVIG) therapy, and large or medium cerebral arterial occlusion has occurred during or 24 hours after the infusion. Thromboembolic events are due to hyperviscosity and may be prevented with a slow infusion rate and good hydration. History of stroke is not a contraindication. Renal failure is a serious complication, and active renal disease is a contraindication. Age over 65 does increase the risk of renal failure, as does diabetes, volume depletion, sepsis, paraproteinemia, and concurrent nephrotoxic drugs, but age alone is not a contraindication. (*Physician's Desk Reference*; Caress et al., *Neurology* 2003)

102. The answer is C. Glycerol reduces intracranial pressure (ICP) within 10 minutes, an effect lasting up to an hour. It increases serum osmolarity transiently. It does cross the blood–brain barrier, and is detected in brain tissue within 30 minutes. (Berger, *JAMA* 2006)

103. The answer is E. No evidence suggests that any of these agents, as well as hyperventilation, reduces ICP or improves outcome in patients with ischemic brain swelling. (Adams)

104. The answer is C. Ancrod is a fibrinolytic agent derived from the venom of the Malaysian pit viper. A double-blinded, randomized trial was reported in 2000. This agent decreased the number of severely disabled patients, with no increase or decrease in mortality. The symptomatic intracranial hemorrhage rate was 5.2%, lower than in the National Institute of Neurological Disorders and Stroke (NINDS) t-PA) trial published in 1995. Fibrinogen levels continue to decrease to their lowest within 12 to 24 hours. Unfortunately, there were administrative issues, including change in the ownership of the company that developed the drug to the clinical trial stage, which interfered with FDA approval and the availability of the agent. A new company was formed and obtained the snake farm. FDA issues are being dealt with, and a follow-up clinical trial is ongoing. The initial trial studied 0 to 3 hours, but the new trial will study later time points in an attempt to increase the duration of the acute treatment window. The European Stroke Treatment with Ancrod Trial (ESTAT)l did not show a positive result with Ancrod treatment, but the majority of the patients in the trial were treated within between 3 to 6 hours. (Sherman, *JAMA* 2000)

105. The answer is D. The Vitamin Intervention for Stroke Prevention (VISP) study was a secondary stroke prevention trial that included patients who had suffered a nondisabling stroke. High or low doses of folic acid, pyridoxine (vitamin B_6), and cobalamin (vitamin B_{12}) were given to lower total homocysteine levels in 3,680 adults. Although high-dose vitamins lowered homocysteine levels more than did low-dose vitamins, no difference was observed in the effect on vascular outcome. A more recent efficacy analysis suggested that there may be some benefit to high-dose treatment in patients with mid-range baseline vitamin B_{12} levels. (Loscalzo, *N Engl J Med* 2006; Spence, *Stroke* 2005; Toole et al. *JAMA* 2004)

106. The answer is E. Metformin is an oral agent used in type II diabetes. This agent can induce lactic acidosis, and all of the choices are risk factors for the development of lactic acidosis. Of concern in the evaluation and treatment of stroke patients is the use of cationic iodine contrast agents for cerebral angiography or CT angiography. The recommendation is that metformin be withheld for at least 48 hours following any procedure requiring iodinated contrast. (Calabrese, *Arch Intern Med* 2002)

107. The answers are A 1, B 3, C 2, D 5, E 4. See Answer 108 for explanation.

108. The answers are A 3, B 2, C3, D 4, E 2, F 2. Drugs that inhibit the platelet-fibrin binding site, the glycoprotein IIb/IIIa receptor, can block the site directly, such as with tirofiban (Aggrastat), abciximab, or eptifibatide, or indirectly through earlier steps in the platelet activation pathway. Aspirin, clopidogrel, and dipyridamole inhibit platelet aggregation through different pathways. Dipyridamole appears to also have other stabilizing effects on the endothelium as well as possible potentiation of nitric oxide and prostacyclin. Danaparoid, a heparinoid, exerts a stronger catalytic effect on the inactivation of factor Xa, mediated by antithrombin III, than on the inactivation of thrombin. Fondaparinux (Arixtra) has the same mechanism of action, but it is a completely synthetic compound, which produces theoretical advantages by its lack of potential antibody production. Enoxaparin and dalteparin, low-molecular-weight-heparins, activate antithrombin III and potentiate the inhibition of coagulation factors Xa and IIa. Factor Xa catalyzes the conversion of prothrombin to thrombin. Argatroban, hirudin, and other direct thrombin inhibitors reversibly bind to the thrombin active site and do not require the cofactor antithrombin III for antithrombotic activity. (Hirsh et al., *Chest* 2001; Patrono et al., *Chest* 2004)

109. The answer is D. Patients who develop heparin-induced thrombocytopenia (HIT) and continue to need anticoagulation should be treated with an IV direct thrombin inhibitor such as argatroban (Novastatin). The oral direct thrombin inhibitor dabigatran is still being tested for safety and efficacy and is not yet approved for clinical use. Unfractionated heparin, low-molecular-weight heparin, and glycoprotein IIb/IIIa inhibitors should not be used in patients with HIT. Patients with HIT can be treated with heparinoids, such as danaparoid. Arixtra, synthetic inhibitor of factor Xa, has not been studied in this situation, but would theoretically be an excellent alternative. (DiNisio, et al., *N Engl J Med* 2005)

110. The answer is A. See Answer 111 for explanation.

111. The answer is B. Some of the older-generation antiepileptic drugs (AEDs), including phenytoin, phenobarbital, and benzodiazepine, but not carbamazepine, have been found to alter or delay functional recovery in animal models of stroke or brain damage. There is concern about their negative influence on functional recovery in stroke patients. Carbamazepine may interact with anticoagulation and interfere with bone health. Treatment with lamotrigine and gabapentin has been suggested for use in stroke patients, because they have not been found to alter post-stroke function. They specifically do not interact with anticoagulants or antiplatelet agents, and they do not interfere with bone health. Gabapentin is the only drug that has been specifically evaluated in stroke patients; it demonstrates a high rate of long-term freedom from seizures. It would be an appropriate medication in a patient who is likely to be on long-term anticoagulation. Levetiracetam is not bound to plasma proteins or metabolized by the liver so INR levels are not altered with this agent, but it has not been specifically studied in stroke patients. (Ryvlin, *Neurology* 2006)

112. The answer is B. A phase IIB trial of patients with intracerebral hemorrhage (ICH) studied various doses of the recombinant factor VIIa with treatment within 4 hours of symptom onset. A beneficial neurologic effect was noted, with significant reduction in hemorrhage size, improved survival, and favorable outcome. The time window in the study may define the therapeutic window, with the suggestion of improved outcome with more rapid treatment. Unfortunately, a more recent trial did not find long-term benefit to the treatment in patients with ICH in general, and the drug's use will probably be restricted to patients with ICH due to warfarin therapy. (Juvela & Kase, *Stroke* 2006; Mayer et al., *N Engl J Med* 2005)

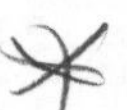

113. The answer is A. The calcium antagonist nimodipine 60 mg, orally every 4 hours for 21 days, decreases the risk of poor outcome from the ischemic complications of subarachnoid hemorrhage–induced vasospasm. Because of a short $t_{1/2}$ (less than 3 hours in patients with normal renal function), a nimodipine dosage interval of every 4 hours is required. Nicardipine is not of benefit in the prevention of ischemic damage from vasospasm. Aminocaproic acid is an antifibrinolytic agent that reduces rebleeding, but at the expense of increased thrombotic events. Intra-arterial therapy, using angioplasty and/or calcium-channel blockers such as verapamil, is used for treatment of symptomatic luminal stenosis from vasospasm. (Suarez et al., *N Engl J Med* 2006)

114. The answer is C. Combination treatment with clopidogrel and aspirin is associated with a statistically significant increased hemorrhage risk in both the Management of Atherothrombosis with Clopidogrel in High-risk patients (MATCH) and Clopidogrel for High Atherothrombotic Risk and Ischemic Stabilization, Management and Avoidance (CHARISMA) trials. In MATCH, 1.3% of patients treated with clopidogrel alone had life-threatening bleeding, as compared with 2.6% using the combination of the two antiplatelet agents. Warfarin anticoagulation is associated with an annual hemorrhage risk of around 2% to 3%. In the European Stroke Prevention Study (ESPS-2) and the European/Australasian Stroke Prevention in Reversible Ischaemia Trial (ESPRIT) trials, the hemorrhage risk associated with the dipyridamole/aspirin treatment was comparable to aspirin alone. Intravenous heparin is rarely indicated for secondary stroke prevention and has an increased hemorrhage risk. (Weinberger, *Drugs* 2005)

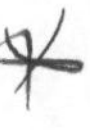

115. The answer is E. The folate, vitamin B_{12}, vitamin B_6 combination lowers homocysteine levels, but no clinical benefit is apparent. The Norwegian Vitamin (NORVIT) trial evaluated 3,745 Norwegian patients with a recent myocardial infarction who were treated with folate and B vitamins (folic acid 0.8 mg, vitamin B_{12} 0.4 mg, vitamin B_6 40 mg). Despite reduction in homocysteine levels, no vascular risk reduction was noted. In the HOPE-2 trial, 5,522 patients with vascular disease or diabetes were randomized to combined treatment with folic acid 2.5 mg, vitamin B_{12} 1 mg, vitamin B_6 50 mg or to placebo. After treatment for an average of 5 years, homocysteine levels were decreased, but no effect on the primary end-point of death from cardiovascular causes, myocardial infarction, and stroke was noted. A treatment effect on the subgroup of stroke was felt to be an overestimate of an effect or a spurious effect. The results of these recent trials, which indicate lack of vascular benefit of lowering homocysteine, confirm the results of older trials showing lack of vascular benefit to folate, vitamin B_6, vitamin B_{12} combinations. Fish oil and vitamin E do not lower homocysteine levels. (Bonaa et al., *N Engl J Med* 2006; Lonn et al., *N Engl J Med* 2006)

116. The answer is C. Digoxin does decrease ventricular rate at rest, but it is more effective when combined with β-blockers. Digoxin is not more effective than placebo in preventing recurrence of atrial fibrillation. Although digoxin is still used in patients with atrial fibrillation, it is no longer considered a first-line agent in its treatment, because more effective agents are available. Digitalis is derived from the foxglove plant. (Fuster et al., *Circulation* 2006)

117. The answer is E. Hormone replacement therapy (HRT) has not been shown to bestow any vascular benefit to any subgroup of postmenopausal women. Primary prevention studies have not shown benefit with HRT in women who are healthy or in women who have vascular risk. The Women's Health Initiative (WHI) found a 44% increased incidence in ischemic, but not hemorrhagic, stroke with estrogen plus progestin treatment of healthy women who were on average a decade into menopause. In women participating in the WHI who were treated with estrogen alone, because of prior hysterectomy, ischemic stroke risk was increased by 39%. In women with increased vascular risk because of coronary artery disease, HRT offered no protection against ischemic stroke, as found in the Heart and Estrogen/Progestin Replacement Study (HERS). Estrogen supplementation has not been shown of benefit in secondary stroke prevention. The Women's Estrogen for Stroke Trial (WEST) was a randomized placebo-controlled trial of women with prior TIA or ischemic stroke to study if 17β-estradiol reduced the rate of recurrent stroke. The results showed that estrogen alone had no overall benefit in preventing recurrent stroke or fatality, but there was an increase in the overall stroke rate in the first 6 months of treatment. The estrogen treated women with nonfatal strokes had worse neurologic deficits compared with women with strokes in the placebo group. (Bushnell et al., *Sem Neurol* 2006)

118. The answer is D. The Stroke Prevention by Aggressive Reduction in Cholesterol Levels (SPARCL) study randomized 4,731 patients with a recent TIA or stroke (ischemic or hemorrhagic), but without history of coronary artery disease, to 80 mg of atorvastatin (Lipitor) or placebo. The patients' initial LDL levels were 100 to 190 mg/dL. The five-year absolute reduction in the risk of the primary endpoint, a first nonfatal or fatal stroke, was 2.2% (95% confidence interval [CI], 0.2–4.2%). Although the risk of ischemic stroke decreased (hazard ratio [HR] 0.78; 95% CI, 0.66–0.94) with treatment, the HR for hemorrhagic stroke was 1.66 (95% CI, 1.08–2.55). The overall mortality was similar in the two treatment groups. The heterogeneity of the patients enrolled in the trial, in terms of stroke etiology and vascular risk, may explain the relatively modest absolute risk reduction with atorvastatin treatment. However, the SPARCL study demonstrated the benefit of statin treatment in secondary stroke risk reduction and is further motivation for initiation of statin treatment after an ischemic stroke. (Amarenco et al., *N Engl J Med* 2006; Kent, *N Engl J Med* 2006)

119. The answer is B. Varenicline (Chantix) is a novel $\alpha 4\beta 2$ nAChR partial agonist that is used for smoking cessation. It was compared to bupropion (Zyban) and to placebo in a study of healthy smokers aged 18 to 75 years. The drug reduced nicotine craving and withdrawal, as well as smoking satisfaction, and was significantly more efficacious than placebo or bupropion. Its most common side effect was nausea. Bupropion is contraindicated in patients with seizures, which may limit its use in patients with cerebrovascular disease. The safety profile of varenicline is more favorable than nicotine-containing products in patients with vascular disease. Hypnosis and a telephone "quit line" may be used in addition to medical therapy. (Gonzales et al., *JAMA* 2006)

120. The answer is A. A meta-analysis of data in breast cancer trials found an 82% percent increase in risk of ischemic stroke and 29% increase in risk of any stroke in women treated with tamoxifen, although the risk of ischemic stroke in these women is small. The other agents have not been shown to be associated with ischemic stroke. Another chemotherapeutic agent with an increased risk of stroke, L-asparaginase, is used to treat leukemias. It is associated with both arterial and venous thrombosis. (Bushnell & Goldstein, *Neurology* 2004)

121. The answer is A. The PROGRESS trial documented a decrease in strokes in patients who received ACE inhibition, whether or not these patients had hypertension. Angiotensin converting enzyme inhibitors rarely produce serious side effects, although persistent dry cough is an annoying side effect that frequently causes patients to discontinue these agents. There is controversy about teratogenic effects of ACE inhibitors, but they have other adverse effects during the 2nd and 3rd trimesters of pregnancy, so they should be discontinued during pregnancy. Angiotensin converting enzyme inhibitors have a nephroprotective effect. (Brunton, Chapter 30; PROGRESS Collaborative Group, *Lancet* 2001)

122. The answer is B. Blood pressure lowering was equal in both treatment groups, but ARB treatment did result in fewer primary end-points as compared to calcium-channel blockade. There were no differences in side effects in the two groups. ARBs and ACE inhibitors were not compared in the MOSES trial. (Schrader et al., *Stroke* 2005)

123. The answer is B. Angiotensin receptor blockers can produce progressive azotemia or acute renal failure in patients with renal function dependent on the renin-angiotensin system. Angiotensin receptor blockers have a lower rate of discontinuation than do ACE inhibitors, because they do not produce cough. Both classes of drugs should be discontinued during pregnancy. There are multiple differences in the enhancement or blockade of production or action of related substances, but it is not known whether the pharmacologic differences between ACE inhibitors and ARBs translate into clinically significant differences in the prevention of stroke or heart disease. Trials comparing the agents head to head are under way. Some ACE inhibitors are much less expensive than ARBs, as there are several generic ACE inhibitors available. (Brunton, Chapter 30)

124. The answer is D. Acute treatment with intravenous unfractionated heparin has not been shown to be of benefit in decreasing death or dependency after an acute stroke. Although it has been used in progressing stroke, its benefit is unproven. Bolus infusion of heparin should not be used in the setting of acute ischemic stroke because of the risk of converting an ischemic stroke to a hemorrhagic stroke. Patients with restricted mobility after a stroke should be treated with prophylactic low-dose subcutaneous heparin or low-molecular-weight heparins or heparinoids to decrease risk of DVT or pulmonary embolism. In the International Stroke Trial (IST), high-dose (12,500 U b.i.d.) subcutaneous heparin was shown to increase death and recurrent ischemic and hemorrhagic stroke risk at 14 days. (Albers et al., *Chest* 2004)

125. The answer is A. The SPARCL study was the first clinical trial to show a reduction of recurrent stroke risk, albeit modest, using statin therapy in patients with recent cerebrovascular disease. The SPARCL study randomized 4,731 patients with a recent TIA or stroke (ischemic or hemorrhagic), but without a history of coronary heart disease, to 80 mg of atorvastatin or placebo. The 5-year absolute reduction in the risk of the primary end-point, a first nonfatal or fatal stroke, was 2.2% (95% CI, 0.2–4.2). The Heart Protection Study found no risk reduction for stroke in those patients with prior cerebrovascular disease, with 10.4% of patients in the group treated with simvastatin and 10.5% of placebo-treated patients suffering a recurrent stroke. The long period between the initial cerebrovascular event and the randomization, and the relatively modest degree of lipid lowering may have factored into the negative results. The CARE, 4S, and LIPID studies showed benefit of statin treatment in the primary prevention of stroke in individuals with cardiovascular, but not cerebrovascular, disease. (Amarenco P, *N Engl J Med* 2006; Heart Protection Collaborative Study Group, *Lancet* 2004; Kent, *N Engl J Med* 2006; Long-Term Intervention with Pravastatin in Ischemic Disease (LIPID) Study Group, *N Engl J Med* 1998; Plehn et al., *Circulation* 1999; Scandinavian Simvastatin Survival Study (4S), *Lancet* 1994)

3 Clinical Stroke Questions

126. Which of the following is characteristically found in patients with Fabry disease?

A. Glaucoma.
B. Proteinuria.
C. Erythema nodosum.
D. Anterior cerebral artery infarcts.
E. Hemangiomas.

127. Each of the following eponymic syndromes is associated with contralateral hemiparesis and what other clinical findings?

A. Millard-Gubler syndrome.	1. Internuclear ophthalmoplegia.
B. Foville syndrome.	2. Oculomotor palsy.
C. Weber syndrome.	3. Facial palsy.
D. Raymond-Cestan syndrome.	4. Facial palsy and lateral gaze paresis.

128. Lifestyle recommendations for ischemic stroke prevention include:

A. Avoidance of a diet rich in fruits, vegetables, and fish.
B. Total abstinence from alcohol.
C. Not smoking but sniffing other people's cigarette smoke.
D. Weight reduction to a body mass index (BMI) in the 19 to 25 kg/m^2 range.
E. Avoidance of exercise for patients with stroke related disability.

129. Sporadic cerebral amyloid angiopathy (CAA):

A. Is a minor cause of nontraumatic intracerebral hemorrhage.
B. Often leads to hemorrhage in the basal ganglia, thalamus, and cerebellum.
C. Is associated with hemorrhage in the parietal lobes more frequently than in the occipital or frontal lobes.
D. Is not associated with increased risk of hemorrhage with anticoagulation in the elderly.
E. Is characterized pathologically by the extracellular deposition of β-amyloid fibrils around leptomeningeal vessels.

130. Which is the most critical aspect of the headache history when a patient presents with suspected subarachnoid hemorrhage (SAH)?

A. Severity of the headache.
B. The presence of neck pain.
C. The acuity of the headache onset.
D. The age of the patient.
E. The gender of the patient.

131. Migraine is most strongly associated with an increased risk of:

A. Hemorrhagic stroke.
B. Myocardial infarction.
C. Ischemic stroke.
D. Cerebral vasospasm.

132. A 68-year-old man with a history of hypertension and smoking was admitted to the hospital with chest pain that had become more frequent and severe over the past few days. He was diagnosed with an anterior wall myocardial infarction due to severe triple-vessel disease and was scheduled for emergent bypass surgery. As part of his preoperative evaluation, he underwent carotid duplex ultrasonography that revealed a right internal carotid lesion producing 65% luminal stenosis. The left carotid system was unremarkable. Despite persistent questioning, the neurology consultant could not elicit any history of neurologic symptoms. The man's neurologic examination was normal. What is the neurologist's most reasonable suggestion to the cardiothoracic surgeon?

A. Cancel the surgery and treat the man with medical therapy only.
B. Perform a right carotid endarterectomy (CEA) and delay the surgery for several weeks.
C. Proceed with the cardiac surgery.
D. Perform synchronous CEA and coronary artery bypass graft procedures.

133. A central midbrain infarct causing a Claude syndrome characteristically involves which structures?

A. The corticospinal tract and oculomotor nerve.
B. The red nucleus and oculomotor nerve.
C. The corticospinal tract, oculomotor nerve, and cerebellothalamic tract.
D. The superior colliculi and oculomotor nerve.

134. Hypertension is a modifiable risk factor for stroke. It is:

A. Present in 24% of adults of all ages in the United States.
B. Less common in African Americans than in those of northern European descent.
C. Higher in Hispanic Americans than in Americans of African descent.
D. Adequately controlled on medications in approximately two-thirds of Americans.

135. Which statement is true about smoking cigarettes?

A. Only malaria and tuberculosis cause as many deaths worldwide as smoking cigarettes.
B. Three years after smoking cessation, the relative risk of dying from coronary heart disease is approximately the same as in an individual who has never smoked.
C. Second-hand smoke is not a risk factor for coronary heart disease.
D. Smoking cigarettes is decreasing in developed countries but increasing in underdeveloped countries.

136. Which of the listed disorders are possible causes of orthostatic hypotension?

A. Parkinson's disease, diabetes, and myasthenia gravis.
B. Diabetes, multiple sclerosis, and pseudotumor cerebri.
C. Parkinson's disease, diabetes, and multiple cerebral infarcts.
D. Cushing's syndrome, renal artery stenosis.

137. The most reliable method for determining systolic blood pressure is:

A. Auscultation of the brachial artery while gradually decreasing the pressure in a mercury blood pressure cuff.
B. Palpation of the radial artery while gradually increasing the pressure of a mercury blood pressure cuff.
C. Auscultation of the brachial artery while lowering the pressure of a non-mercury blood pressure cuff.
D. Ausculatation of the radial artery while gradually lowering the pressure of a mercury blood pressure cuff.

138. Which of the following statements best describes primary angiitis of the central nervous system (PACNS)?

A. A benign form of PACNS may not need immunosuppressive treatment.
B. PACNS can be ruled out by normal catheter angiography.
C. PACNS is often accompanied by fever, weight loss, and malaise.
D. A pathognomonic abnormality is seen on magnetic resonance imaging (MRI).
E. An abnormal single-photon emission tomography (SPECT) scan is specific for PACNS.

139. A 68-year-old man underwent graft repair of a descending thoracic aortic aneurysm. To decrease risk of perioperative paraplegia, a lumbar cerebrospinal fluid drainage catheter was inserted into the subarachnoid space after induction of anesthesia. Lumbar pressure was kept at 12 mm Hg or less with fluid drainage. A day after surgery, while he was in the intensive care unit, the man had a focal seizure with residual left-sided weakness. What do you think happened?

A. Hypoxic encephalopathy.
B. Right frontal subdural hematoma.
C. Right middle cerebral artery (MCA) territory ischemic stroke.
D. Anterior spinal artery stroke.
E. Right epidural hematoma.

140. Match the granulomatous vasculitis with its most likely patient. Use each answer only once.

A. Takayasu's arteritis.
B. Giant-cell arteritis.
C. Wegener's granulomatosis.
D. Churg-Strauss syndrome.

1. Fifty-year-old an with nasal polyps and asthma.
2. Seventy-year-old woman with malaise and headaches.
3. Thirty-year-old woman with malaise and headaches.
4. Fifty-year-old man with nose bleeds and a cough.

141. Match the multiorgan vasculitic disorder that may affect the central nervous system (CNS) with one of its non-CNS areas of involvement. Use each answer only once.

A. Wegener's granulomatosis.
B. Behçet's disease.
C. Polyarteritis nodosa.
D. Sjögren syndrome.
E. Churg-Strauss syndrome.

1. Nerve and muscle.
2. Airway sinuses.
3. Genitalia.
4. Salivary and lacrimal glands.
5. Eosinophilia.

142. As compared to sporadic aneurysms, familial intracranial aneurysms that cause SAH:

A. Are more likely to occur in the posterior circulation.
B. Rupture at an earlier age.
C. Are rare in Finnish men as compared to men of other nationalities.
D. Are less likely to be multiple.
E. Are more likely to be on the anterior communicating artery.

143. Use of the Boston Criteria for the diagnosis of CAA:

A. Requires postmortem pathologic examination of the brain for definite diagnosis.
B. Allows the possible diagnosis in patients of any age.
C. Allows the probable diagnosis after a single hemorrhage.
D. Results in a low specificity for the diagnosis of probable CAA.
E. Results in a greater frequency of ApoE alleles with definite CAA, as compared to with probable CAA.

144. Which vascular risk factor, when present in a patient with a transient ischemic attack (TIA), indicates increased very early risk of an ischemic stroke?

A. Elevated cholesterol.
B. Diabetes.
C. Cigarette smoking.
D. Family history of stroke.
E. Peripheral arterial disease.

145. Which of the following statements best describes obstructive sleep apnea (OSA)?

A. The stroke risk associated with OSA is associated with an increased incidence of hypertension.
B. People with OSA are less likely to have atrial fibrillation (AF) than are people without OSA.
C. The association of OSA with stroke is explained by a single known mechanism.
D. Central sleep apnea is common after stroke.
E. Sleep apnea prevalence after stroke is independent of stroke location.

146. Match the cerebrovascular disorder with its best race or ethnic association. An answer may be used more than once.

A. Familial cerebral amyloid angiopathy.
B. Moyamoya syndrome.
C. Sickle cell disease.
D. Familial cavernous malformations.
E. Ischemic stroke associated with phosphodiesterase 4D polymorphism.

1. Japanese children.
2. African American children.
3. Hispanic American individuals.
4. Icelandic adults.

147. A 52–year-old woman was admitted within an hour of the sudden onset of right hemiparesis. She had hypertension treated with ramipril (Altace). Intravenous tissue plasminogen activator (t-PA) was administered within 2 hours of onset of stroke symptoms, and she was admitted for evaluation. On the way to the stroke unit from the emergency department, she was sent to the cardiology suite for a transesophageal echocardiogram. When the patient arrived on the stroke unit, the nurse noted that the right side of her tongue and mouth were swollen; you were called to evaluate her. What did you conclude was the most likely cause of her orolingual swelling?

A. The nurse did not record the patient's history of collagen injection of her lips for cosmetic reasons.
B. The cardiologist traumatized the tongue and mouth during the echocardiogram.
C. The patient has orolingual angioedema as a complication of thrombolysis.
D. The patient just has a large tongue and big lips.
E. The transport person did not report the bee sting of the patient's mouth that occurred in the elevator.

148. Eales disease is an idiopathic obliterative vasculitis that primary affects which area of the body?

A. Liver.
B. Kidney.
C. Retina.
D. Peripheral nerve.
E. Lung.

149. What is the most common neurologic manifestation of hepatitis C virus (HCV) infection?

A. Ischemic stroke.
B. Encephalopathy.
C. Intracerebral hemorrhage.
D. Peripheral neuropathy.
E. Spinal cord infarct.

150. Which of the following best describes reversible cerebral vasoconstriction syndromes (RCVS)?

A. Patients with RCVS are predominantly male.
B. Vascular imaging using catheter angiography, computed tomography angiography (CTA), and magnetic resonance angiography (MRA) are generally normal in RCVS.
C. The MRI or computed tomography (CT) scan of the brain in RCVS may show minor SAH, parenchymal hemorrhage, or vasogenic edema.
D. Reversible cerebral vasoconstriction syndromes are the same as PACNS.
E. Reversible cerebral vasoconstriction syndromes should be treated with immunosuppressive agents.

151. A 40-year-old woman has a mechanical mitral valve. Because of a pharmacy mix-up in her medication, her international normalized ratio (INR) went to 5.8 and she sustained a right frontal intracerebral hemorrhage (ICH). She improved neurologically, and her CT showed that the hemorrhage was stable. When would you restart warfarin?

A. As soon as the INR can be corrected.
B. In less than a week.
C. In 1 to 2 weeks.
D. In 1 to 2 months.
E. Never.

152. What are the systolic (SBP) and diastolic (DBP) blood pressures above which treatment of elevated blood pressure is recommended in acute ischemic stroke, in the absence of end-organ damage or anticipated thrombolysis?

A. SBP 240 mm Hg and DBP 140 mm Hg.
B. SBP 220 mm Hg and DBP 120 mm Hg.
C. SBP 200 mm Hg and DBP 120 mm Hg.
D. SBP 180 mm Hg and DBP 100 mm Hg.
E. SBP 160 mm Hg and DBP 100 mm Hg.

153. A 71-year-old man presented to the emergency department an hour after the sudden onset of right hemiparesis. His elevated blood pressure was treated with intravenous labetalol, and he was given t-PA intravenously within the 3-hour window. What is the recommended upper limit for systolic and diastolic blood pressures during and after his thrombolytic therapy?

A. SBP 220 mm Hg and DBP 120 mm Hg.
B. SBP 200 mm Hg and DBP 100 mm Hg.
C. SBP 185 mm Hg and DBP 110 mm Hg.
D. SBP 180 mm Hg and DBP 105 mm Hg.
E. SBP 160 mm Hg and DBP 100 mm Hg.

154. Which of the following is the most common complication of hypertensive, hypervolemic, hemodilution (triple-H) therapy in aneurysmal SAH?

A. Aneurysmal rebleeding.
B. Hydrocephalus.
C. Delayed cerebral ischemia.
D. Congestive heart failure.
E. Deep vein thrombosis (DVT).

155. Which of the following clinical trials demonstrated that oral anticoagulation with warfarin was more effective than aspirin therapy in preventing a second stroke in patients with a noncardioembolic stroke?

A. The European/Australian Stroke Prevention in Reversible Ischaemia Trial (ESPRIT).
B. The Stroke Prevention in Reversible Ischemia Trial (SPIRIT).
C. The Warfarin Aspirin Recurrent Stroke Study (WARSS).
D. The Warfarin-Aspirin Symptomatic Intracranial Disease (WASID) trial.
E. None of the above.

156. The European Stroke Prevention Study (ESPS) 2 compared the combination of aspirin (25 mg) with modified-release dipyridamole (200 mg), taken twice daily, to aspirin 25 mg, taken twice a day alone. What was the relative risk reduction (RRR) in secondary stroke for patients on the combination treatment versus aspirin alone?

A. 6%.
B. 12%.
C. 23%.
D. 40%.

157. Spinal dural arteriovenous fistula (SDAVF):

A. Is the most common spinal vascular disease.
B. Is found more frequently in women than in men.
C. Is a congenital disorder found predominantly in younger individuals.
D. Generally presents with the sudden onset of paraplegia.
E. Is associated with thrombophilia.

158. The Columbia Arteriovenous Malformation (AVM) databank categorizes AVMs based on presentation (hemorrhagic or incidental) and anatomic characteristics (location, draining vein). What is the average annual re-rupture rate for an AVM that has hemorrhaged at presentation in a deep location with deep drainage versus the annual rupture rate for an AVM discovered incidentally without these risk factors?

A. 52% versus 30%.
B. 40% versus 10%.
C. 34% versus 1%.
D. 12% versus 0.5%.

159. Which statement best describes eclampsia?

A. Eclampsia is a disorder defined as preeclampsia and new-onset seizures occurring during the last trimester of pregnancy.
B. Elevated blood pressure in the patient with eclampsia should be treated with an angiotensin-converting enzyme (ACE) inhibitor prior to delivery.
C. The MRI in eclampsia may show posterior increased signal intensity on fluid-attenuated inversion recovery (FLAIR) consistent with cytotoxic edema.
D. Eclampsia may be associated with hemolysis, elevated liver enzymes, and low platelet counts.
E. Seizures due to eclampsia are best treated with intravenous phenytoin.

160. Which order best ranks the highest to lowest annual risk of recurrent hemorrhage in these causes of intracranial hemorrhage?

A. Cerebral amyloid angiopathy (CAA); developmental venous anomaly (DVA); cavernous malformation.
B. Hypertension (HTN); CAA; intracerebral aneurysm.
C. Arteriovenous malformation (AVM); DVA; CAA.
D. CAA; HTN; DVA.
E. Cavernous malformation; DVA; HTN.

161. The Mechanical Embolus Removal in Cerebral Ischemia (MERCI) retriever:

A. Is a Food and Drug Administration (FDA)-approved device for restoration of blood flow in patients experiencing an acute ischemic stroke due to large vessel occlusion.
B. Uses intravascular ultrasound technology to disrupt the embolus prior to removal.
C. Showed recanalization rates in a clinical trial that were equivalent to historical controls.
D. Is absolutely contraindicated in combination with t-PA treatment.
E. Is available and appropriate for most patients with an acute ischemic stroke.

162. A 68-year-old man called his internist to report that he had two episodes of transient right-sided weakness and speech difficulty in the past week, lasting about 15 minutes each. The last episode occurred 2 days ago. When the internist told him to go to the emergency department, he walked three blocks uptown to the nearest hospital. There he told the triage nurse that the chest pain he was having in the emergency department felt just like it did last night when he opened his wife's charge card bill. His CT scan of the head, electrocardiogram (ECG), and carotid ultrasound were all normal. What is the appropriate treatment for this man?

A. Suggest that he take an aspirin and follow-up with a cardiologist, a neurologist, and a divorce attorney next week as an outpatient.
B. Admit him for a cardiac and cerebrovascular evaluation, and start aspirin and clopidogrel.
C. Admit him for a cardiac and cerebrovascular evaluation, and start aspirin and sustained-release dipyridamole.
D. Admit him for a cardiac and cerebrovascular evaluation and start intravenous heparin.

163. Which German composer, with high blood pressure, smoking, and probable hyperlipidemia, had recurrent episodes of right arm weakness and speech difficulty, as well as loss of vision in his left eye?

A. Robert Schumann.
B. Georg Fredrich Handel.
C. Joseph Hayden.
D. Ludiwg van Beethoven.
E. Felix Mendelssohn.

164. Match the neurocutaneous disorder (vascular phakomatosis) with its most characteristic orbital vascular lesion. An answer may be used more than once.

A. Sturge-Weber syndrome.
B. Von Hippel-Lindau disease.
C. Wynburn-Mason syndrome.
D. Osler-Weber-Rendu syndrome.
E. PHACE syndrome.

1. Retinal hemangioblastoma.
2. Retinal/orbital arteriovenous malformation.
3. Choroidal hemangioma.
4. Conjunctival telangiectasias.

165. All the following are associated with the formation of carotid cavernous fistulae (CCFs). Which one is the most common cause of CCF?

A. Aneurysm of the cavernous internal carotid artery.
B. Motor vehicle accidents.
C. Transsphenoidal resection of the pituitary.
D. Pseudoxanthoma elasticum.
E. Ehlers-Danlos syndrome.

166. Which of the following statements best describes moyamoya syndrome?

A. Moyamoya-like changes have been described in association with sickle cell disease, pseudoxanthoma elasticum, and neurofibromatosis type 1.
B. Children with moyamoya syndrome present most frequently with seizures and cerebral hemorrhage due to vessel rupture.
C. The main manifestations of moyamoya in adults are TIAs and ischemic strokes.
D. Most causes are familial, with an autosomal dominant pattern of inheritance.
E. Internal carotid artery (ICA) occlusion generally occurs just distal to the bifurcation.

167. Homocystinuria:

A. Is associated with a dietary deficiency of vitamins B_6, B_{12}, and folate.
B. Is associated with plasma homocysteine levels of 15 to 100 μmol/L.
C. Most commonly results from disturbances in the conversion of homocysteine to methionine.
D. May be a risk factor for ischemic stroke in the general population.
E. Can cause stroke through atherosclerosis, thromboembolism, small-vessel disease, or arterial dissection.

168. Match the location of the unruptured cerebral aneurysm and its most common prodromal symptom.

A. Posterior communicating artery.
B. Cavernous carotid artery.
C. Supraclinoid carotid artery.
D Middle cerebral artery
E. Posterior inferior cerebellar artery.

1. Cranial nerve VI palsy.
2. Bitemporal hemianopia.
3. Cranial nerve III palsy.
4. Posterior neck pain.
5. Retro-orbital pain.

169. Match the thalamic region with its most characteristic clinical syndrome. Use each answer only once.

A. Anterior territory.
B. Paramedian territory.
C. Inferolateral territory.
D. Posterior territory.

1. Apathy, amnesia, disorganization of speech output ("palipsychism").
2. Sensory loss, visual field deficits.
3. Ataxia, sensory loss, hemiparesis.
4. Decreased arousal, vertical gaze paresis, personality change.

170. Which of the following best describes emergency management of patients with spontaneous ICH?

A. The hypoxic patient should be intubated and ventilated to PCO_2 below 25 mm Hg.
B. Sodium nitroprusside should be used for blood pressure control.
C. The mean arterial pressure (MAP) should be maintained at or below 130 mm Hg in patients with a history of hypertension.
D. Fluids are optimally managed with a solution of 5% dextrose in water.
E. Serum osmolality should be kept <280 mmol/kg.

171. Which of the following statements best describes the association between vascular disease and systemic lupus erythematosus (SLE)?

A. SLE is a risk factor for the development of atherosclerotic vascular disease.
B. Pregnant women with SLE have a decreased risk of preeclampsia.
C. Cerebrovascular disease in patients with SLE is generally independent of the presence of antiphospholipid antibodies.
D. Lupus patients who have seizures are less likely to have vascular events and antiphospholipid antibodies than are lupus patients without seizures.
E. The majority of patients with antiphospholipid antibody syndrome eventually develop SLE.

172. Which of the following is the most common CNS manifestation of SLE?

A. Primary generalized seizures.
B. Migraine headaches.
C. Cerebritis.
D. Aseptic meningitis.
E. Movement disorders.

173. Moyamoya disease:

A. Is an inflammatory vasculopathy.
B. Is a small vessel vasculopathy.
C. Exclusively affects individuals of Asian descent.
D. Produces a characteristic "puff of smoke" on cerebral angiography.
E. Is seen exclusively in children.

174. Fibromuscular dysplasia (FMD) is:

A. A vasculopathy that is never familial.
B. Generally an endothelial disorder.
C. Associated with an increased risk of subarachnoid hemorrhage.
D. Most often seen as focal tubular stenosis on angiography.
E. Affects only intracranial arteries.

175. The most common manifestation of cavernous malformations is:

A. Lobar cerebral hemorrhage.
B. Subarachnoid hemorrhage.
C. Seizures.
D. Headaches.

176. The duration of a TIA is most often:

A. Under 1 minute.
B. Five to 60 minutes.
C. One to 24 hours.
D. Over 24 hours.

177. Severe headache at the onset of a focal neurologic deficit:

A. Is most compatible with migraine with aura.
B. Is essentially diagnostic of ICH.
C. Can be consistent with ischemic stroke.
D. Should be evaluated by immediate MRI scanning of the brain.

178. Spastic dysarthria:

A. Occurs only following strokes in the posterior circulation.
B. Presents as hypernasal speech with imprecise articulation.
C. Is frequently accompanied by inappropriate tearfulness.
D. Is rarely associated with caudate lesions.

179. Sudden onset of painless brachial monoparesis with hyporeflexia is:

A. Most likely a brachial plexopathy or plexitis.
B. Consistent with a small stroke in the contralateral MCA territory.
C. Consistent with a small stroke in the contralateral vertebral artery territory.
D. Peripheral, as demonstrated by the hyporeflexia.

180. Crossed sensory deficits:

A. Can occur in lateral medullary (Wallenberg) infarcts.
B. Are always related to spinal cord lesions.
C. Are generally accompanied by urinary incontinence.
D. All of the above.

181. A 62-year-old woman with no history of neurologic problems developed nausea 24 hours after a radical mastectomy. She was treated with 4 mg droperidol (Inapsine) intravenously. Twenty minutes later, she suddenly noted uncontrolled movements of the left arm and leg. These movements were described as choreiform by the consulting neurologist.

A. These movements were most likely caused by droperidol and should be treated with diphenhydramine (Benadryl).
B. The most likely diagnosis is Wilson's disease with acute symptoms precipitated by recent anesthesia.
C. A perfusion CT will likely show decreased perfusion in the right subthalamic nucleus.
D. An MRI will likely show metastatic tumor in the right hemisphere.

182. A 83-year-old woman presented to the stroke clinic, describing "foggy vision in the left eye" that lasted most of the previous day. Her physician drew a circle on a piece of paper and asked her to put the numbers in, making a clock face. The patient put all the numbers in the right side of the circle. The most likely diagnosis is:

A. Left ophthalmic artery territory stroke with loss of vision on the left.
B. Right posterior cerebral artery (PCA) stroke.
C. Left PCA stroke.
D. Alzheimer dementia with apraxia.

183. A 72-year-old woman had been an avid gardener for years, but presented to her physician with problems in her vision associated with gardening. One sunny day, she went out to pull dandelions. She noted that within a couple of minutes the vision in her right eye faded, and images were dim in the right compared to the left. There was no associated headache. She stated that her husband suggested perhaps she was trying to avoid weed pulling, but she felt this was unlikely as she had always liked to pull weeds. Visual field testing in the office was normal. The most likely diagnosis is:

A. Malingering.
B. Glaucoma.
C. Right carotid occlusion.
D. Cerebral vasculitis with vasospasm.

184. A 62–year-old woman was hospitalized with acute onset of left hemiparesis with a National Institute of Health Stroke Scale (NIHSS) score of 5. She was therapeutically anticoagulated with heparin and then warfarin after atrial fibrillation was found on ECG. She had a good recovery, but 3 months later had a secondarily generalized seizure. She was seizure-free for 3 years on carbamazepine, 200 mg t.i.d. with a NIHSS score of 9 to11. Which of the following statements is correct?

A. She should be maintained on lifetime anticonvulsant therapy.
B. If her electroencephalogram (EEG) does not show epileptiform discharges, her anticonvulsants can be discontinued because she has been seizure-free for 3 years.
C. She should be changed to a seizure medication that does not interact with warfarin.
D. Warfarin should have been discontinued when she developed the seizure disorder 3 years earlier, because seizures are a contraindication to warfarin therapy.

185. A 32-year-old woman with a right MCA stenosis had MRI evidence of strokes distal to the stenosis and TIAs that began to break through both platelet inhibition and anticoagulation therapies. A successful angioplasty was performed, and the patient was followed with serial transcranial Doppler (TCD) imaging. Within 2 years, the right MCA velocities had increased to near preangioplasty levels, and an angiogram revealed an 80% stenosis that was much longer than the original atherosclerotic plaque, involving the entire M1 segment of the MCA. The next step in this patient's evaluation is:

A. Follow the patient until clinical symptoms occur.
B. Immediate surgery with anastomosis of the right superficial temporal artery to the M2 segment of the right MCA.
C. Transcranial Doppler with carbon dioxide inhalation or IV acetazolamide.
D. Administration of antihypertensive agents.

186. Which statement is true about vascular dementia?

A. The differentiation between vascular dementia and Alzheimer's dementia is reliably made by MRI scan.
B. The only treatment for vascular dementia is prevention of new ischemic damage.
C. Computed tomographic scanning of the brain is the diagnostic test of choice.
D. Cholinesterase inhibition may improve memory function in patients with Alzheimer's disease and vascular dementia.

187. A 58-year-old hypertensive man was found comatose and brought to the emergency department. He was unresponsive and had decerebrate posturing, along with pinpoint pupils. The most likely diagnosis is:

A. Narcotic overdose.
B. Hypertensive crisis.
C. Pontine hemorrhage.
D. Cardiac arrest.

188. Which of the following categories of cerebral hemorrhage is most commonly associated with CAA?

A. Putaminal hemorrhage.
B. Lobar hemorrhage.
C. Cerebellar hemorrhage.
D. Intraventricular hemorrhage.
E. Pontine hemorrhage.

189. A 42-year-old white man with no history of headaches developed sudden onset of severe headache during intercourse. Within 2 minutes, his wife noted dysarthria and inability to move his left side. He was taken to the emergency department, where he complained of the worst headache of his life, arriving 35 minutes after headache onset. On neurologic examination, he was alert with a spastic left hemiplegia and dysarthria. The CT scan was negative for hemorrhage. Blood counts and coagulation studies were within normal limits. The next intervention should be:

A. A spinal tap to rule out SAH.
B. A cerebral angiogram to rule out cerebral vasculitis.
C. Intravenous t-PA.
D. A triptan for acute severe migraine with hemiplegic aura.

190. Which of the following describes posterior circulation disease?

A. Vertebrobasilar ischemia frequently presents with a single symptom or sign.
B. Patients with cerebellar infarction not involving the brainstem do not have hemiparesis or hemisensory loss.
C. Vertigo is a common symptom seen in isolation in posterior circulation ischemia.
D. Dissection of the vertebral artery is most common in the middle portion.
E. Ischemia of the lateral medullary tegmentum is rarely caused by disease of an intracranial vertebral artery.

191. A 67-year-old man is evaluated in the emergency department for intravenous thrombolysis of his acute ischemic stroke. His family is very concerned about the risk of ICH as a result of thrombolytic therapy. Which of the following characteristics of this patient is the most reassuring for a low risk of symptomatic hemorrhagic conversion?

A. Leukoaraiosis and old lacunes on his CT scan.
B. Low levels of low-density lipoprotein (LDL) cholesterol on admission.
C. Current smoking history.
D. A NIHSS score of 12.

192. Which of the following statements best describes stroke risk and pregnancy?

A. Ischemic stroke risk is increased in the third trimester of pregnancy.
B. Ischemic stroke risk is increased after delivery.
C. Pregnancy is not associated with an increased risk of stroke.
D. Ischemic stroke risk is increased in the first two trimesters of pregnancy.
E. Intracerebral hemorrhage is much less likely to occur during pregnancy, than is cerebral infarction.

193. Which is an appropriate risk factor reduction goal for diabetic patients with cerebrovascular disease?

A. Hemoglobin A1C ≤7%.
B. LDL cholesterol ≤100 mg/dL.
C. Fasting glucose <200 mg/dL.
D. Three drinks or less per day for women.
E. Exercise every so often.

194. 71–year-old man presented to the emergency department with sudden onset of upper thoracic back pain and paresthesias in both arms. He had a loss of pain and thermal sensation below C6, but position sensation was preserved. Distal weakness of both arms was present. Useful diagnostic studies to guide potential treatment include:

A. Sedimentation rate, VDRL, spinal tap, and transesophageal echo.
B. Spinal angiogram.
C. Magnetic resonance imaging of the upper thoracic and lower cervical cord.
D. Radiographs of the thoracic spine.

195. Which statement is true about the Hunt and Hess classification of SAH?.

A. Patients with grade IV SAH have stupor or hemiparesis or both.
B. Grade IV most often correlates with bleeding limited to the subarachnoid space on CT scan.
C. Patients with hemorrhages of grades IV and V may have a normal acute head CT scan.
D. Patients with grade I SAH always have subarachnoid blood seen on head CT scan.
E. Patients with grade I SAH frequently have bilateral Babinski signs.

196. Which of the following statements regarding aneurysms of the cavernous carotid artery is correct?

A. Most of these aneurysms present acutely with rupture.
B. These aneurysms should be treated with ligation of the internal carotid artery when discovered incidentally.
C. Cavernous carotid artery aneurysms mainly occur in older women.
D. These aneurysms are rarely bilateral.
E. Endovascular treatment is associated with significant morbidity.

197. Which of the following best describes the diagnosis of a SDAVF?

A. Spinal fluid analysis is generally normal.
B. Myelography is rarely helpful.
C. A homogeneous increase in T2 signal in the central cord is present on MRI.
D. Cord diameter is always normal in the area of the T2 signal abnormality.
E. Abnormal vessels around the spinal cord on MRI are difficult to distinguish from pulsation artifact.

198. Cerebral dural arteriovenous (AV) fistulae:

A. Are easily diagnosed on CT or MRI.
B. Are most often caused by venous outflow obstruction or venous sinus thrombosis.
C. Have a rupture rate of <0.2% per year.
D. Are congenital lesions.
E. Are almost always asymptomatic.

199. The wife a United States President assumed control of the presidency after her husband suffered a stroke. Which president was no longer able to govern the country after his stroke?

A. Chester A. Arthur.
B. Millard Fillmore.
C. Woodrow Wilson.
D. Richard M. Nixon.
E. John Quincy Adams.

200. A patient with a MCA stroke and an infarct volume of 9 cm^3 or more on diffusion-weighted MRI

A. Will have an NIHSS score that varies 1 to 3 points depending on the side of the lesion.
B. Will have a possibility of approximately 20% of having an NIHSS score as low as 0 to 5 with a right hemispheric lesion.
C. Will have a lower NIHSS score with a left hemispheric lesion.
D. Is at risk for hemorrhagic transformation from t-PA.

201. Restenosis following CEA:

A. Is a common cause of ipsilateral cerebral ischemia following endarterectomy.
B. Is most often a reaccumulation of atherosclerotic plaque.
C. Is generally caused by myointimal hyperplasia.
D. Progresses to carotid occlusion in approximately 20% of patients.

202. Which statement is true about patch graphs with CEA?

A. A long arteriotomy is a strong indication for a patch graft.
B. An autologous vein graft is associated with fewer degenerative changes than is an arterial graft.
C. Aneurysmal dilatation is a potential complication of patch grafting.
D. Patch grafts are not useful in conjunction with endarterectomy.

203. Heparin usage in endarterectomy:

A. Is the best method for preventing thrombus formation during the procedure.
B. Is important for thrombus prevention in the early postoperative period.
C. Should not be used either during surgery or in the early postoperative period.
D. Is given routinely for the prevention of postoperative DVT.

204. A 53-year-old woman presented to the emergency room with an acute onset of visual field loss in the right lower quadrant. The CT scan was normal, but MRI scan showed an area of restricted diffusion in the left occipital lobe, along with several hyperintense lesions (6–12 mm) on T2WI and FLAIR images. Her electrocardiogram (EKG) was normal. Routine blood work was ordered, and the lab called a panic value with an extremely elevated eosinophil count. The test most likely to establish the cause of the patient's stroke would be:

A. Allergy testing.
B. Cardiac echo.
C. Carotid duplex.
D. Antinuclear antibody (ANA).

205. Which of the following is consistent with a persistent vegetative state?

A. Intact bladder and bowel functioning.
B. Sleep-wake cycles.
C. Consistent eye opening to verbal stimuli.
D. Absence of any cranial nerve reflexes.
E. Unawareness of the environment for 3 weeks after brain injury.

206. Which of the following parameters is part of the diagnostic criteria for metabolic syndrome?

A. Fasting blood sugar greater than 110, elevated LDL, elevated body mass index (BMI).
B. Waist circumference greater than 40 inches for women, reduced high density lipoprotein (HDL), elevated C-reactive protein (C-RP).
C. Reduced HDL, elevated triglycerides, elevated fasting blood sugar (above 110).
D. Elevated triglycerides, elevated LDL, hemoglobin A1C above 7.

207. According to the National Institute of Neurological Disorders and Stroke (NINDS) rt-PA Stroke Study published in December 1995, which of the following is a predictor of symptomatic ICH after thrombolytic treatment?

A. Age of the stroke patient.
B. Higher NIHSS score at baseline.
C. Higher Barthel Index at baseline.
D. Protocol violations.
E. Stroke subtype.

208. Giant-cell arteritis:

A. Occurs at a similar rate in men and women.
B. Has an average yearly incidence in Caucasians of 18:100,000 over age 50.
C. Is associated with an erythrocyte sedimentation (ESR) rate of over 50 in 98% of cases.
D. Usually only produces unilateral visual loss, even when untreated.

209. Which of the following cerebrovascular disorders is associated with Hodgkin's disease?

A. Subarachnoid hemorrhage.
B. Primary angiitis of the CNS (PACNS).
C. Cerebral venous thrombosis.
D. Epidural hematoma.
E. Subdural hematoma.

210. Transient global amnesia (TGA):

A. Is never associated with a headache.
B. Produces a characteristic abnormality on EEG.
C. Is much more common in people with traditional vascular risk factors.
D. May be related to a transient disturbance of hippocampal CA-1 neurons.
E. Causes long-term neurocognitive deficits.

211. Spinal epidural hematomas:

A. Never occur spontaneously.
B. Can occur associated with anesthetic procedures.
C. Are always treated with surgery.
D. Are best diagnosed by myelogram.
E. Should be investigated using a spinal angiogram.

212. A medical student was asked to remove the central venous catheter from a patient who was in the intensive care unit after multiple orthopedic injuries from a motor vehicle accident. The man was about to be sent to the surgical floor and was sitting in a wheelchair ready for transfer. Almost immediately after the student pulled out the catheter, the man became unresponsive and slumped over in the wheelchair. He became apneic with hypotension, but his vital signs were quickly stabilized. The patient remained lethargic. What happened?

A. The man had a syncopal episode from the pain of catheter removal.
B. A fat embolus dislodged from a long-bone fracture and caused a cerebral infarct.
C. An air embolus caused multiple cerebral infarcts.
D. The man was overmedicated for pain.

213. A 46-year-old woman with melanoma resected from her chest wall 3 years ago presented to the emergency department with a week of a severe right parietal headache. Her only other complaint in addition to the headache was progressively worsening shortness of breath. Her neurologic examination showed only left upper extremity drift. The radiology resident reported that the CT scan showed a right subdural hematoma. What do you think is the cause of her subdural?

A. A fender-bender accident last month.
B. Trauma from bumping her head playing tennis a week ago.
C. Excessive use of aspirin for her migraine headache.
D. A misreading of a meningioma on CT scan by an inexperienced resident.
E. Bleeding from a dural metastasis.

214. A 40-year-old man had a cardiac arrest as a result of a heroin overdose. He suffered severe cerebral anoxic damage and was ventilated in the intensive care unit for several months for multisystem failure. Very gradually, he improved and was extubated. In the rehabilitation facility, he regained use of his arms and legs that had been severely deconditioned due to prolonged bedrest. However, his gait was markedly impaired by an inability to fully extend his hips and knees. What test would best diagnose his joint stiffness?

A. An electromyogram-nerve conduction study.
B. A MRI of his lumbar spine.
C. Radiographs of his hips and knees.
D. A MRI of his brain.

215. Which of the following statements best describes CEA in women?

A. Benefit from CEA for asymptomatic internal carotid artery stenosis is independent of gender.
B. Restenosis rates are higher in women than men.
C. The Asymptomatic Carotid Atherosclerosis Study (ACAS) indicated that CEA reduced the 5-year event rate by 66% in women.
D. Perioperative stroke and death rate in women are similar for both symptomatic and asymptomatic CEA.
E. Restenosis is more common in older, as compared to younger, women.

216. Which of the following statements best describes the results of the Women's Health Study?

A. Low-dose aspirin decreased recurrent stroke risk in women with prior ischemic stroke.
B. Low-dose aspirin protected women of all ages against myocardial infarction and vascular death.
C. Myocardial infarction was more common than ischemic stroke in the placebo group.
D. Treatment with vitamin E decreased ischemic stroke risk.
E. Low-dose aspirin protected women against a first stroke.

217. Which of the following best describes stroke risk in women?

A. Hormone replacement therapy in healthy women in clinical trials has been protective against cerebrovascular disease.
B. Estrogen plus progestin replacement in postmenopausal women increases both ischemic and hemorrhagic stroke risk.
C. In the 6 weeks postpartum, the increase in relative risk of ischemic stroke is greater than the increase in relative risk of hemorrhagic stroke.
D. Women have a lower lifetime risk of stroke than do men.
E. Stroke risk decreases with an increasing level of physical activity.

218. According to the NINDS rt-PA Stroke Study published in December 1995, what is the benefit of thrombolytic therapy?

A. An absolute increase in favorable outcome of 11% to 13% at 3 months.
B. A 30% greater likelihood of minimal or no benefit at 24 hours.
C. An improvement in NIHSS score by 4 or more points at 24 hours.
D. A significant decrease in mortality at 3 months.
E. A decrease in asymptomatic intracranial hemorrhage.

219. Aspirin used in primary prevention of ischemic stroke:

A. Is of no benefit in women.
B. Increases hemorrhagic stroke risk in men.
C. Improves vascular mortality.
D. Has no effect on major bleeding.
E. Is of benefit in both men and women.

220. The best screening test for the development of vasospasm following SAH is:

A. Cerebral angiography.
B. Magnetic resonance angiography.
C. Transcranial Doppler.
D. Computed tomography angiography (CTA).

221. Arteriovenous malformations (AVMs) are:

A. Congenital lesions.
B. Developmental lesions.
C. Most often symptomatic in the sixth or seventh decade.
D. Accompanied by seizures as the most common and serious complication.
E. Generally diagnosed when they present with subdural hemorrhage.

222. Venous angiomas (developmental venous anomalies) are:

A. Hereditary venous anomalies.
B. Common in the spinal cord.
C. Infrequent causes of cerebral hemorrhage.
D. Treated surgically.
E. A major cause of headaches.

223. A 76-year-old man underwent surgery for a thoracic aortic aneurysm. When he awakened from anesthesia, he reported numbness and inability to move both legs. A T8 sensory level to pain was found on neurologic examination. The most likely cause of these symptoms is:

A. Coarctation of the aorta.
B. Vascular malformation of the thoracic cord.
C. Spinal cord infarct.
D. Vasculitis.
E. Transverse myelitis.

224. Spinal cord infarcts are most frequently associated with occlusions of the:

A. Anterior spinal artery.
B. Posterior spinal artery.
C. Venous drainage of the spinal cord.
D. Artery of Adamkiewicz.

225. Which one of the following statements best describes the risk for cervical arterial dissection?

A. All types of Ehlers-Danlos syndrome (EDS) are equally at risk for dissection.
B. Catheter angiography is the recommended diagnostic procedure for all patients with arterial dissection.
C. Spinal manipulative therapy (SMT) is more closely associated with carotid than vertebral arterial dissection.
D. Spinal manipulative therapy may exacerbate pre-existing dissections.
E. Increase in neck or head pain after spinal manipulative therapy is always inconsequential.

226. A 78-year-old woman presents to the emergency department with the sudden onset of right hemiparesis and difficulty with expressive language, onset 20 minutes ago. She was brought in by the paramedics who reported that she was getting her nails done when she suddenly stopped speaking and could no longer hold up her arm. She was unable to speak, but a phone call to her family doctor provided details of her medical history. Which of the following pieces of information from her doctor made you consider her ineligible for intravenous thrombolysis by NINDS criteria?

A. She has a seizure disorder for which she takes Depakote.
B. She had a hip replacement 3 weeks ago.
C. She has atrial fibrillation for which she takes warfarin, with an INR of 1.8 in the emergency department.
D. A recent MRI with gradient recovery imaging showed multiple small areas of hypointensity.
E. She had an ischemic stroke 4 months ago.

227. Which of the following statements about stroke in human immunodeficiency virus (HIV)-infected patients is true?

A. Combination antiretroviral treatment has been associated with the development of metabolic syndrome and increased risk of vascular events.
B. Cardiac disease is common in patients in the later stages of HIV infection and may be an etiology for stroke.
C. Protein S deficiency and antiphospholipid antibodies are the most common hematologic abnormalities.
D. A variety of infectious agents are associated with vasculitis causing stroke.
E. All of the above.

228. A 56-year-old man who was taking warfarin for atrial fibrillation was seen in the Coumadin clinic and was found to have an INR of 4.3 using finger-stick testing. The most appropriate immediate intervention is:

A. Oral vitamin K as an outpatient.
B. Hospital admission for IV vitamin K.
C. Hold warfarin for 1 week.
D. Hold warfarin for 1 day.

229. The nurse in the Coumadin clinic told the patient in Question 228 to hold the Coumadin for 2 days. No venipuncture was done. That evening, the patient presented to the emergency department with severe lumbar back pain, with radiation down the right buttocks and into the lateral right leg. He had a decreased right ankle jerk but no other abnormalities on neurologic examination. Immediate blood work revealed an INR of 4.8 and a normal hemoglobin. The next step in this patient's care should be:

A. An MRI of the LS spine.
B. A lumbar puncture.
C. Outpatient care with strict bed rest and narcotic analgesics.
D. An angiogram of the spinal cord.

230. A 22-year-old weight-lifter presented in the outpatient clinic with complaints of episodic difficulty with speaking. He described four events over the last 3 weeks, lasting for 1 to 2 minutes, of difficulty completing sentences. His weightlifting buddies had noticed this and asked him what the matter was. He told them he had slept poorly and it was just fatigue. He reported no head or neck pain. The patient appeared healthy and very muscular. He was 5'10" tall and weighed 240 pounds, all of which appeared to be solid muscle. Neurologic examination was normal. The next piece of useful information in this setting would be most likely obtained by:

A. Further history.
B. Blood and urine toxicology screen.
C. Blood evaluation for creatinine kinase (CK) level.
D. Magnetic resonance imaging scanning with diffusion weighted imaging (DWI).

231. A 22-year-old woman, with a history of snorting crack, presented to the emergency department with inability to open her left eye. She stated that 2 weeks previously, while using cocaine with friends, she developed pain behind her left eye. She became frightened and stopped her cocaine use. In spite of this, the pain worsened and, over the last 3 days, her left eyelid became progressively droopy. On examination, she had complete ptosis on the left and a dilated pupil. She had good lateral movement of the left eye, but movement in other directions was restricted. The most likely necessary intervention will be:

A. Urgent surgery.
B. Massive doses of corticosteroids.
C. Mestinon.
D. Antibiotics.

232. A 22-year-old man presented with headache and problems using his computer. The previous day at work, he had sudden onset of clumsiness in his right hand and was unable to use his computer with both hands. This was accompanied by a mild headache. Several weeks earlier, he had had an erythematous rash that he attributed to allergies. He had hyperreflexia and slowing of fine motor coordination in the right upper extremity. Pupils were 3 mm and reactive. Spinal fluid analysis revealed a protein of 84 and 24 white blood cells, all mononuclear. He had acute multiple infarcts on MRI, and cerebral angiography revealed multifocal narrowing consistent with vasculitis. His VDRL screen was negative. The most likely cause of the patient's signs and symptoms is:

A. Primary angiitis of the CNS.
B. Lyme disease.
C. Paradoxical emboli from a patent foramen ovale (PFO).
D. Herpes encephalitis.

233. A 24-year-old HIV-positive man presented to the emergency department with right arm weakness and incoordination. He had been well until the past 3 weeks, when he developed headaches, fevers, and fatigue. On neurologic examination, he had hyperreflexia in the right arm with mild weakness and ataxia of that limb. He was somnolent, falling asleep when not stimulated. His temperature was 38.5°C, and his blood pressure was normal. In the emergency room, he had a generalized seizure. An MRI scan showed an acute infarct in the left basal ganglia, along with mild hydrocephalus and enhancement of the basal leptomeninges. There was cerebrospinal fluid (CSF) pleocytosis, with 78 white cells, all mononuclear; a protein of 110; and a glucose of 36. Acid-fast bacillus (AFB) staining was negative, and no bacteria were seen on staining of the spinal fluid. This picture is most consistent with:

A. Tuberculous meningitis.
B. Bacterial meningitis.
C. Systemic lupus erythematosus.
D. Cerebral vasculitis.
E. Infective endocarditis.

234. Which statement about cerebral malaria is true?

A. Steroids are useful to decrease vascular inflammation.
B. Most patients have multiple clinical strokes.
C. Cerebral malaria usually presents with encephalopathy and seizures.
D. Brain damage is rarely due to vascular disease.

235. A 36-year-old IV drug abuser presented with ataxia. His MRI showed three acute ischemic lesions in multiple vascular territories. *Staphylococcus aureus* endocarditis was diagnosed on blood cultures. He was treated with appropriate antibiotics, but he had two additional events that were documented as recurrent cerebral ischemia. Repeat echocardiogram showed his ejection fraction had decreased from 55% to 42%. The next step should be:

A. Anticoagulation.
B. Antiplatelet medications.
C. Urgent surgical valve replacement.
D. Intravenous digoxin.

236. Blindness as a complication of giant-cell arteritis is generally caused by:

A. Occlusion of the posterior ciliary artery.
B. Occlusion of the central retinal vein.
C. Calcarine cortex infarct.
D. Papilledema.

237. Common causes of stroke in SLE include:

A. Cerebral vasculitis.
B. Infective endocarditis.
C. Libman-Sacks endocarditis.
D. Protein C deficiency.

238. A patient with mononeuritis multiplex who develops multiple cerebral infarcts and is positive for antineutrophilic cytoplasmic antibodies (ANCA) most likely has:

A. Wegener's granulomatosis.
B. Giant-cell arteritis.
C. Granulomatous angiitis of the CNS.
D. Polyarteritis nodosa.

239. Patients with Ehlers-Danlos syndrome are at risk for:

A. Subarachnoid hemorrhage.
B. Cerebral vasculitis.
C. Cerebral arterial thrombosis.
D. Cerebral venous thrombosis.

240. A healthy 37-year-old woman, in her thirty-fourth week of an uneventful pregnancy, awoke with severe thoracic back pain. Getting out of bed, she discovered that both legs were weak and she was unable to stand. In the emergency department, she was noted to have abdominal distention and was catheterized for over a liter of urine. She had a T6 sensory level and a flaccid paraparesis. What therapeutic intervention should be considered for the most likely cause of her presentation?

A. Emergent neurosurgical consultation.
B. Intravenous methylprednisolone.
C. Emergent radiation therapy consultation.
D. Intravenous antibiotics.
E. Emergent psychiatry consultation.

241. According to the North American Symptomatic Carotid Endarterectomy Trial (NASCET) results, what is the absolute risk reduction of ipsilateral stroke at 2 years with surgery for patients with symptomatic carotid stenosis of equal to or greater than 70%?

A. 6%.
B. 17%.
C. 23%.
D. 35%.
E. 42%.

242. Which of the following statements best describes the results of the Warfarin-Aspirin Symptomatic Intracranial Disease (WASID) Trial?

A. The rate of myocardial infarction was lower with treatment with warfarin than with aspirin.
B. Aspirin at 325 mg daily showed benefit over warfarin in preventing vascular death.
C. Warfarin showed no benefit over aspirin in preventing ischemic stroke, brain hemorrhage, or nonstroke vascular death.
D. Warfarin and aspirin had equivalent rates of overall adverse events in the trial.
E. The actual mean duration of follow-up was 36 months.

243. Which of the following conditions is associated with *lower* risk of impending ischemic stroke related to internal carotid stenosis?

A. Poststenotic narrowing.
B. Plaque ulceration.
C. Contralateral internal carotid occlusion.
D. Male gender.
E. Transient hemispheric symptoms.

244. Which of the following best describes the benefits of CEA for symptomatic moderate (50%–69%) stenosis, according to the results of NASCET?

A. There is significant benefit from a CEA performed 2 to 3 years after the clinical symptoms.
B. The risk of ipsilateral stroke dropped to about 2% per year after endarterectomy.
C. There was a gradient of benefit according to deciles of stenosis.
D. The surgical group was more likely to die from a myocardial infarction.
E. Right-sided carotid artery disease and contralateral occlusion were risk factors for poor outcome.

245. Match the skin lesion with the associated unusual stroke syndrome. Use each answer only once.

A. Livedo racemosa.	1. Sneddon syndrome.
B. Erythematous papulosis.	2. Kawasaki syndrome.
C. Livedo reticularis.	3. Kohlmeier-Degos disease.
D. Epidermal nevus.	4. Epidermal nevus syndrome.
E. Desquamating exanthema and leukoencephalopathy.	5. Diffuse meningocerebral angiomatosis.

246. A 35-year-old woman with a low-grade astrocytoma underwent resection and radiation therapy. Five years later, she began having transient episodes of right-sided weakness and speech difficulty, not resolving with antiplatelet or antiepilepsy drugs. She also noted new-onset headaches and intermittent confusion. Several months later, she developed a right hemiparesis, with an MRI showing enhancement of the cortical ribbon in the left parietal region. The hemiparesis and MRI lesion resolved in 3 weeks. What is the most likely explanation for this woman's symptoms?

A. Cerebral autosomal dominant arteriopathy with subcortical infarcts and leukoencephalopathy (CADASIL).
B. Mitochondrial encephalomyopathy lactic acidosis and stroke-like symptoms (MELAS).
C. Familial hemiplegic migraine (FHM).
D. Posterior reversible encephalopathy syndrome (PRES).
E. Stroke-like migraine attacks after radiation therapy (SMART).

247. Which of the following best describes cerebral vasospasm?

A. Cerebral vasospasm is a common cause of cerebral infarction, not associated with subarachnoid hemorrhage.
B. In the setting of SAH, cerebral vasospasm appears at 3 to 4 days after a single hemorrhage.
C. Subarachnoid hemorrhage–induced cerebral vasospasm usually resolves at 6 to 8 days after a single hemorrhage.
D. The risk of cerebral vasospasm in SAH is independent of the Fisher Scale.
E. Nimodipine decreases cerebral vasospasm and improves outcome after SAH.

248. The most common cause of cerebral infarction associated with cocaine use is:

A. Vasoconstriction.
B. Vasculitis.
C. Cardiac emboli.
D. Enhanced platelet aggregation.
E. Large-vessel occlusion.

249. Strokes due to chronic Chagas disease are most often caused by:

A. Intracerebral hemorrhage.
B. Arterial dissection.
C. Cardiac embolization.
D. Cerebral arteritis.
E. Subarachnoid hemorrhage.

250. Which statement best describes unruptured intracranial aneurysms?

A. Autopsy and angiographic studies indicate an unruptured intracranial aneurysm frequency of 2% to 5%.
B. Anterior circulation aneurysms are more likely to have poor surgical outcome than are posterior circulation aneurysms.
C. Age of the patient has no effect on surgical or endovascular outcome in patients with unruptured aneurysms.
D. The presence of a previous ruptured intracranial aneurysm does not impact the risk of an unruptured aneurysm.
E. Size and location of the unruptured intracranial aneurysm do not impact treatment outcome.

251. Which statement best describes our knowledge of ruptured intracranial aneurysms?

A. Computed tomography angiography (CTA) is a less useful imaging modality than MRA for patients with a SAH.
B. The International Subarachnoid Aneurysm Trial (ISAT) compared the 1-year death and disability outcome with clipping versus coiling strategies.
C. No difference in 1-year outcome between clipping and coiling strategies was seen in the ISAT.
D. The rebleeding risk in the coiled group after 1 year was approximately 2% per patient year.
E. The ISAT has answered all major questions about surgical versus endovascular treatment of ruptured intracranial aneurysms.

252. A 46-year-old female had onset of headaches and multifocal neurologic deficits that progressed over 6 months. Magnetic resonance imaging showed multifocal small hyperintensities on T2 images. Spinal fluid had a mildly elevated protein and no pleocytosis. Cultures, including TB and fungi, were negative. Bilateral, multifocal stenoses were present on cerebral angiography. Meningeal biopsy revealed a mononuclear vascular infiltrate with focal areas of vascular necrosis. The patient began to improve clinically a week before the biopsy. What is the appropriate course of action?

A. Observation, because the process may be remitting spontaneously.
B. Cyclophosphamide (Cytoxan).
C. Prednisone.
D. Combination of Cytoxan and prednisone.

253. Robert Louis Stevenson wrote of the threat of sudden death, "All our lives long, we may have been about to break a blood vessel...and that has not prevented us from eating dinner, no, nor from putting money in the Savings Bank." He had chronic respiratory complaints with recurrent episodes of pulmonary hemorrhage. The writer died at age 44, in Samoa, of probable cerebral hemorrhage. His mother had pulmonary hemorrhages and what appeared to be a stroke at age 38 years. What disease is Stevenson suspected to have had?

A. Hereditary hemorrhagic telangiectasia (HHT, Osler-Weber-Rendu).
B. Von Hippel-Lindau disease.
C. Sturge-Weber syndrome.
D. Moyamoya syndrome.
E. Amyloid angiopathy.

254. Which of the following best describes surgical treatment of patients with ICH?

A. Early surgery after an ICH improves outcome, as noted in the Surgical Trial in Intracerebral Hemorrhage (STICH) study.
B. The STICH study evaluated the benefit of surgery for spontaneous infratentorial hemorrhage.
C. Comatose patients with ICH in the basal ganglia or thalamus are likely to benefit from clot removal.
D. Surgery may benefit a patient with a cerebellar hematoma larger than 3 cm in diameter and impaired consciousness.
E. Most patients with spontaneous ICH undergo clot removal.

255. Which congenital cutaneovascular syndrome is characterized by multiple intracranial arterial and venous CNS malformations?

A. Neurofibromatosis.
B. Osler-Weber-Rendu disease.
C. Ehlers-Danlos syndrome.
D. Sturge-Weber syndrome.
E. Marfan syndrome.

256. Which statement best describes the risk of stroke in women, as compared to men?

A. Women are more likely to have a stroke than a myocardial infarction.
B. Girls have more strokes than boys.
C. Fewer women than men die of stroke each year.
D. Stroke is more common in women under the age of 80.
E. Incidence of stroke is greater in women in their 60s and 70s.

257. A 19-year-old man was brought to the emergency department by police. He was found wandering aimlessly, confused, and exhibiting bizarre behavior. He had little facial expression. His speech was slow and enunciation was poor. A CT scan demonstrated bilateral and symmetrical globus pallidus hypodensity. Blood and urine toxicology screen was negative. The most likely diagnosis is:

A. Cocaine abuse.
B. Ischemic stroke.
C. Venous sinus thrombus.
D. Carbon monoxide poisoning.
E. Schizophrenia.

258. According to practice parameters on prediction of outcome in comatose survivors after cardiopulmonary resuscitation, which of the biochemical markers performed within 1 to 3 days after resuscitation is the most valuable in predicting poor prognosis?

A. Serum neuron-specific enolase (NSE).
B. Serum S100.
C. Cerebrospinal fluid CK brain isoenzyme.
D. Cerebrospinal fluid lactate.
E. Serum lactate.

259. According to practice parameters on prediction of outcome in comatose survivors after cardiopulmonary resuscitation, which of the following laboratory tests performed within 1 to 3 days after resuscitation is the most valuable in predicting poor prognosis?

A. Electroencephalogram.
B. Somatosensory evoked potentials.
C. Visual evoked potentials.
D. Brainstem evoked potentials.
E. Computed tomography scanning.

260. Which of the following statements best describes angiography in patients with SAH?

A. A follow-up second catheter angiogram should always be performed if the initial one is negative for aneurysm.
B. Catheter angiography has been supplanted by MRA.
C. Catheter angiography in SAH patients is a harmless procedure.
D. Patients with perimesencephalic hemorrhage on CT scanning usually have a vertebrobasilar circulation aneurysm on catheter angiography.
E. The sensitivity of CTA is about 95% compared to catheter angiography.

261. A complication seen late after recovery from SAH is:

A. Hydrocephalus.
B. Anosmia.
C. Loss of hearing.
D. Low back pain.

262. Acute posterior multifocal placoid pigment epitheliopathy (APMPPE):

A. Is a known viral infection of the retina.
B. May cause strokes or aseptic meningitis in young patients.
C. Is not associated with radiographic or pathologic evidence of vasculitis.
D. Is treated with lifelong immunosuppressive agents.
E. Has an autosomal recessive inheritance.

263. An 83-year-old woman with diabetes and chronic atrial fibrillation is on warfarin, oral hypoglycemics, and digoxin. She presents to the emergency room with hallucinations that began 4 days earlier and have gradually worsened. Heart rate was 38 and irregular, with no ischemic changes on EKG. Temperature was normal. The patient had no nuchal rigidity. Blood counts and electrolytes, including serum glucose, were all normal, and her INR was 2.8. A CT scan of the brain was negative for blood. The test most likely to define the etiology of the hallucinations is:

A. Electroencephalogram.
B. Spinal tap.
C. Digoxin level.
D. Blood cultures.
E. Blood and urine toxicology screen.

264. Which statement is true about PACNS?

A. Antinuclear antibody is generally positive.
B. Spinal fluid always has pleocytosis.
C. If angiography is positive for segmental narrowing in multiple vessels bilaterally, treatment can be given without biopsy.
D. Although angiitis can be missed on biopsy because of the patchy involvement of the disease process, biopsy should be considered.
E. An underlying viral process is the most likely etiology.

265. A 19-year-old man fell while waterskiing, immediately noting pain in the right neck and behind the right eye. His friends took him to the emergency department, where the resident noted a mild right ptosis, which was clearly not present on his driver's license photo. Eye movements were full and conjugate. Pupillary size was 3 mm on the right, 4 mm on the left, with asymmetry most noticeable in the dark. Both pupils were round and reactive to light. The most appropriate first test is:

A. Urine test for cocaine.
B. Magnetic resonance angiography, CTA, or carotid duplex.
C. Carotid angiogram.
D. Chest CT.

266. Which of the following best describes an internuclear ophthalmoplegia (INO) due to an ischemic stroke?

A. An INO does not present as an isolated or predominant stroke symptom.
B. An INO is characterized by abduction impairment with contralateral adduction nystagmus.
C. The lesion causing the INO can be in the pons or midbrain.
D. The functional prognosis of the patient with an isolated INO is poor.
E. An INO is never accompanied by a skew deviation or gaze paresis.

267. Which statement best describes mycotic aneurysms?

A. Many mycotic aneurysms become smaller or disappear over time.
B. They are congenital.
C. They are unlikely to produce SAH.
D. They are unlikely to occur at arterial bifurcations.
E. They only occur in the brain.

268. A 45-year-old man underwent an allogenic hematopoietic stem cell transplant for acute myelogenous leukemia. He was treated with tacrolimus for immunosuppression to prevent graft-versus-host disease. He developed pneumonia and was admitted to the hospital for IV antibiotics. He was pancytopenic. The nurse who came into his room to check vital signs found him unresponsive, with left gaze deviation and left-sided tonic–clonic movements. The CT scan of the brain showed bilateral hypodensities in the parieto-occipital lobes. He was loaded with intravenous levetiracetam (Keppra) because of concern about the hematosuppressive effects of other medications to treat his seizures. What is the cause of this man's symptoms?

A. Tuberculous meningitis.
B. Basilar artery dissection.
C. Posterior reversible encephalopathy syndrome (PRES).
D. Disseminated intravascular coagulopathy (DIC).
E. Herpes encephalitis.

269. Match the autosomal dominant disorder associated with increased stroke risk with its genetic defect. Use each answer only once.

A. Marfan syndrome.
B. Ehlers-Danlos syndrome type IV.
C. Neurofibromatosis type 1.
D. Cerebral autosomal dominant arteriopathy with subcortical infarcts and leukoencephalopathy (CADASIL).
E. Osteogenesis imperfecta.

1. Notch 3 (19q12).
2. Type III collagen (2q31).
3. α1 or α2 chain of type I collagen.
4. Neurofibromin (17q11.2).
5. Fibrillin-1 (15q21.1).

270. Match the disorder associated with increased stroke risk with its most usual inheritance pattern. Use each answer only once.

A. Fabry disease.
B. Mitochondrial encephalomyopathy, lactic acidosis, and stroke-like episodes (MELAS).
C. Pseudoxanthoma elasticum.
D. Familial cardiomyopathies.
E. Cerebral amyloid angiopathy.

1. Maternal.
2. X-linked.
3. Autosomal recessive.
4. Sporadic.
5. Autosomal dominant.

271. According to established guidelines, which of the following populations should be routinely screened for extracranial carotid stenosis?

A. All patients undergoing coronary artery bypass grafting.
B. Patients with isolated dizziness.
C. Patients with symptomatic peripheral vascular disease.
D. Patients with renal artery stenosis.
E. Patients with abdominal aortic aneurysms.

272. Which of the following statements best applies to patients undergoing radiotherapy for head and neck malignancy?

A. Patients should be screened for extracranial carotid disease prior to radiotherapy.
B. The risk of carotid disease decreases with time after radiotherapy.
C. Carotid endarterectomy is much preferable to carotid stent placement for radiation-induced stenosis.
D. Patients should be screened 10 years after unilateral or bilateral irradiation.
E. A clear relationship has been established between dose and duration of radiotherapy and risk and degree of carotid disease.

273. In published studies, which of the following statements best applies to restenosis after carotid artery stenting?

A. Standardized definitions for restenosis have been used in the published clinical trials.
B. Restenosis is almost always associated with recurrent symptoms.
C. Higher rates of restenosis have been observed with self-expanding stents, as compared to balloon angioplasty and balloon-expanding stents.
D. Restenosis is in the range of 1% to 18.5%.

274. Least benefit is associated with CEA in which subgroup of symptomatic patients in the NASCET and the European Carotid Surgery Trial (ECST) studies?

A. Men.
B. Patients older than 75 years.
C. Patients operated within 2 weeks of diagnosis.
D. Patients with retinal ischemia.
E. Patients with an ischemic stroke.

275. A 61-year-old man with paroxysmal atrial fibrillation, not on an anticoagulant, went to the emergency department after he sliced his thumb cutting a bagel for breakfast. While being sutured, he had a sudden onset of right-sided weakness and a right visual field cut. The MRI scanner was immediately available, and a left anterior choroidal artery infarct was noted on DWI. The neuroradiologist also reported that multiple small cortical black dots were present on gradient echo T2*-weighted MRI sequences. Which statement best describes his therapy?

A. Intravenous thrombolysis is associated with unacceptable hemorrhage risk.
B. He should be given intravenous thrombolysis, and he should be put on antiplatelet therapy.
C. He should be given intravenous thrombolysis, and he should be put on long-term anticoagulant therapy.
D. Thrombolysis, antiplatelet therapy, and anticoagulation are all contraindicated.

276. In patients who have an untreated brain AVM, which of the following is the major predictor of future hemorrhage?

A. Arteriovenous malformation size.
B. Hemorrhagic initial presentation.
C. Exclusively deep venous drainage.
D. Female gender.
E. Associated aneurysm.

277. Which of the following symptom groups results from infarction of the lateral medulla?

A. Contralateral hemiplegia, contralateral loss of position and vibration sense.
B. Ipsilateral deviation of the tongue and nystagmus.
C. Ipsilateral Horner's syndrome, ipsilateral loss of pain and thermal sense on the face.
D. Contralateral loss of pain and thermal sense on the body and contralateral ataxia.

278. A 74-year-old woman underwent emergent coronary artery bypass graft surgery for increasing angina at rest. Postoperatively she was noted to be lethargic, with bilateral upper arm weakness. An MRI scan was obtained. What is its most likely diagnosis?

A. Bilateral brachial plexus avulsion injuries from perioperative traction.
B. Bilateral MCA infarcts on DWI.
C. Bilateral medial thalamic lesions on DWI.
D. Small linear cortical and white matter lesions in the high frontal area bilaterally.
E. Normal MRI of the brain.

279. Which of the following statements best describes our knowledge of Lp(a):

A. Increased Lp(a) levels are independent of increased levels of LDL cholesterol (LDL-C).
B. Levels of Lp(a) are independent of gender and race/ethnicity.
C. Levels of Lp(a) correlate with hemorrhagic stroke risk.
D. Screening for Lp(a) levels has been shown to impact patient management.
E. The specific population at ischemic stroke risk with elevated Lp(a) levels is still unclear.

280. A 71-year-old right-handed man with atrial fibrillation had the sudden onset of right hemiplegia and a dense right homonymous hemianopic defect. His speech was intact. The CT scan of the head was negative within 2 hours. Carotid ultrasonography showed patent vessels. Which vessel is most likely to be occluded?

A. Middle cerebral artery.
B. Anterior cerebral artery.
C. Posterior cerebral artery.
D. Anterior choroidal artery.
E. Lenticulostriate arteries.

281. According to the Seventh Report of the Joint National Committee on Prevention Detection, Evaluation, and Treatment of High Blood Pressure (the JNC 7 Report), published in 2003, what is the lifetime risk of hypertension for a normotensive person aged 55 years?

A. 50%.
B. 60%.
C. 70%.
D. 80%.
E. 90%.

282. Which one of the following patients is best treated with long-term warfarin anticoagulation?

A. A healthy 55-year-old man with two episodes of paroxysmal atrial fibrillation and a normal transesophageal echocardiogram.
B. A 66-year-old woman with two episodes of symptomatic paroxysmal atrial fibrillation and a transesophageal echocardiogram that shows mild left ventricular hypokinesis.
C. A 32-year-old woman, who is pregnant, with a past history of cerebral venous thrombosis and activated protein C resistance.
D. A 78-year-old man who had a second stroke on aspirin, with an MRA that shows MCA stenosis.
E. An 81-year-old woman, who awoke from surgery to replace a broken femoral head, with an MRI that showed multifocal acute infarcts and pulmonary infiltrates.

283. Which was statement best describes perioperative stroke?

A. Most strokes in patients undergoing carotid and cardiac surgery are due to hypoperfusion.
B. Hemorrhage is a common etiology of perioperative stroke.
C. The combination of coronary artery bypass surgery and valve replacement has about the same stroke risk as valve replacement alone.
D. Aortic atherosclerosis does not increase the risk of perioperative stroke with cardiac bypass surgery.
E. Atrial fibrillation is rarely the cause of stroke after cardiac surgery.

284. Which condition is associated with familial intracranial aneurysms?

A. Polycystic ovary disease.
B. Polycystic kidney disease.
C. Inflammatory bowel disease.
D. Rheumatoid arthritis.
E. All of the above.

285. A 23-year-old woman was on a treadmill exercising after a stressful day at work when she developed a sudden severe frontal headache with nausea and lightheadedness. Her trainer drove her to an emergency department, where her neurologic examination showed only a woman in moderate distress from a headache and stiff neck. An emergent CT scan was interpreted as negative. Which of the following statements is true?

A. The woman probably had a migraine headache induced by exercise and relief from stress.
B. The CT scan should be repeated with intravenous contrast.
C. A lumbar puncture should be performed even though the CT scan was negative.
D. A subcutaneous injection of sumatriptan should be given for symptomatic relief.
E. An MRI of brain should be ordered.

286. A 36-year-old man was working in a grocery store, stocking shelves on the graveyard shift. He was carrying boxes when he developed the sudden onset of a severe headache. He dropped the boxes, and a coworker came to his aid. He began to vomit, and the coworker called 911. In the emergency department, he was found to have a bitemporal field defect. The most likely diagnosis is:

A. Subarachnoid hemorrhage.
B. Lobar hemorrhage in the right occipital lobe.
C. Pituitary apoplexy.
D. Cluster headache.

287. Acute postanoxic myoclonus:

A. Responds to traditional anticonvulsant medications.
B. Is correlated with paroxysmal EEG activity.
C. Has no prognostic value.
D. Is described as "Lance-Adams syndrome."
E. May respond to high doses of benzodiazepines.

288. A 34-year-old woman came to the office with her husband, who complained that she no longer seemed to notice when he was talking to her and that she had been acting strangely. She had recently lost her job as a bookkeeper after some financial problems in her records were noted. Two recent motor vehicle accidents, where she hit the car in front of her, resulted in suspension of her driver's license. Her only complaint was of vertigo. Mental status testing showed difficulty with word retrieval and memory, and she appeared disinhibited. Vision appeared impaired, although her field testing was inconsistent. An ophthalmologic evaluation showed branch retinal artery occlusions bilaterally. Hearing testing revealed bilateral sensorineural hearing loss. Ataxia with left-sided weakness on examination was noted. What suspected diagnosis should you note on the request for an MRI of the brain?

A. Cogan syndrome.
B. Susac syndrome.
C. Syphilis.
D. Lupus erythematosus.
E. Multiple sclerosis.

289. An MRI was ordered on this patient. What would you expect the findings to be, given your clinical suspicion?

A. Diffuse meningeal enhancement.
B. No findings except for incidental sinusitis.
C. Multiple foci of high T2 signal intensity and contrast enhancement in gray and white matter.
D. Multifocal microhemorrhages.
E. Confluent white matter areas of high T2 signal intensity, with sparing of gray matter.

290. Preoperative consultation on a 48-year-old man was requested because of a history of vertigo, accompanied by nausea and vomiting. The patient recounted abrupt onset of vertigo, gait instability, and tinnitus several months ago, which was episodic but becoming more frequent. He reported decreased hearing, with difficulty using a phone in his right ear. The patient is lying motionless in the hospital bed with the lights off. On examination, his eyes are injected and his visual acuity is decreased. He has decreased hearing bilaterally. He protests having to walk but when coerced, his gait is ataxic and he gets short of breath. What operation is scheduled for the next day?

A. Inguinal hernia repair.
B. Hair plugs.
C. Aortic valve replacement.
D. Ventriculo-peritoneal shunt.
E. Renal transplant.

291. Which group includes the major risk factors for ICH in young adults?

A. Hypertension, anticoagulation, cerebral amyloid angiopathy.
B. Hypertension, vascular malformations, substance abuse.
C. Trauma, cerebral amyloid angiopathy, vascular malformations.
D. Anticoagulation, trauma, eclampsia.
E. Cerebral vasculitis, substance abuse, reperfusion injury.

292. Which of the following statements best describes early findings in intracerebral hemorrhage?

A. Bleeding in patients with ICH is completed within minutes of symptom onset.
B. Neurologic deterioration occurring during the first 24 hours after hemorrhage is mainly due to progressive cerebral edema.
C. Increase in size of ICH is commonly noted during the first 24 hours after symptom onset.
D. Early increase in hemorrhage volume is not associated with clinical deterioration.
E. Location is a significant predictor of early change in volume of hemorrhage.

293. Which statement best describes risk of spontaneous ICH?

A. Treatment of chronic hypertension has minimal impact on risk of ICH.
B. Risk of recurrent hemorrhage is greater with chronic hypertension than with cerebral amyloid angiopathy.
C. The recurrent hemorrhage risk associated with cerebral amyloid angiopathy may be increased by the presence of ε2 and ε4 alleles of the apolipoprotein E gene.
D. Intracerebral hemorrhage risk is not increased by excessive alcohol use.
E. Serum total cholesterol level greater than 160 mg/dL is associated with an increased hemorrhage risk.

294. A 28-year-old woman, 24 weeks pregnant, was brought into the emergency department with right hemiparesis and moderate dysphasia, with onset 20 minutes ago. Her husband reported that she had been in a fender-bender motor vehicle accident a week prior, with lateral neck pain and tenderness lasting for a couple of days. Her blood pressure was 138/88. Her NIHSS score was 16. A CT scan did not show any acute changes, and blood work was unremarkable. Which best describes the therapeutic options?

A. She should be considered for treatment with intravenous thrombolysis as quickly as possible within 3 hours.
B. Intravenous thrombolysis is absolutely contraindicated because of suspected internal carotid dissection.
C. Intravenous thrombolysis is absolutely contraindicated because of her pregnancy.
D. No acute stroke-specific therapy should be offered.
E. She should be treated with a loading dose followed by a maintenance infusion of heparin.

295. A 34-year-old woman delivered a healthy infant after an uneventful 38-week pregnancy. Four days after delivery, she developed a headache that gradually increased in severity. In the emergency department, she had a generalized tonic–clonic seizure. Her blood pressure was 124/86. She was lethargic after the seizure and did not move her right arm spontaneously. No peripheral edema was found on examination, and urine was negative for protein. A CT scan was negative for acute changes. Of the following, which is the most likely diagnosis?

A. Eclampsia.
B. Preeclampsia.
C. Posterior reversible encephalopathy syndrome.
D. Postpartum cerebral angiopathy.
E. Subarachnoid hemorrhage.

296. Which of the following statements best describes ICH and pregnancy?

A. Risk of ICH is increased in the immediate postpartum period.
B. Intracerebral hemorrhage causes less than 1% of all death related to pregnancy.
C. Risk of ICH is increased in the third trimester.
D. Risk of ICH is not influenced by maternal blood pressure history.
E. Pregnancy does not increase ICH risk.

297. You see a 42-year-old woman in the emergency department at 8 AM who awoke from sleep at 7 AM with a right hemiparesis and aphasia. Her husband reports that she walked to the bathroom at 6 AM and then told him that she was going back to sleep. The CT scan was negative for hemorrhage or ischemia. Which of the following is a contraindication to giving intravenous t-PA?

A. Her husband gave her an aspirin, 325 mg, before he called 911.
B. Her NIHSS score is 19.
C. She has idiopathic thrombocytopenic purpura (ITP) with a platelet count of 45,000.
D. Her blood pressure was 190/100 but decreased to 170/90 with 10 mg of intravenous labetalol.
E. The timing of her stroke onset is unknown.

298. A 78-year-old man with a history of hypertension, diabetes, hyperlipidemia, and smoking presented to the emergency department with 3 hours of nausea, vomiting, dizziness, and blurry vision. A CT scan of the brain was negative. His neurologic examination appeared unremarkable until he got up from lying on the stretcher to go to the bathroom and fell to the floor. What would be the most appropriate next step?

A. Send the patient home with an antiemetic and instructions to call the family doctor within the next 2 to 3 days.
B. Obtain an MRI of the brain and an MRA of the brain and neck vessels.
C. Admit the patient to the hospital with acute onset of vertigo and order nursing checks every 6 hours.
D. Do a lumbar puncture to rule out SAH.
E. Obtain a carotid ultrasound in the emergency department.

299. Several hours after running the New York Marathon in 4.5 hours, a young woman complained of a headache of increasing severity. She became progressively more lethargic before she was brought to the emergency department. She has no significant past medical history and is on no medications except for oral contraceptives. A CT scan with contrast showed an empty delta sign. Which test should be part of her evaluation?

A. Activated protein C resistance (Factor V Leiden mutation).
B. Transesophageal echocardiogram.
C. Liver function tests.
D. Transthoracic echocardiogram.
E. Holter monitor.

300. Familial hemiplegic migraine type 1:

A. Is rarely associated with permanent cerebellar symptoms.
B. Generally consists of reversible motor weakness without other neurologic symptoms.
C. Affects women more frequently than men.
D. Has been associated with a mutation of the *CACNA1A* gene encoding a subunit of a voltage-dependent neuronal calcium channel.
E. Is an inherited autosomal recessive migraine subtype.

301. A 78-year-old woman complains of an intermittent bitemporal headache and neck pain. Her hair is disheveled, and she has lost weight because of aching in her face when she eats. Which noninvasive test will suggest her diagnosis with greatest accuracy?

A. Erythrocyte sedimentation rate (ESR).
B. C-reactive protein (C-RP).
C. Von Willebrand factor.
D. Oculoplethysmography (OPG).

302. Which of these statements best describes the headache associated with an ischemic stroke?

A. The headache is more commonly associated with posterior than anterior circulation ischemia.
B. The headache is more commonly associated with lacunar than nonlacunar infarcts.
C. The headache is more commonly associated with cardioembolic than atherothrombotic stroke.
D. The severity of the headache correlates with the size of the infarction.
E. None of the above.

303. A 34-year-old woman developed a progressively severe headache in the second trimester of an otherwise uneventful pregnancy. After bilateral leg weakness was noted, she was admitted to the hospital for evaluation. She had a tonic–clonic seizure on the way to the CT scanner. Subtle hypodensity and small hemorrhages were noted in the high frontal regions bilaterally on the CT scan. The most likely diagnosis is:

A. Postpartum cerebral angiopathy.
B. Eclampsia.
C. Spinal cord epidural hemorrhage.
D. Venous infarction.
E. Posterior reversible encephalopathy syndrome (PRES).

304. What is the most appropriate therapy for this woman?

A. Intravenous unfractionated heparin followed by warfarin.
B. Intravenous hydration followed by warfarin.
C. Intravenous unfractionated heparin followed by subcutaneous low-molecular-weight heparin.
D. Intravenous hydration followed by aspirin.
E. Oral antibiotics followed by subcutaneous low-molecular-weight heparin.

305. Lack of correlation with reduction in ischemic stroke risk was found with which individual component of a healthy lifestyle, in the Women's Health Study (WHS)?

A. Abstinence from smoking.
B. Body mass index less than 22 kg/m^2.
C. Exercise four or more times/week.
D. Alcohol consumption of 4 to 10.5 drinks per week.
E. Diet high in fiber and polyunsaturated fats and low in trans fat and glycemic load.

306. Which vascular event is increased in women with migraine with aura?

A. Ischemic stroke.
B. Myocardial infarction.
C. Angina.
D. Coronary revascularization.
E. All of the above.

307. Patients with von Hippel-Lindau syndrome often have which type of cancer?

A. Astrocytoma.
B. Sarcoma.
C. Hepatoma.
D. Clear-cell carcinoma of the vagina.
E. Renal cell carcinoma.

308. In patients with thrombosis of the major cerebral veins and sinuses, more than one structure is generally involved. Which of these structures is most commonly affected in cerebral venous thrombosis?

A. Jugular veins.
B. Cortical veins.
C. Straight sinus.
D. Transverse sinuses.
E. Superior sagittal sinus.

309. What is the most common cause of bilateral external ophthalmoplegia?

A. Miller-Fisher syndrome.
B. Guillain-Barré syndrome.
C. Midbrain-thalamic infarcts.
D. Pituitary apoplexy.
E. Trauma.

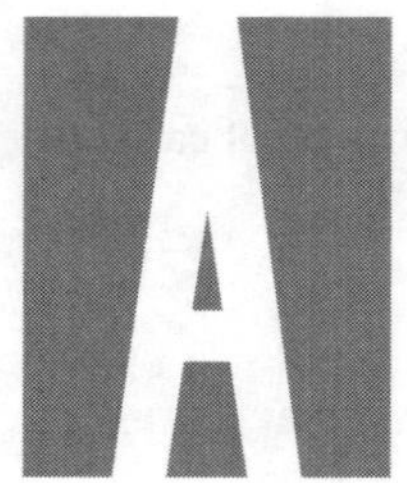

Clinical Stroke Answers

126. The answer is B. Fabry disease is an X-linked recessive lysosomal storage disorder, due to deficient activity of α-galactosidase A (α-Gal A), which leads to accumulation of globotriaosylceramide in vascular endothelium. Globotriaosylceramide accumulation in the vasculature of the kidney, heart, cornea, and brain may lead to renal failure, myocardial infarction, and ischemic stroke at an early age, because of vascular occlusion and a prothrombotic state. The ischemic strokes tend to occur in the posterior circulation, involving both large and small vessels. Characteristic skin (angiokeratomas) and ocular (corneal opacities) lesions, as well as a painful peripheral neuropathy, are also found in many affected patients. Fabry disease should be considered in unexplained ischemic stroke in young patients, especially when vertebrobasilar territory infarction is seen in combination with proteinuria. (Rolfs et al., *Lancet* 2005)

127. The answers are A 3, B 4, C 2, D 1. The syndromes of Millard-Gubler, Foville, and Raymond-Cestan result from lesions in the pons affecting the corticospinal tract and additional structures. A lesion of the medial pons involving emerging fibers of the abducens nerve and the corticospinal tract causes ipsilateral abducens palsy and contralateral hemiparesis. The lesion may extend laterally and involve the fibers of the facial nerve, causing ipsilateral peripheral facial paresis (Millard-Gubler syndrome). Dorsal expansion into the pontine tegmentum involving the paramedian pontine reticular formation abolishes the ability to turn toward the side of the lesion, leading to conjugate gaze paralysis and ipsilateral peripheral facial paresis (Foville syndrome). A lesion involving the corticospinal tract and the medial longitudinal fasciculus causes contralateral hemiparesis and an internuclear ophthalmoplegia, with loss of adduction on the side of the lesion (Raymond-Cestan syndrome). The combination of unilateral oculomotor palsy and contralateral hemiparesis (Weber syndrome) results from a lesion of the cerebral peduncle and the oculomotor nerve in the basal midbrain. (Silverman et al., *Arch Neurol* 1995)

128. The answer is D. A Mediterranean diet and occasional fish can decrease ischemic stroke risk. The famous "J-shaped curve" dictates that about two drinks per day for men and one drink per day for nonpregnant women may be considered for stroke risk reduction. Even secondary smoke may increase stroke risk. Weight reduction to a body mass index (BMI) in the 19 to 25 kg/m^2 range decreases stroke risk factors. Exercise should be encouraged, including as tolerated for patients after stroke. (Sacco et al., *Stroke* 2006)

129. The answer is E. Sporadic cerebral amyloid angiopathy (CAA) is common in elderly individuals and is often found in association with Alzheimer's disease. Pathologically, there is deposition of β-amyloid peptide (A-β) in the tunica media of cerebral blood vessels, with gradual infiltration of the blood vessel and the surrounding neuropil. Cerebral amyloid angiopathy is a major cause of nontraumatic intracerebral hemorrhage in the elderly. Risk of hemorrhage is increased with anticoagulation. The occipital and frontal lobes are the most frequent sites of CAA-related hemorrhage, with subcortical hemorrhages rarely seen. Multiple cortical microhemorrhages may be seen on the gradient echo (GRE) sequence on magnetic resonance imaging (MRI). (Attems, *Acta Neuropathol* 2005)

130. The answer is C. A subarachnoid hemorrhage (SAH) is the most devastating cause of a headache of apoplectic onset. Other conditions that can cause a thunderclap headache include "crash migraine," intracerebral hemorrhage, pituitary apoplexy, exertional headache, and benign thunderclap headaches. Neck pain may be present with either migraine or SAH. Although SAH has been described as "the worst headache of my life," the pain may be severe to moderate, with the main characteristic being its sudden onset. Migraine and SAH both are more common in middle-aged women. (Oleson et al., Chapter 109)

131. The answer is C. Patients with migraine headaches, especially migraine with aura, have an increased incidence of ischemic stroke. In women aged less than 45 years, the risk of stroke is increased threefold associated with migraine without aura and sixfold in women with migraine with aura. The increased risk may be related to platelet aggregation, vasoreactivity of extracerebral vessels, or an increased incidence of patent foramen ovale. There may be an increased incidence of myocardial infarction in migraine patients, but the relationship is less clear than with ischemic stroke. Hemorrhagic stroke is not clearly associated with migraine headaches. Although changes in blood vessel diameter may play a role in migraine headaches, it is primarily a neurovascular disorder modulated by brainstem nuclei. (Olesen et al., Chapter 64)

132. The answer is C. Coexistent internal carotid and coronary artery stenosis increases the risk for intraoperative ischemic stroke with cardiac surgery, but operative management of carotid artery disease prior to cardiac surgery is controversial. In general, treatment of the acutely symptomatic lesion is suggested with coexistent carotid and coronary artery disease. In this case, the man has severe symptomatic coronary artery disease with asymptomatic moderate carotid artery disease. Proceeding with the cardiac surgery while minimizing perioperative hypotension and bypass time are appropriate. Synchronous or staged surgical procedures may be considered when there is symptomatic and/or severely stenotic disease of both internal carotid and coronary arteries. Carotid stenting is an option to decrease stroke risk associated with cardiac surgery. Synchronous carotid stenting and cardiac surgery may be an acceptable strategy for appropriate high-risk patients. (Newman et al., *Lancet* 2006)

133. The answer is B. An infarct of the red nucleus and the cerebellothalamic fibers (contralateral ataxia and tremor) and oculomotor nerve (ipsilateral eye movement paresis with down and out deviation and dilated pupil) produces a Claude syndrome. The cortical spinal tract and oculomotor nerve are involved in the medial midbrain (Weber) syndrome, with contralateral hemiplegia and ipsilateral eye movement paresis and dilated pupil. A larger lesion of both the central and medial midbrain produces the Benedikt syndrome, involving the cortical spinal tract, oculomotor nerve, the red nucleus, and the cerebellothalamic tract. The superior colliculi and oculomotor nerve are involved in the Parinaud syndrome, generally caused by a compressive lesion in the pineal region. (Haines, *Neuroanatomy*)

134. The answer is A. Hypertension is not only more common in African Americans than in whites but, at approximately 32% the prevalence of hypertension in Americans of African descent, is among the highest in the world. The prevalence of hypertension is 22.6% in Mexican Americans and 23.3% in non-Hispanic whites. About three-quarters of Americans with hypertension are inadequately controlled on medications. (Fuster, Chapter 2)

135. The answer is B. Smoking causes more deaths worldwide than tuberculosis and malaria combined. Second-hand smoke increases the risk of cardiovascular death by up to 30%. Although smoking decreased from 1981 to 1991 in most developed countries, smoking is again on the rise. In the United States, the prevalence of smoking is over 20% in adults. (Fuster, Chapter 2)

136. The answer is C. Parkinson's disease may produce orthostatic hypotension on a neurogenic basis, and the medications used to treat Parkinson's disease also may cause orthostatic hypotension. Many central nervous system (CNS) disorders contribute to orthostatic hypotension on a neurogenic basis, including multiple sclerosis, multiple cerebral infarcts, and multiple system atrophy. Other disorders contribute to orthostatic hypotension by producing an autonomic neuropathy, such as diabetes. Myasthenia gravis and pseudotumor cerebri (idiopathic intracranial hypertension) do not produce orthostatic hypotension. Orthostatic hypotension is a common problem encountered in stroke patients, because they often have multiple contributing factors with their concomitant medical disorders and polypharmacy. Cushing's syndrome and renal artery stenosis are both causes of hypertension. (Fuster, Chapter 40)

137. The answer is B. Palpation of the radial artery while gradually increasing the pressure in a blood pressure cuff gives an accurate systolic blood pressure, determined by the point at which the pulse can no longer be palpated. The possibility of an auscultatory gap reduces the accuracy of auscultation in some patients. Mercury columns have been extremely accurate, but it is of interest that environmental concerns in some countries do not allow mercury in the workplace. Calibration of nonmercury blood pressure cuffs every 6 months (against mercury columns) is important to assure accuracy. The radial artery is easily palpated but not amenable to auscultation. (Fuster, Chapter 61)

138. The answer is A. Benign angiitis of the CNS may be a form of primary angiitis of the central nervous system (PACNS), although it has been classified recently as a reversible cerebral vasoconstriction syndrome. It has a benign clinical course, presenting with headache and focal neurologic deficit. Although a focal area of involvement may be seen on catheter angiography, sedimentation rate and spinal fluid are generally unremarkable. Vasospasm has been suggested to explain the angiographic picture. Because of a nonprogressive, monophasic course, treatment with immunosuppressive therapy may not be indicated. Primary angiitis of the central nervous system generally presents with headaches followed by focal neurologic deficits. Rarely, is it accompanied by fever, weight loss, and malaise. Catheter angiography shows beading, occlusion, or luminal irregularity in 60% to 80% of patients with PACNS. Because PACNS predominantly involves small vessels, up to 40% of patients may have negative angiography. MRI abnormalities include ischemic lesions, leptomeningeal enhancement, hemorrhage, mass lesion, or diffuse white matter disease. The MRI can also be normal. There are multiple causes of an abnormal single-photon emission tomography (SPECT) scan other than PACNS. (West, *Curr Rheum Rep* 2003)

139. The answer is B. A lumbar drain can be used to decrease the risk of paraplegia due to an anterior spinal artery infarct, not an uncommon complication of thoracic aorta repair. Lumbar cerebral spinal fluid drainage can be used preventatively during surgery or postoperatively if an anterior spinal artery infarct occurs, although its efficacy is not entirely clear. A subdural hematoma can complicate the removal of spinal fluid, either from a lumbar puncture or a lumbar drain, because of shifting of cranial contents with stretching and rupture of subdural bridging veins. This man had a right frontal subdural hematoma presenting as a seizure with a postictal paresis. (Cheung et al., *Ann Thorac Surg* 2005)

140. The answers are A 3, B 2, C 4, D 1. Takayasu's arteritis characteristically affects young women, who present with nonspecific systemic symptoms including fatigue and headaches. They develop inflammatory changes of the aorta and its main branches, with bruits and asymmetric blood pressures. Women with giant-cell arteritis are older when they present with nonspecific systemic symptoms followed by inflammatory changes to medium- and large-sized cranial vessels. Wegener's granulomatosis consists of necrotizing granulomatous changes in the upper and lower respiratory tract and pulmonary vessels, as well as necrotizing glomerulitis. Patients present with nonspecific symptoms, and upper airway and pulmonary symptoms. Patients with Churg-Strauss syndrome, a rare systemic necrotizing granulomatous vasculitis, have a history of allergic rhinitis with nasal polyps, asthma, eosinophilia, and elevated levels of immunoglobulin (Ig) E. (Marquez et al., *Curr Rheum Rep* 2003)

141. The answers are A 2, B 3, C 1, D 4, E 5. Wegener's granulomatosis consists of necrotizing granulomatous changes in the upper and lower respiratory tract and pulmonary vessels, as well as necrotizing glomerulitis. Behçet's disease is a rare multiorgan disorder characterized by recurrent oral and genital ulcers, uveitis, and arthritis, with meningoencephalitis in some patients. Polyarteritis nodosa is a generalized vasculitis involving medium and small vessels in multiple visceral organs, including muscle, and peripheral nerve. Polyarteritis nodosa with involvement of the vasa nervorum may present as a mononeuritis multiplex. Sjögren syndrome is a disorder of cellular and humoral immunity that involves exocrine glands, including lacrimal and salivary glands, and peripheral nerves. Patients with Churg-Strauss syndrome, a rare systemic necrotizing granulomatous vasculitis, have a history of allergic rhinitis with nasal polyps, asthma, eosinophilia, and elevated levels of IgE. (Graham & Lantos, Chapter 6; Marquez et al., *Curr Rheum Rep* 2003)

142. The answer is B. Familial predisposition is a strong risk factor for the development of intracranial aneurysms. Approximately 10% of patients with aneurysmal SAH have a familial clustering. In comparison to sporadic aneurysms, familial aneurysms appear to rupture at an earlier age and are more often located on the middle cerebral artery (MCA). Some studies conclude that familial aneurysms are larger at time of rupture, with worse outcome. The incidence of SAH in Finland is three times higher than in other parts of the world and, unlike in the United States, Finnish men are more affected by SAH than are Finnish women. Although there are some discordant studies, familial aneurysms are more likely to be multiple. (Ruigrok et al., *Neurology* 2004)

143. The answer is A. The Boston Criteria can be used to diagnose CAA with varying degrees of certainty. Possible CAA (only one lobar hemorrhage) and probable CAA (multiple lobar hemorrhages) are categories for patients age 55 years or older, without other cause of intracerebral hemorrhage. Pathologic diagnosis can be made by biopsy (probable CAA with supporting pathology) or postmortem examination (definite CAA). There is a high degree of clinical and pathologic correlation with probable CAA. The ApoE allele frequency is the same with probable CAA and pathologically proven CAA, indicating the validity of the criteria. (Smith & Greenberg, *Curr Athero Rep* 2003)

144. The answer is B. Prognostic scores (ABCD, California) have been used to predict the short-term risk of stroke after transient ischemic attack (TIA). The five factors that predict increased risk are: (a) age greater than or equal to 60 years, (b) blood pressure greater than or equal to 140/90 mm Hg, (c) unilateral weakness or speech impairment without weakness, (d) duration of TIA greater than or equal to 60 minutes, and (e) diabetes. Patients with these criteria are at increased short-term risk of ischemic stroke after a TIA. This may reflect specific pathology or the accuracy of the diagnosis of TIA in patients with these vascular risk factors. (Johnston et al., *Lancet* 2007)

145. The answer is E. Obstructive sleep apnea (OSA) syndrome is associated with an increased risk of stroke or death from any cause, independent of other risk factors including hypertension. There appears to be an association between atrial fibrillation (AF) and OSA, perhaps because of hypoxemia and hypercarbia, which promote arrhythmias. Multiple mechanisms, including a prothrombotic state, inflammation, oxidative stress, and cerebral hemodynamics, link OSA to increased stroke risk. Obstructive sleep apnea, not central sleep apnea, is found commonly after stroke and is associated with worse stroke outcome. No difference in sleep apnea prevalence is noted based on location of the stroke. Treatment of OSA with continuous positive airway pressure (CPAP) lowers blood pressure, but the evidence for improved stroke outcome with CPAP is unclear at this time. (Brown, *Sem Neurol* 2006; Yaggi et al., *N Engl J Med* 2005)

146. The answers are A 4, B 1, C 2, D 3, E 4. An association between ischemic stroke and the phosphodiesterase 4D and *ALOX5AP* genes has been found by linkage analysis in Icelandic families. With further study, the association may be found in other populations. A familial form of CAA, with lobar hemorrhage occurring at a younger age than in the sporadic form, has been found in Icelandic and Dutch families. Although moyamoya syndrome and Takayasu's vasculitis are found in patients of multiple nationalities, they are more common in the Japanese population. Familial cavernous malformations are also found in patients of multiple ethnic backgrounds, but are more often found in Hispanic American families. Sickle cell disease is mainly found in African Americans. (Dichgans, *Lancet Neurol* 2007; Mohr et al., Chapter 33 and Chapter 69)

147. The answer is C. Orolingual angioedema may be seen in patients on angiotensin-converting enzyme (ACE) inhibitors and is also a rare, but potentially life-threatening complication of thrombolysis with alteplase/tissue plasminogen activator (t-PA). In patients on ACE inhibitors who are treated with t-PA, orolingual angioedema may occur on the side of the paresis before spreading bilaterally. The mechanism for this lateralized orolingual angioedema may be increased bradykinin production by the thrombolysis and reduced clearance by the ACE inhibitor. The angioedema may be life-threatening, with need for emergent airway protection. (Engelter et al., *J Neurol* 2005)

148. The answer is C. Eales disease is an idiopathic obliterative vasculitis that primarily affects the peripheral retina. Inflammation of the retinal vessels is generally bilateral, leading to retinal and disc neovascularization, vascular sheathing, branch retinal vein occlusion, and vitreous hemorrhage. Visual acuity is progressively compromised by the retinal pathology. Laser photocoagulation can be used to forestall vision loss. Neurologic involvement in Eales disease is rare. Multiple etiologies of the disorder have been proposed. (Atmaca et al., *Ocular Immunol Inflamm* 2002)

149. The answer is D. The most common neurologic complication in hepatitis C virus (HCV)-infected patients is a peripheral neuropathy, occurring in up to 50% of patients. Almost half of patients with chronic HCV infection are cryoglobulin positive. Hepatitis C virus infection and mixed cryoglobulinemia vasculitis–related peripheral neuropathy can range from a pure sensory axonopathy to mononeuritis multiplex, with sensory progressing to motor deficits. Neurocognitive deficits and fatigue can be seen in patients with HCV, but chronic infection is not generally associated with encephalopathy. Ischemic stroke and intracerebral hemorrhage occur rarely associated with HCV infection. The etiology of ischemic stroke appears to be small- and medium-sized vessel vasculitis, based on angiographic and pathologic case reports. (Cacoub et al., *AIDS* 2005)

150. The answer is C. Reversible cerebral vasoconstriction syndromes (RCVS) is a group of disorders, distinct from PACNS, characterized by the sudden onset of headache with clear sensorium and focal neurologic deficits. By definition, vascular imaging shows vasoconstriction, but multiple abnormalities are generally seen on brain imaging. Patients with RCVS are more often female, as distinct from PACNS, which more often afflicts men. Because the clinical course is generally benign, treatment with immunosuppressive agents is not warranted but calcium channel blockers can be used to relieve the headache and decrease vasospasm. (Bernstein, *Curr Treat Options Cardiovasc Med* 2006)

151. The answer is C. Although the specific clinical and radiographic situation may dictate the timing of reinstituting warfarin after intracerebral hemorrhage (ICH) with warfarin in the setting of a mechanical heart valve, review of the literature and expert opinion suggest that the warfarin may be started in 7 to 14 days. According to some recommendations, once the international normalization ratio (INR) is normalized, subcutaneous heparin for venous prophylaxis may be instituted as necessary. (Aguilar et al., *Mayo Clin Proc* 2007)

152. The answer is B. Current guidelines recommend withholding antihypertensive therapy for acute ischemic stroke unless there is end-organ damage or anticipated thrombolysis, or if the blood pressures are greater than systolic blood pressure (SBP) of 220 mm Hg or diastolic blood pressure (DBP) of 120 mm Hg. These numbers are based on the upper limit of cerebral autoregulation. (Rose & Mayer, *Neuro Crit Care* 2004)

153. The answer is D. Intravenous thrombolysis should not be given unless blood pressure can be easily and consistently maintained below a SBP of 185 mm Hg and DBP of 110 mm Hg. During and after intravenous t-PA administration, BP control is stricter, with targets for therapy dropping 5 mm Hg. Blood pressure should be monitored and treated to maintain levels at or below the target using labetalol if possible. (Rose & Mayer, *Neuro Crit Care* 2004)

154. The answer is D. Congestive heart failure and myocardial ischemia are the most common complications of triple-H therapy. Because triple-H therapy is used to treat symptomatic cerebral vasospasm, to avoid delayed cerebral ischemia after the aneurysm is obliterated, rebleeding is not a common complication. Hydrocephalus and deep vein thrombosis (DVT) are not complications of the therapy but may occur in SAH. (Rose & Mayer, *Neuro Crit Care* 2004)

155. The answer is E. No randomized controlled clinical trial has shown superiority of warfarin over aspirin in secondary stroke prevention in patients without cardioembolic strokes. Patients with strokes due to high-grade extracranial internal carotid artery stenosis were excluded from the studies. There was no therapeutic benefit to high-intensity anticoagulation in the Stroke Prevention in Reversible Ischemia Trial (SPIRIT) (INR target 3.0–4.5) or to medium-intensity anticoagulation in the European/Australian Stroke Prevention in Reversible Ischaemia Trial (ESPRIT) and Warfarin Aspirin Recurrent Stroke Study (WARSS) (INR target 2.0–3.0) evaluations. There was significantly increased hemorrhagic risk with anticoagulation seen in SPIRIT and ESPRIT. Daily doses of aspirin ranged from 30 to 325 mg in ESPRIT, to 1,300 mg in the Warfarin-Aspirin Symptomatic Intracranial Disease (WASID) trial. Multiple studies have shown that, in the absence of a cardiac source of embolization or other specific indication, warfarin therapy to prevent recurrent cerebral ischemia of arterial origin is generally not warranted. (ESPRIT Study Group, *Lancet Neurol* 2007)

156. The answer is C. The combination of aspirin (25 mg) with modified-release dipyridamole (200 mg) taken twice daily was compared to its individual components and placebo in the European Stroke Prevention Study (ESPS) 2 trial. The treatment showed a 37% relative risk reduction (RRR) versus placebo, and 23% RRR versus aspirin at the 2-year follow-up point. (Diener et al., *J Neuro Sci* 1996)

157. The answer is A. Spinal dural arteriovenous fistula (SDAVF), the most common of all spinal vascular diseases, accounts for about 70% of all spinal arteriovenous malformations. It is an acquired disorder, with a mean age at diagnosis of about 60 years. It is seen more commonly in men. Spinal dural arteriovenous fistula may present with multiple sclerosis–like symptoms, for which it may be mistaken in young women. The myelopathic symptoms are generally slowly progressive or stepwise, and diagnosis is often delayed. The SDAVF is predominantly located in the lower thoracic and upper lumbar regions. The etiology of this necrotizing myelopathy appears to be impairment of venous outflow causing an increase in venous pressure around the cord. There is no association with thrombophilia. (Koch, *Curr Opin Neurol* 2006)

158. The answer is C. The rupture rate of an arteriovenous malformation (AVM) is highly variable depending on its characteristics and presentation. A newly discovered AVM should be evaluated by angiography to determine its location and drainage pattern, to assess risk of rupture and determine appropriate treatment. The majority of AVMs are discovered without signs of hemorrhage, and they tend to have a relatively benign natural history as compared with the risk of invasive management. A Randomized Trial of Unruptured Brain AVMs (ARUBA) is an ongoing study, randomizing patients with unruptured brain AVMs to medical management versus best interventional therapy. The results of ARUBA may help to select those patients with unruptured AVMs who can be treated with best results. (Stapf et al., *Curr Opin Neurol* 2006)

159. The answer is D. Although eclampsia is defined as hypertension, proteinuria greater than 3 g/24 hour, and seizures occurring after 20 weeks of gestation, about 30% of cases of eclampsia occur during labor and delivery, and approximately 20% of cases occur up to 4 weeks after delivery. Short-term use of ACE inhibitors immediately prior to delivery has unclear risk, but chronic use of ACE inhibitors during pregnancy has been associated with fetal and neonatal death as well as birth defects, including oligohydramnios, fetal skull hypoplasia, intrauterine growth retardation, and pulmonary hypoplasia. In general, use of an ACE inhibitor during any stage of pregnancy should be avoided. Although the MRI does show abnormal fluid-attenuated inversion recovery (FLAIR) signals posteriorly in eclampsia, this is due to vasogenic, not cytotoxic, edema. A subtype of eclampsia is known as HELLP (Hemolysis, Elevated Liver enzymes, and Low Platelet counts) syndrome. Seizures in eclampsia are best treated with intravenous magnesium sulfate, using a 5- to 6-g intravenous bolus and 1 to 2 g/hour continuous intravenous infusion. (Ringelstein & Knecht, *Curr Opin Neurol* 2006)

160. The answer is D. The trick to answering this question is realizing that the annual recurrent hemorrhage risk for cerebral amyloid angiopathy (CAA) is very high (10.5%), whereas the annual recurrent hemorrhage risk for developmental venous anomaly (DVA; also known as venous angioma) is very low (0.15%). The annual recurrent hemorrhage risk for hypertension is approximately 2% depending on blood pressure control. The annual recurrent hemorrhage risk for an AVM ranges from 4% to 34%, depending on its characteristics. The annual recurrent hemorrhage risk for a cavernous malformation is approximately 4.5%. (Qureshi et al., *N Engl J Med* 2001; Stapf et al., *Curr Opin Neurol* 2006)

161. The answer is A. The Mechanical Embolus Removal in Cerebral Ischemia (MERCI) retriever is a Food and Drug Administration (FDA)-approved device for restoring blood flow in patients experiencing an acute ischemic stroke. It does not use ultrasound but is an angiographically applied clot retriever that has a corkscrew-like design. When used in one clinical trial within 8 hours of symptom onset, recanalization was seen in 48% of patients in whom it was used. This compares with a historical control recanalization rate of 18%. Although there was an almost 8% symptomatic intracerebral hemorrhage rate, there was an increase in good outcome and a decrease in mortality with recanalization. Although the MERCI retriever may be considered in combination with t-PA use, with unclear risks or benefits, it has generally been used on patients ineligible for thrombolysis. Use of the device requires a skilled and experienced neuro-interventionalist operating under optimal circumstances, and the device is not generally available. (Smith et al., *Stroke* 2005)

162. The answer is B. This man is having TIAs and should be admitted for evaluation of vascular disease. His angina is triggered by minimal stress, because his wife usually pays cash so he does not notice her spending and the Manhattan blocks going uptown are quite short. Noncardioembolic TIAs in the setting of unstable angina or a non-Q wave myocardial infarction (MI) should be treated with the combination of aspirin and clopidogrel. There is no indication for heparin to decrease stroke risk; and aspirin and sustained-release dipyridamole would not be indicated for acute coronary syndrome. (Johnston et al., *Ann Neurol* 2006)

163. The answer is B. Georg Fredrich Handel was said to suffer from a "paraletick" disorder with right hand weakness, at age 52 in 1737, and then progressive loss of vision in his left eye in 1750, consistent with left internal carotid artery disease. Joseph Hayden is suspected to have had subcortical vascular dementia with gait disturbance and change in cognition and behavior. Felix Mendelssohn died in 1847, at age 38 after several strokes. Robert Schumann had a focal dystonia of his right hand, and Ludwig van Beethoven is thought to have died of chronic lead poisoning. (Bougousslavsky & Boller, 2005)

164. The answers are A 3, B 1, C 2, D 4, E 3. Sturge-Weber syndrome and the *p*osterior fossa malformations, facial *h*emangiomas, *a*rterial cerebrovascular, *c*ardiovascular, *e*ye anomalies (PHACE) syndrome are both associated with choroidal hemangiomas. The facial capillary malformation characteristic of Sturge-Weber syndrome is present at birth, and grows commensurate with the child; but the infantile facial hemangioma seen in PHACE is inconspicuous at birth with rapid neonatal growth then slow regression. Hemangioblastomas, occurring in the brain, spinal cord, and retina, are characteristic of Von Hippel-Lindau disease. Osler-Weber-Rendu syndrome, or hereditary hemorrhagic telangiectasia, causes telangiectasias of the skin and mucous membranes. Conjunctival telangiectasias are common. Wyburn-Mason syndrome is associated with large tortuous arteries and veins forming arteriovenous communications (racemose) in the retina and through to the optic nerve. (Kupersmith, Chapter 4; Heyer et al., *Pediatr Neurol* 2006)

165. The answer is B. Carotid cavernous fistulae (CCFs) are acquired pathologic direct shunts from the cavernous portion of the internal carotid artery (ICA) into the enveloping cavernous sinus. The majority (80%) results from trauma, mostly motor vehicle accidents. Surgical causes include endarterectomy, angioplasty, and transsphenoidal surgery. Causes of spontaneous CCFs arising from weakness in the wall of the cavernous ICA include Ehlers-Danlos syndrome, pseudoxanthoma elasticum, aneurysm, fibromuscular dysplasia, and a persistent embryologic trigeminal artery. (Kupersmith, Chapter 2)

166. The answer is A. In the Japanese population, about 10% of cases of moyamoya are familial with a multifactorial inheritance. Children generally present with TIAs, often bilaterally, evolving into cerebral infarcts and seizures. Cerebral hemorrhage occurs more frequently in adults. Stenosis or occlusion occurs in the terminal portions of the ICA or in the proximal middle or anterior cerebral arteries. (Fukui et al., *Neuropathy* 2000)

167. The answer is E. Homocystinuria and homocysteine plasma concentrations of >100 μmol/L are associated with autosomal recessive enzyme deficiencies that cause stroke, mental retardation, lens abnormalities, and skeletal deformities in children. The most common cause of homocystinuria is deficiency of cystathionine β-synthase, a key enzyme in the degradation of homocysteine. Strokes can occur before age 30 through atherosclerosis, thromboembolism, small-vessel disease, or arterial dissection. Homocystinuria is distinguished from hyperhomocysteinemia (plasma homocysteine levels of 15–100 μmol/L), which is a risk factor for stroke in the general population and is associated with a dietary deficiency of vitamins B_6, B_{12}, and folate. Hyperhomocysteinemia most commonly results from disturbances in the conversion of homocysteine to methionine by a pathway that requires the formation of methylated derivatives of folate. (Dichgans, *Lancet Neurol* 2007)

168. The answers are A 3, B 1, C 2, D 5, E 4. A posterior communicating artery aneurysm, and less commonly an internal carotid artery aneurysm, may present with a third nerve palsy with an enlarged pupil. The cavernous sinus contains cranial nerves III, IV, V1, V2, and VI, as well as the internal carotid artery and sympathetic chain. Aneurysms of the intracavernous carotid present with sixth nerve paresis more commonly than third nerve paresis and may be accompanied by a Horner's syndrome. A bitemporal visual field deficit is due to chiasmal compression, generally from a supraclinoid internal carotid artery aneurysm, although a bitemporal visual field deficit may be seen with anterior cerebral and anterior communicating aneurysms. Pain may rarely be a presenting symptom for an expanding unruptured aneurysm, with periorbital pain seen with MCA aneurysms and posterior neck pain seen with posterior inferior cerebellar artery (PICA) aneurysms. (Ropper & Brown, 2005)

169. The answers are A 1, B 4, C 3, D 2. The thalamic nuclei are involved in multiple functions, including arousal, pain perception, motor control, sensation, language, cognition, mood, and motivation. The territory of the thalamic infarct dictates which functions are impaired. Anterior territory infarcts (about 12% of thalamic infarcts) interrupt limbic projections and produce the "anterior behavioral syndrome" with apathy, amnesia, and disorganization of speech output. Paramedian infarcts (about 35% of thalamic infarcts) cause decreased arousal, particularly if the lesion is bilateral, and impaired learning and memory, as well as personality and behavioral changes after the decreased consciousness has resolved. Inferolateral territory strokes (about 45% of thalamic infarcts) produce contralateral hemisensory loss, hemiparesis, and hemiataxia, followed by pain syndromes that are more common with right thalamic lesions. Posterior lesions (about 8% of thalamic infarcts) result in visual field deficits due to involvement of the lateral geniculate body, as well as variable sensory loss, weakness, dystonia, tremors, and occasionally amnesia and language impairment. (Carrera & Bogousslavsky, *Neurology* 2006; Schmahmann, *Stroke* 2003)

170. The answer is C. Blood pressure control of patients with ICH is controversial; extreme hypertension should be treated initially with caution, to avoid excessive reduction in cerebral perfusion pressure that might precipitate ischemia in the perihematomal zone. The American Stroke Association guidelines suggest that the mean arterial pressure (MAP) should be maintained at or below 130 mm Hg in patients with a history of hypertension. The patient should be ventilated to a P_{CO_2} of 30 to 35 mm Hg to lower intracranial pressure (ICP) 25% to 35% in most patients. Failure of elevated ICP to respond to hyperventilation indicates a poor prognosis. Sodium nitroprusside should be avoided because of its tendency to cause cerebral vasodilatation and increased ICP. Fluids should be managed with isotonic saline, avoiding hyperglycemia that could be detrimental to the injured brain. Serum osmolality should be kept >280 mmol/kg, and hyperosmolality (300–320 mmol/kg) may be used in the setting of significant perihematomal edema and mass effect. Hyperosmolality may be achieved with hypertonic saline or mannitol, (Broderick et al., *Stroke* 1999; Mayer & Rincon, *Lancet Neurol* 2005)

171. The answer is A. Cardiovascular risk is increased, independent of vascular risk factors, in patients with systemic lupus erythematosus (SLE). Atherosclerosis develops prematurely, related to the vascular and endothelial damage associated with the chronic inflammatory process. Increased vascular risk is seen in patients with SLE alone, but risk is increased with the combination of SLE and elevated antiphospholipid antibodies titers. Pregnant women with SLE, especially those with renal disease, have a greater risk of complications of pregnancy including preeclampsia. Epilepsy is more common in patients with both SLE and antiphospholipid antibodies than in patients with lupus alone. Patients with antiphospholipid syndrome and epilepsy are more likely to have cardiac valvular disease. Epilepsy appears to be correlated with focal ischemic events such as stroke and TIAs. Primary antiphospholipid syndrome rarely progresses to SLE, although the combination increases the risk of arterial thrombosis and death. (D'Cruz et al., *Lancet* 2007)

172. The answer is A. Systemic lupus erythematosus may induce 16 different clinical syndromes of the CNS. The most common clinical manifestation is seizures. A relationship does not appear to exist between SLE and migraine. The use of the term *cerebritis*, inflammation of the brain, is misleading because it does not describe a pathologic or radiologic entity in SLE. Aseptic meningitis is probably heterogeneous in origin and is an infrequent manifestation. Movement disorders, including chorea and parkinsonism, are seen associated with SLE. (Futrell et al., *Neurology* 1992; Jennekens & Kater, *Rheumatology* 2002)

173. The answer is D. "Moyamoya" refers to dilated small-vessel collaterals that produce the appearance of a "puff of smoke" on angiography. Although the small-vessel collaterals are dilated, the vasculopathy affects large vessels as well, including the internal carotid, middle cerebral, and anterior cerebral arteries, producing stenosis or even occlusion of these vessels. The vasculopathy is noninflammatory. Although it is more common in individuals of Japanese descent, it can occur in any ethnic group, in both adults and children. It can result in hemorrhage in adults, often intraventricular. (Osborn)

174. The answer is C. Fibromuscular dysplasia (FMD) is a vasculopathy with an increased incidence of cerebral aneurysms, thus it can be associated with subarachnoid hemorrhage. Fibromuscular dysplasia can be either familial or sporadic. It is most often an abnormality of the media, although the intima and adventitia can be involved. The angiographic picture is most commonly a "string of pearls" with multifocal narrowing, occurring in approximately 80% of cases. Less commonly, there may be unifocal or multifocal tubular stenosis. Fibromuscular dysplasia is most common in carotid and vertebral arteries, both extracranial, along with renal arteries. Intracranial vessels are less often affected. (Mettinger et al., *Stroke* 1982)

175. The answer is C. Cavernous malformations, collections of blood-filled vascular spaces without brain or smooth muscle tissue in their interstices, are generally asymptomatic. They can be sporadic or familial. Their main clinical manifestation is seizures, which occur when associated cortical dysplasia is present. The hemorrhage associated with these lesions can be symptomatic, or asymptomatic noted incidentally on MRI. A cavernous malformation may be associated with a developmental venous anomaly (venous angioma). Association with headaches is coincidental. Cavernous malformations are relatively frequent incidental finding on MRI or autopsy. (Osborn)

176. The answer is B. Most TIAs last 30 to 60 minutes, with amaurosis fugax often lasting 5 to 10 minutes. The initial definition of a TIA emphasized a duration of under 24 hours, with episodes lasting longer than 24 hours being defined as stroke. Even though the formal definition of a TIA includes episodes lasting up to 24 hours, in practicality almost all TIAs have resolved or markedly improved within 30 to 60 minutes. This is of practical importance in consideration of t-PA administration. If a patient has a focal neurologic deficit that has not resolved or nearly resolved in 60 minutes, this is most likely a stroke and the patient should be considered for t-PA therapy. Reports of neurologic symptoms lasting less than 1 minute are difficult to interpret and are generally considered nonspecific. (Albers et al., *N Engl J Med* 2002)

177. The answer is C. Headache, even severe headache, may occur in 18% to 40% of ischemic strokes. Although headache can occur with ICH, it is not an invariable accompaniment. The immediate imaging study is generally a computed tomography (CT) scan, rather than an MRI, because CT is faster and more readily available. Headaches and focal neurologic deficits can be due to migraine with aura, but this is a diagnosis based on past history of such events, an appropriate history, and a negative evaluation for ischemic and hemorrhagic stroke. (Ginsberg, Chapter 68)

178. The answer is C. Pseudobulbar palsy includes spastic dysarthria and emotional incontinence. Spastic dysarthria can occur with strokes in the anterior or posterior circulation and is particularly associated with multiple cortical or subcortical strokes. Spastic dysarthria with behavioral changes can occur with caudate infarcts. Flaccid dysarthria—hypernasal speech with poor articulation—can be caused by ischemia in the posterior circulation producing lower motor neuron lesions affecting cranial nerves VII, IX, X, XII. Spastic dysarthria also includes poor articulation, but the vocal quality is harsh. (Ginsberg, Chapter 68)

179. The answer is B. Brachial monoparesis when caused by ischemia is almost always caused by occlusion of an MCA branch. Hyporeflexia does not always indicate a lower motor neuron or cerebellar lesion, because acute stroke often presents with hyporeflexia with delayed development of hyperreflexia and spasticity. Brachial plexus lesions can produce a flaccid monoparesis, but these are unlikely to be of sudden onset unless trauma is involved, which can easily be clarified by history. These are much more likely to be painful. (Ginsberg, Chapter 68)

180. The answer is A. The lateral medullary syndrome is generally caused by ischemia of the PICA. It produces ipsilateral facial anesthesia and contralateral thermoanalgesia on the body. The Brown-Sequard syndrome is a hemilesion of the spinal cord that produces ipsilateral loss of position sensation with contralateral loss of pain and temperature sensation. Although crossed sensory findings can occur with spinal cord lesions, these syndromes are rare. Urinary incontinence is an unlikely accompaniment of crossed sensory deficits. (Currier, *Neurology* 1961)

181. The answer is C. The most likely diagnosis is an acute infarction in the right basal ganglia. A dystonic reaction to neuroleptics and antinausea medicines can occur 10 to 30 minutes following IV injections, but is generally bilateral. Similarly, Wilson's disease is associated with bilateral movement disorders and generally occurs at a younger age. Wilson's disease is a gradually progressive disease. Metastatic breast cancer in the basal ganglia could produce contralateral hemichorea, but brain metastases are late complications of breast cancer that would generally occur years after diagnosis. (Lee, *Mov Disord* 1995)

182. The answer is B. Infarcts of the right posterior cerebral artery (PCA) classically produce constructional apraxia and the omission of features on the left side of a drawing. It is not uncommon for a patient with a defect in the left visual field to describe it as a visual problem "in the left eye." The clinician must be wary in this instance and determine whether a patient has covered each eye to determine if a field defect is monocular or homonymous. A left ophthalmic artery infarct would cause a loss of vision in the left eye, but the clock face drawing should be normal. A left PCA stroke would produce vision problems on the right and would be less likely to produce constructional apraxia, which is typically associated with right hemispheric lesions. A patient with Alzheimer's disease can have construction difficulties, but the definite neglect of the right side of the drawing is clearly a focal lesion. (Ginsberg, Chapter 71)

183. The answer is C. Hypoperfusion of the retina produces a classic syndrome of visual dulling or loss on exposure to bright light. This is thought to be caused by inadequate blood flow to satisfy the high metabolic demand of the retina when exposed to bright light. Malingering is unlikely in this patient, who enjoys weeding, and should never be the first consideration when a well-described syndrome explains the patient's reported symptoms. Glaucoma does produce visual loss, but tends to be associated with pain and is unlikely to produce transient recurring visual loss. Vasospasm producing visual loss has been difficult to document, and the association with sunlight would lead away from this answer. (Furlan, *Arch Neurol* 1979)

184. The answer is A. Patients who have onset of seizure following a stroke have 20% to 40% chance of recurrent seizures, making lifetime treatment advisable. The ability to stop anticonvulsant medications in some young individuals with idiopathic seizures who are seizure free for years on medications does not apply to the post-stroke seizure patient. Carbamazepine does interact with warfarin, but in this patient who has been stable on both of these medications for 3 years, there is no need to change to a more expensive anticonvulsant. The continuation of warfarin was appropriate because of the high risk of recurrent stroke in atrial fibrillation. Uncontrolled seizures would be a relative contraindication to warfarin, but this patient's seizures have been easily controlled on a single agent. Warfarin therapy increases the risk of hemorrhagic complications of seizure, which may be another indication for lifetime anticonvulsant therapy. (Ginsberg, Chapter 77)

185. The answer is C. Transcranial Doppler (TCD) with carbon dioxide or acetazolamide (Diamox) is a test for vasomotor reserve, which decreases in critical low-flow states. Alternate diagnostic methods include positron emission tomography (PET) with oxygen extraction fraction, which would be elevated in low-flow states. Computed tomography perfusion studies before and after Diamox challenge can also be useful. An extracranial to intracranial (EC-IC) bypass is not useful if vasomotor reserve is adequate distal to the stenosis. Preliminary evidence has suggested the possibility of benefit from EC-IC bypass in patients with low vasomotor reserve, and a trial of this group of patients is under way.

Administration of antihypertensive agents is contraindicated in potential low-flow states. Sometimes reactive hypertension does occur in low-flow states, and the treatment is to restore perfusion, not to lower blood pressure. In cases with moderate or low blood pressure, midodrine (ProAmatine) can be used in the short term to support blood pressure and protect perfusion. (Adams et al., *Neurosurg Clin N Am* 2001)

186. The answer is D. Anticholinesterase medication, initially used in Alzheimer's disease, is now been approved by the FDA for use in multi-infarct or vascular dementia. The MRI is not always reliable for the diagnosis of vascular dementia, because other disorders, such as *c*erebral *a*utosomal *d*ominant *a*rteriopathy with *s*ubcortical *i*nfarcts and *l*eukoencephalopathy (CADASIL), can have a similar MRI picture. Although CT may demonstrate vascular lesions, MRI is much more sensitive for multiple small vascular lesions. The diagnosis of vascular dementia is not made on imaging alone, but is a combined clinical and imaging diagnosis. Certainly, the prevention of new vascular lesions is important in patients with vascular dementia, but anticholinesterase medication now provides the possibility of symptomatic treatment. (Roman, *Med Clin N Am* 2002)

187. The answer is C. Coma and pinpoint pupils are classic findings with large pontine hemorrhages. Patients with pontine hemorrhage may be quadriplegic and have decerebrate or decorticate posturing. The pinpoint pupils are useful to differentiate pontine hemorrhage from narcotic overdose and cardiac arrest. Hypertensive crisis rarely presents with coma, and again pinpoint pupils would not be present unless the hypertension was associated with pontine hemorrhage. (Kushner, *Neurology* 1985)

188. The answer is B. Lobar hemorrhages are frequently associated with amyloid angiopathy. Putaminal, pontine, and cerebellar hemorrhages are most often related to hypertension. Intraventricular hemorrhage is most often caused by ruptured intracranial aneurysm. (Attems, *Acta Neuropath* 2005)

189. The answer is C. This patient had an acute right MCA stroke and is a candidate for t-PA therapy. The "worst headache of his life" is not always indicative of SAH. Small amounts of subarachnoid blood can be missed on CT, but this will not be associated with an acute focal neurologic deficit. A deficit this large could be associated with a ruptured aneurysm if it ruptured into brain tissue, but that would be easily visible on CT scan. Delayed neurologic deficits from vasospasm generally occur 3 days or later following SAH. In addition, vasospasm is associated with large amounts of subarachnoid blood and would be unlikely to occur in a patient without subarachnoid or intraventricular blood on the acute CT scan. In an older patient with no prior headache history, migraine with hemiplegic aura would be unusual, and triptans are contraindicated in patients with hemiplegic migraine. (Ginsberg & Bougousslavsky, Chapter 108)

190. The answer is B. Posterior-circulation disease rarely causes only one symptom. Patients with pure cerebellar infarction may present with dizziness, vertigo, blurred vision due to nystagmus, difficulty walking due to ataxia, and hypotonia, but they do not have hemiparesis or hemisensory loss. Dissection of the vertebral artery occurs most commonly in those portions that are most freely movable. These areas are the first portion between the origin and the entrance to the intervertebral foramina, as well as the third portion around the upper cervical vertebrae. (Savitz, *N Engl J Med* 2005)

191. The answer is D. Leukoaraiosis and old lacunes on CT scan, low levels of low-density lipoprotein (LDL) cholesterol on admission, current smoking history, and very high National Institute of Health Stroke Scale (NIHSS) score are all risk factors for symptomatic hemorrhagic transformation after thrombolysis for acute ischemic stroke. A patient with an NIHSS score of 12 would have a low risk of hemorrhagic transformation and a greater probability of favorable outcome than a patient with a higher NIHSS score. (Bang et al., *Neurology* 2007; Palumbo et al., *Neurology* 2007)

192. The answer is B. The risk of stroke in pregnancy, both ischemic and hemorrhagic, is unclear, with estimates in the range of four to 11 cerebral infarctions and five to nine hemorrhagic strokes per 100,000 births. Greater risk of cerebral infarction and hemorrhagic stroke is found in the postpartum period as compared to the prepartum trimesters. Kittner et al. reviewed data from the Baltimore-Washington Cooperative Young Stroke Study and found that for cerebral infarction, the adjusted relative risk during pregnancy was 0.7 (95% confidence interval [CI], 0.3 to 1.6), but increased to 8.7 (95% CI, 4.6 to 16.7) for the postpartum period (after a live birth or stillbirth). For ICH, the adjusted relative risk was 2.5 (95% CI, 1.0 to 6.4) during pregnancy, but 28.3 (95% CI, 13.0 to 61.4) for the postpartum period. The risks of cerebral infarction and intracerebral hemorrhage were increased in the 6 weeks after delivery but not during pregnancy itself. The French Stroke in Pregnancy Study Group also found that the risk of cerebral infarction or ICH was higher during the postpartum period than during any trimester of pregnancy. (Kittner et al., *N Engl J Med* 1996; Sharshar, *Stroke* 1995)

193. The answer is A. Diabetic patients with cerebrovascular disease should be maintained as normoglycemic as possible with a hemoglobin A1C ≤ 7%. The LDL-cholesterol target should be less than 70 mg/dL because these patients are in the high-risk category for LDL management. The alcohol target for women should be one drink a day (men are allowed slightly more), and exercise should be for 30 minutes most days. (Sacco, *Stroke* 2006)

194. The answer is A. These signs and symptoms are most compatible with an acute spinal cord infarct. Common causes of spontaneous spinal cord infarction include emboli from the aortic arch, giant-cell arteritis, tuberculosis, sarcoidosis, and both viral and fungal infections. Syphilis, although an unlikely cause in HIV-negative patients, can be easily ruled out. Spinal fluid can be investigated for acid-fast bacilli, herpes viruses, and fungi, along with Lyme disease. Spinal arterial atherosclerosis is rare. Spinal angiography is technically more difficult and has more complications than cerebral angiography, so it is rarely utilized. An MRI of the spinal cord might show an infarct but would not give specific information that would guide acute treatment. Radiographs could show subluxation, which can be a cause of spinal cord infarct in patients with rheumatoid arthritis, but this occurs in the late stage of that disorder. A patient with rheumatoid arthritis who presents with possible spinal cord symptoms should have plain films of the neck. (Ginsberg, Chapter 111)

195. The answer is A. In the Hunt and Hess classification, there is progressive worsening of clinical status with higher numerical values. The full classification is grade I, no symptoms or mild headache; grade II, moderate to severe headache; grade III, mild decreased level of consciousness and/or focal neurologic deficit (excluding cranial nerve III palsy); grade IV, stupor or hemiparesis; and grade V, coma. Bleeding confined to the subarachnoid space would be associated with grades I and II. Particularly in patients with grade I, the amount of subarachnoid blood may be low enough that it does not show on CT scan. In these patients lumbar puncture may be necessary to establish the diagnosis. Grade II will almost always have subarachnoid blood visible on CT and blood on CT is always seen in grade III. Grades IV and V will generally have subarachnoid, along with intraventricular or intraparenchymal, blood, so these SAHs will always be detected by CT scan of the brain. (Hunt & Hess, *J Neurosurg* 1968)

196. The answer is C. Most aneurysms of the cavernous portion of the internal carotid artery present with diplopia, decreased visual acuity, headache, and facial pain. The rare presentation with hemorrhage can lead to carotid-cavernous fistula or epistaxis. Treatment of both symptomatic and asymptomatic aneurysms is controversial, ranging from surgical resection to endovascular obliteration to no intervention. Cavernous carotid artery aneurysms are more common in older women and are frequently bilateral. Endovascular treatment is associated with a low rate of transient neurologic complications. (Goldenberg-Cohen, et al. *J Neurol Neurosurg Psychiatry* 2004)

197. The answer is C. Unlike cerebral dural fistulae, spinal dural arteriovenous fistula (SDAVF) rarely rupture, although a basilar SAH can occur due to leakage of a cervical fistula. Spinal fluid may show nonspecifically increased protein in three-quarters of patients with SDAVF. Abnormal vessels appear as filling defects in the subarachnoid space on myelogram. A multilevel cord abnormality with swelling is seen on T2-weighted MRI. Subarachnoid flow void seen along the posterior cord on T2 weighted images and vascular enhancement on T1 imaging can be easily distinguished from pulsation artifact. (Koch, *Curr Opin Neurol* 2006)

198. The answer is B. Dural arteriovenous (AV) fistulae are acquired lesions. They are thought to form from neovascularization in the setting of a thrombosis or obstruction of a venous sinus or a cerebral vein. They occur most often near the transverse and sigmoid sinuses, but they can occur at other venous sites including the vein of Galen. Presenting symptoms include pulsatile tinnitus, proptosis, chemosis, and well as seizures and progressive neurologic deficits. The risk of rupture is about 2% per year depending on site and hemodynamics. They are typically seen poorly on CT. Magnetic resonance imaging may detect dilated veins and feeding arteries, but cerebral arteriography with selective external carotid artery injection is most appropriate for diagnosis. (Brown, *Mayo Clin Proc* 2005)

199. The answer is C. Presidents Richard M. Nixon, Millard Fillmore, Chester A. Arthur, and John Quincy Adams suffered strokes after they left office. President Woodrow Wilson suffered his first stroke in 1919, when he developed word-finding difficulty, headache, and left-sided weakness during a speech to rally support for the League of Nations. Until he left office in 1921, President Wilson had emotional and cognitive problems that left him unable to fulfill the obligations of the presidency. Access to him was controlled by his wife, Edith Galt Wilson, who kept his condition secret from the public and Congress and made decisions in his place. (Fields & Lemak, 1989)

200. The answer is B. With the NIHSS scale, higher scores correlate with more severe neurologic deficits. Because the points given for communication difficulties produce higher NIHSS scores with dominant lesions, there can be a surprisingly low NIHSS score for patients with right hemispheric lesions. When patients with lesions of 9 cm^3 or more on diffusion-weighted MRI were compared, eight of 37 patients with a right hemispheric stroke had a NIHSS score of 0 to 5. Only one of 39 patients with the same size lesion in the left hemisphere had such a low NIHSS score. This weighting of the dominant hemisphere must be kept in mind when the NIHSS score is used as an inclusion or exclusion criterion, as well as when it is used to correlate acute stroke severity with functional outcome. A 9 cm^3 stroke is not a high risk for hemorrhage with TPA. (Fink et al., *Stroke* 2002)

201. The answer is C. Myointimal hyperplasia generally produces a smooth lesion that is not a high risk for future stroke. Progression to occlusion occurs in approximately 4% of patients. (Strandness, Chapter 2)

202. The answer is C. A short arteriotomy is preferred for patch grafting. Long or side patch grafts are associated with increased risk of aneurysmal dilatation. Autologous arterial patches have fewer degenerative changes than do venous grafts. They are seldom used because veins are more accessible as a grafting material. (Strandness, Chapter 16)

203. The answer is A. A combination of local and systemic heparin is usually used during endarterectomy and is considered the best method for preventing thrombotic complications. The complications of postoperative heparin outweigh the potential benefits. Uncomplicated carotid endarterectomy (CAE) does not produce significant DVT risk, as patients are are ambulatory immediately. (Strandness, Chapter 17)

204. The answer is B. The idiopathic hypereosinophilic syndrome is a spectrum of leukoproliferative diseases that result in a sustained increase in eosinophil production. About half of these patients have neurologic symptoms, including embolic stroke, diffuse encephalopathy, and mononeuritis multiplex. The first stage of the disorder is generally asymptomatic, although cardiac damage is occurring. The second stage involves the development of endocardial thrombi, which can be seen on 2–D echocardiography. The third stage results in myocardial fibrosis. (Rich, Chapter 56)

205. The answer is B. A persistant vegetative state (PVS) is a vegetative state present for 1 month after brain injury. The vegetative state is characterized by the absence of awareness of self or the environment. The patient in a PVS has preserved sleep-wake cycles but has no behavioral response to any stimuli and has no language comprehension or expression. Patients are incontinent and require skilled nursing care. Unlike patients who are brain dead, cranial nerve reflexes are variably preserved in a vegetative state. (The Multi-Society Task Force on PVS, *N Engl J Med* 1994)

206. The answer is C. The metabolic syndrome is a combination of abnormal body measurements and laboratory tests. The diagnosis requires any three of the following: fasting blood sugar greater than 110, waist circumference greater than 40 inches for men or greater than 35 inches for women, elevated triglycerides, reduced high-density lipoprotein (HDL), and hypertension. Elevated LDL, elevated C-reactive protein (C-RP), and elevated HgA1C are often present, but these parameters do not constitute part of the diagnostic criteria. Central obesity, as defined by waist circumference, not an elevated BMI, is a diagnostic criterion. These patients are at high risk for developing type II diabetes, coronary artery disease, and stroke. (Wannamethee et al., *Arch Intern Med* 2005)

207. The answer is B. Patients with symptomatic ICH during the first 36 hours after treatment with t-PA had more severe neurologic deficits at baseline (median NIHSS score 20, range 3–29) than did the study population as a whole (median NIHSS score 14; range 1–37). The only other correlate with increased symptomatic ICH (present in 6.4% of t-PA treated patients) was CT evidence of cerebral edema at baseline, seen in 9% of the patients with ICH but only 4% of the study population as a whole. Although protocol violations were correlated with hemorrhage risk in papers published later about regional use of t-PA, protocol violations were rare in the National Institute of Neurological Disorders and Stroke (NINDS) study. Likewise, age and stroke subtype were not risks for hemorrhage with treatment. (National Institute of Neurological Disorders and Stroke, *N Engl J Med* 1995)

208. The answer is B. Giant-cell arteritis has a yearly incidence of 18:100,000 in individuals over age 50 in Olmsted County, Minnesota, according to epidemiologic data from the Mayo Clinic. Women are twice as likely to be affected as men. Reports of normal sedimentation rates vary from 7% to 20%. In the Mayo Clinic series, 5.4% had an erythrocyte sedimentation rate (ESR) of less than 40, and 10.8% had an ESR less than 50. Visual loss, which occurs in 20% of patients, often occurs early in the course of the disease. Without treatment the other eye generally becomes affected within 1 to 2 weeks. (Salarani, *N Engl J Med* 2002)

209. The answer is B. Primary angiitis of the CNS (PACNS) may present prior to the diagnosis of Hodgkin's disease, or it may be noted after diagnosis and treatment of the malignancy. Hodgkin's disease associated PACNS may involve the brain or spinal cord. Outcome is a function of response to treatment of the underlying malignancy. (Rosen et al., *Neurosurgery* 2000)

210. The answer is D. An older adult with transient global amnesia (TGA) suddenly develops selective retrograde and antegrade amnesia, lasting generally less than 24 hours. Recovery of memory is complete, except for the period of time of the event. Attacks are differentiated from seizures or TIAs by their length and the specificity of the deficit. An individual is unlikely to have a repeat attack, although one can occur rarely. A headache may be noted during the episode, and migraine has been suggested as a cause. Speculation about the pathogenesis of TGA also includes association with physical or emotional stress and cerebral venous congestion. Although focal ischemia may factor into the etiology of TGA, patients generally lack the traditional vascular risk factors such as hypertension and hypercholesterolemia. Transient global amnesia does not increase risk of ischemic stroke. Transient global amnesia is a benign, short-lived memory disorder, related to transient disturbance of hippocampal CA-1 neurons, without structural and neuropsychological sequelae. (Bartsch et al., *Brain* 2006; Roach, *Arch Neurol* 2006)

211. The answer is B. Spinal epidural hematomas can occur spontaneously or associated with antiplatelet or anticoagulant therapy. They may occur after spinal or epidural anesthesia, and rarely after lumbar puncture, especially in patients at risk for bleeding. Although most cases are treated with surgery, in a patient with a small hematoma without cord compression, surgery may not be necessary. The diagnosis of a spinal epidural or subdural hematoma is made by MRI imaging of the spine. (Matsumura et al., *Spine J* 2007)

212. The answer is C. This man's central venous catheter was removed in an upright position, resulting in a paradoxical venous air embolus to his brain. This may occur with failure of a spontaneous collapse or thrombotic obliteration of the catheter tract with introduction of air into the venous system. The air can embolize within the venous system during insertion, disconnection, or removal of the catheter. Cardiovascular collapse, respiratory failure, cerebral ischemia, and even death, can occur in patients with air embolism. A central venous catheter should be removed with the patient in the Trendelenburg position. Patients may be treated with supplemental or hyperbaric oxygen after air embolization, although the neurologic consequences can still be permanent. (Peter & Saxman, *Medsurg Nurs* 2003)

213. The answer is E. This woman has bleeding from a dural metastasis. Dural metastases result from direct extension of skull metastases or from hematogenous spread. They are found at autopsy in about 10% of patients with advanced systemic cancer and may be clinically asymptomatic. When they bleed, these metastases can present as subdural hematomas. The dural metastasis may be mistaken for a meningioma on imaging. The prognosis in this patient is poor, because her chest radiograph showed extensive infiltration with tumor. (Laigle-Donadey et al., *J Neurooncol* 2005)

214. The answer is C. This man has heterotopic ossification (HO), which is caused by ectopic bone formation in muscles and soft tissue near large joints. Heterotopic ossification causes pain, joint swelling, limitation of movement, and joint dysfunction. It is a complication that affects a small number of patients who recover from prolonged immobility from critical illnesses, such as spinal cord injury, traumatic brain injury, and cerebral anoxia. The diagnosis is generally made through radiographs of the affected joints, although changes may be seen early on MRI of the clinically impaired joints. No effective treatments are available. (Hudson & Brett, *Crit Care* 2006)

215. The answer is B. Clinical trials have shown that the risk of perioperative stroke or death after CEA is approximately 3% in asymptomatic patients and up to 6% when associated with symptomatic carotid disease. Women appear to have a higher rate of stroke and death after CEA in general and benefit less than men do from surgery for stroke risk reduction. However, results of studies vary depending on the length of follow-up and definition of the vascular event. Women benefit from CEA performed for symptomatic carotid artery disease. But, the benefit of carotid surgical revascularization for asymptomatic disease in women is less certain. The results of the Asymptomatic Carotid Atherosclerosis Study (ACAS) indicated that CEA reduced the 5-year event rate by 66% in men, but only by 17% in women.

Restenosis rates are consistently higher in women than in men. Smaller vessel size and increased vessel redundancy in women may contribute to their increased restenosis risk. Variability in surgical technique and in the definition of restenosis complicates the prediction of risk of postoperative restenosis and occlusion. A younger age has been shown to be a risk factor for restenosis, perhaps reflecting a more virulent form of atherosclerotic disease. (Hugl et al., *Ann Vasc Surg* 2006)

216. The answer is E. The Women's Health Study (WHS), the first primary prevention trial of aspirin therapy specific to women, found that low-dose aspirin (100 mg every other day) protected women against a first stroke, but generally offered no protection against myocardial infarction (MI) or vascular death. Women aged 65 years and older accounted for only 10% of the WHS population but experienced 31% of the major cardiovascular events in the trial. This older subgroup did show a significant benefit from aspirin in the prevention of primary cardiovascular events, including ischemic stroke and myocardial infarction. Although vitamin E showed virtually no benefit, this older age group did show a decrease in MIs and cardiovascular death on vitamin E. Among women in the placebo group of WHS, more strokes than MIs occurred (266 vs. 193), with a stroke to MI ratio of 1.4:1, as compared with the ratio of 0.4:1 among men in the Physicians' Health Study. Secondary prevention is not addressed in this study. (Burling, *Clev Clin J Med* 2006; Ridker et al., *N Engl J Med* 2005)

217. The answer is E. Clinical trials (the Women's Health Initiative, the Heart and Estrogen/Progestin Replacement Study, the Women's Estrogen for Stroke Trial) indicate that estrogen plus progestin, as well as estrogen alone, provide no cerebrovascular protection. The Women's Health Initiative found estrogen and progestin replacement in postmenopausal women increased ischemic stroke risk by 44%, without effect on hemorrhagic stroke. Postpartum, the risk of hemorrhagic stroke is increased compared to ischemic stroke. The Baltimore Washington Cooperative Young Stroke Study found an increase in ischemic stroke in the postdelivery period of 8.7-fold, but the increase in hemorrhagic stroke was 28.3–fold. Because of their survival advantage, women have a higher lifetime risk of stroke than men. In the Nurses' Health Study, relative risk for total stroke progressively decreased with increasing level of physical activity. (American Heart Association Statistics Committee and Stroke Statistics Subcommittee, *Circulation* 2006)

218. The answer is A. The NINDS trial found that patients treated with t-PA were at least 30% more likely to have minimal or no disability at 3 months, as measured by the outcome scales (absolute increase in favorable outcome of 11%–13%), as compared to placebo-treated patients. There was no statistically significant difference in mortality at 3 months between the two groups. In part 1 of the study there was no significant improvement in the predetermined end-point of improvement in NIHSS score of 4 or more points at 24 hours after stroke onset, although 24-hour benefit was seen in the post hoc analysis of other time points. Rates of asymptomatic ICH were similar in the treated (5%) and placebo (4%) groups. (National Institutes of Neurologic Disorders and Stroke rt-PA Stroke Study Group, *N Engl J Med* 1995)

219. The answer is B. Multiple clinical trials verify the benefit of aspirin therapy in the reduction of recurrent ischemic stroke in both men and women. However, aspirin's benefit in primary prevention of ischemic stroke is less clear. Gender differences further complicate the benefit of aspirin in primary prevention. Women appear to benefit from aspirin for prevention of a first stroke, an effect that is not as striking in men. The pathophysiologic mechanisms for the perceived clinical difference is not clear, but it may reflect differences in aspirin metabolism or aspirin resistance, as well as gender differences in the incidence of stroke and MI.

A sex-specific meta-analysis of aspirin therapy for the primary prevention of cardiovascular events evaluated studies of aspirin in over 95,000 individuals, including 51,342 women. The analysis noted women had fewer MIs but increased strokes, as compared to men. Aspirin therapy was associated with a 24% reduced rate of ischemic stroke (OR 0.76; 95% CI, 0.63–0.93; $p = 0.02$) with no apparent effect on hemorrhagic stroke in women. In men, aspirin had no significant effect on ischemic stroke risk but was associated with a significantly increased risk of hemorrhagic stroke. Both men and women showed increased major bleeding and no improvement in mortality associated with aspirin. (Berger et al., *JAMA* 2006)

220. The answer is C. Transcranial Doppler is fast and noninvasive, and the test can be done in the intensive care unit. This makes it possible to do daily monitoring in patients with SAH. Magnetic resonance angiography has the major disadvantage of transportation to the scanner, time away from ICU care, and longer duration of the procedure. Cerebral angiography is invasive and is not performed as a screening test. Computed tomography angiography is emerging as a more sensitive and specific test than MRA. With the recent advent of multislice portable CT scanners that can be taken to the ICU, the relative merits of computed tomography angiography (CTA) and TCD as a screen for vasospasm will need future evaluation. With the drawback of iodine contrast in CTA, patients needing repeat studies may be best followed by TCD. (Ginsberg & Bogousslavsky, Chapter 108; Joo et al., *Minim Invasive Neurosurg* 2006; Masdeu et al., *Eur J Neurol* 2006)

221. The answer is A. Arteriovenous malformations (AVMs) are congenital, not developmental, lesions. They most often become symptomatic during the second to fourth decades, although symptoms can occur in children or in the elderly. Seizures are a common problem in these patients, but the most common and serious symptoms are related to cerebral hemorrhage. Hemorrhage is generally intraparenchymal; less usually subarachnoid or intraventricular; but rarely subdural. (Ginsberg & Bogousslavsky, Chapter 109)

222. The answer is C. Venous angiomas are developmental venous anomalies composed of a radial arrangement of white matter medullary veins draining into a transcerebral central draining vein. They occur most often in the cerebral hemispheres and very rarely occur in the spinal cord, brainstem, or thalamus. They are the most common incidental vascular anomalies found in the brain and are not associated with cerebral hemorrhages or seizures. Surgical resection interrupts venous drainage and produces venous infarction, so this approach is contraindicated. They are generally asymptomatic and do not require treatment. They do not cause headaches. (Ginsberg & Bogousslavsky, Chapter 109)

223. The answer is C. Iatrogenic spinal cord infarcts can occur after surgical procedures involving the aorta, producing an anterior spinal artery infarct. Vascular malformations of the spinal cord can also produce spinal cord infarcts, but this is generally associated with a stepwise progression of symptoms over time. Coarctation of the aorta and vasculitis of spinal arteries can cause cord infarcts, unrelated to a surgical procedure. Postoperative transverse myelitis is unlikely. (Ginsberg & Bogousslavsky, Chapter 111)

224. The answer is A. The most frequent infarcts of the spinal cord generally involve all or part of the territory of the anterior spinal artery, the single artery lying in the anterior median fissure of the cord. Posterior spinal artery infarcts are rare, probably because there are multiple feeding vessels to these paired posterior arteries, which run along the posterior lateral aspect of the spinal cord. Venous infarcts of the cord may be related to vascular malformations such as spinal dural arteriovenous fistulae or to a coagulopathy. The artery of Adamkiewicz arises from the lumbar and/or intercostal arteries, generally on the left, at the T8 to L1 vertebral level. In about 30% of individuals, it originates on the right. It joins the anterior spinal artery and supplies the anterior lower two-thirds of the spinal cord. (Ginsburg & Bogousslavsky, Chapter 111)

225. The answer is D. Ehlers-Danlos syndrome (EDS) is a clinically and biochemically heterogenous group of connective tissue disorders with hyperextensible skin, joint hypermobility, and easy bruising. Ehlers-Danlos syndrome type IV, with mutations in the *COL3A1* gene, which encodes chains of type III procollagen, is associated with arterial dissection and rupture. Catheter angiography and anticoagulation in these patients may increase risk of arterial dissection and rupture, as well as bleeding. Spinal manipulative therapy (SMT) is an independent risk factor for vertebral artery dissection, according to a case control study of patients with cervical artery dissection. Spinal manipulative therapy may exacerbate pre-existing cervical dissections, so patients should be screened for symptoms of dissection prior to chiropractic treatment. An exacerbation of neck or head pain after SMT may indicate a treatment-related dissection. (North et al., *Ann Neurol* 1995; Smith et al., *Neurology* 2003)

226. The answer is C. The neurologist's evaluation of the individual risk and the potential benefit should be used to evaluate contraindications to treatment using t-PA. Seizure at the onset of an ischemic stroke could potentially complicate the interpretation of the neurologic examination and, as such, may be a contraindication to t-PA treatment. This is especially true if the differentiation between postictal paresis and cerebral infarct is uncertain. Major surgery within 14 days is a contraindication to t-PA treatment, although the neurologist and the surgeon may need to determine what constitutes major surgery. Anticoagulation treatment with an INR >1.7 is an exclusion criterion. Evidence of microhemorrhages may indicate a possible diagnosis of cerebral amyloid angiopathy and an increased risk for lobar hemorrhage; however, their presence does not necessarily indicate a contraindication to t-PA. The degree of increased risk of t-PA in patients with microhemorrhages is unknown. Patients with an ischemic stroke within the past 3 months should not be given t-PA treatment, although a small infarct with transient deficits may not present a significant risk compared to potential benefit. (Albers et al., Chest 2004; National Institutes of Neurologic Disorders and Stroke rt-PA Stroke Study Group, *N Engl J Med* 1995)

227. The answer is E. In HIV-infected patients, the presence of stroke, either clinically evident or noted incidentally, ranges from 6% to 34%. Mechanisms are variable, with disproportionate cardioembolic disease, infectious vasculitis, and hematologic abnormalities. Infections associated with HIV-related stroke include syphilis, tuberculosis, aspergillosis, varicella infection, as well as bacterial endocarditis. (Ortiz et al., *Neurology* 2007)

228. The answer is D. In the absence of bleeding complications, oral vitamin K is not recommended for an INR of 4.3. Intravenous vitamin K should be reserved for a seriously elevated INR with active bleeding. Even in this setting, fresh frozen plasma is preferable and will more quickly reverse the coagulopathy. The exception to this might be in a patient with congestive heart failure, in whom volume overload from fresh frozen plasma could worsen the heart failure. Warfarin should be held for 1 or 2 days, but 1 week without warfarin is excessive and will result in complete loss of effective anticoagulation in most patients. (Sachdev et al., *Am J Health Syst Pharm* 1999)

229. The answer is A. The most likely cause of the acute onset of back pain and radicular symptoms in a patient with supra-therapeutic anticoagulation is a spinal epidural hematoma. Magnetic resonance imaging is the best diagnostic test and should be done emergently, because these hematomas can expand and produce irreversible spinal cord or nerve damage. Lumbar puncture is contraindicated in a patient who is anticoagulated, and it would provide no useful diagnostic information in this setting. Bed rest and narcotic analgesics may be appropriate therapy for a radiculopathy from a protruding lumbar disc, but an epidural hematoma may require urgent surgical intervention to prevent subsequent paraplegia and loss of bowel and bladder control. The patient should be admitted for reversal of his anticoagulation and evaluation for surgery. An angiogram of the spinal cord provides no diagnostic information regarding spinal epidural hematoma. (Ginsberg & Bogousslavsky, Chapter 112)

230. The answer is A. In a young weight-lifter with intermittent focal neurologic symptoms, a careful history should be taken for substance use. Because many of the substances used by weight-lifters and other athletes to enhance performance, such as over-the-counter sympathomimetics and creatine supplements, are not necessarily illegal and are not measurable through routine blood and urine toxicology screens, the history will be most sensitive for potential substances that can be associated with TIA and stroke. A creatine kinase (CK) level would also not give this information. Although the diffusion weighted imaging (DWI) sequence might show an abnormality anatomically correlated with his TIA symptoms, the scan would not determine the etiology of his transient symptoms. (Ginsberg & Bogousslavsky, Chapter 114)

231. The answer is A. This patient had an expanding cavernous ICA aneurysm producing a compressive third nerve palsy. (The most frequently described location of an aneurysm that produces a third nerve palsy is the posterior communication artery, although cavernous, basilar, superior cerebellar, and posterior cerebral artery aneurysms can also cause a third nerve palsy. These are complete III palsies, with both extraocular muscle evaluation, ptosis, and a dilated pupil with no reaction to light.) Because these can rupture, urgent treatment is necessary. The patient should be kept as comfortable and calm as possible to reduce the possibility of aneurysm rupture. Computed tomography angiography or MRA scanning, followed by urgent cerebral angiography and surgery, are recommended. Corticosteroids are not helpful. Mestinon would be used for myasthenia gravis, which can produce ptosis and restricted extraocular muscle function, but pain and a dilated pupil do not fit this diagnosis. Infection requiring antibiotics is far less likely in this setting than is an aneurysm. (The actual patient in this case had a large cavernous carotid aneurysm and was taken to surgery the same day. As the clip was being placed, the aneurysm ruptured. Although she had a stormy postoperative course, she had an unusually good recovery and became a campaigner against cocaine use in the community. The moral of the story is that happy endings are not limited to fairy tales.) (Howington et al., J *Nerosurg* 2003)

232. The answer is B. Lyme disease is caused by a tick-borne spirochete, *Borrelia burgdorferi*. Erythema chronicum migrans occurs early and is followed in weeks or months by neurologic symptoms. Cerebral infarcts are caused by an inflammatory vasculopathy, which can appear identical on angiography to other types of vasculitides. Primary angiitis of the CNS (PACNS) is less likely because of the association with the rash weeks prior to the development of neurologic symptoms. But again, the spinal fluid and angiographic findings are consistent with PACNS. Paradoxical emboli from PFO would be very unlikely to produce this much inflammatory change in the spinal fluid. Herpes encephalitis generally shows temporal lobe abnormalities on the MRI with unremarkable angiography. (Ginsberg & Bogousslavsky, Chapter 117)

233. The answer is A. The acid-fast bacillus (AFB) stain was negative, but this will be negative in at least half of patients with tuberculous meningitis. Fever, strokes, seizures, and altered levels of consciousness are classic clinical manifestations of tuberculous meningitis. Hydrocephalus and enhancement of the basal meninges are classic imaging findings. Tuberculosis has undergone a resurgence in this country in individuals with acquired immune deficiency syndrome (AIDS). Bacterial meningitis can also cause fevers, strokes, seizures, and altered consciousness, but would generally have more white cells with a neutrophilic predominance. Lupus can also produce a similar clinical picture, but generally there would be a prior history of lupus-like symptoms and no enhancement of the basal meninges. The hypoglycorrhachia would be unusual for CNS lupus. Cerebral vasculitis is associated with cerebrospinal fluid (CSF) pleocytosis, but rarely hypoglycorrhachia. Infective endocarditis is associated with strokes and seizures, but does not produce hydrocephalus or meningeal enhancement. (Breen et al., *Drugs* 2006; Ginsberg & Bogousslavsky, Chapter 117)

234. The answer is C. Cerebral malaria presents as an acute encephalopathy in the setting of infection with *Plasmodium falciparum*. It is a vascular disorder, and diffuse petechial hemorrhages in the subcortical white matter are commonly found on autopsy. Despite this, most patients do not suffer clinical stroke-like episodes, and cerebral malaria commonly presents with fever, stupor progressing to coma and seizures. The most common treatment is chloroquine. Steroids are contraindicated because they worsen the outcome. (Ginsberg & Bogousslavsky, Chapter 117)

235. The answer is C. Several series have documented improved outcome in patients with a combination of medical and surgical therapy when heart failure develops during bacterial endocarditis. Another indication for surgical therapy is failure of antibiotic therapy to control embolic events. Anticoagulation is generally contraindicated in patients with endocarditis. Staphylococcal infections have the highest risk of hemorrhagic conversion of cerebral infarcts. There is no role for antiplatelet agents in the treatment of infective endocarditis. Intravenous digoxin will be of no value in this setting. (Mylonkis et al., *N Engl J Med* 2001)

236. The answer is A. The occlusions leading to infarcts of the retina and/or optic nerve occur in the central retinal artery or in the posterior ciliary artery. Venous occlusions are not part of the pathology of giant-cell or temporal arteritis. Although any medium or large vessel in the body may be affected by this systemic angiitis, posterior circulation infarcts are rarely the cause of blindness in giant-cell arteritis. Disk swelling with giant-cell arteritis may be indistinguishable from that associated with increased ICP but it occurs after vision loss. (Ginsberg & Bogousslavsky, Chapter 118)

237. The answer is C. The most common cause of stroke in SLE in this list is verrucous (Libman-Sacks) endocarditis. Infective endocarditis can occur, but is relatively infrequent; although infections must always be considered, particularly in patients on immunosuppressive medications. Cerebral vasculitis is rare in SLE. Protein C deficiency is not described as a complication of SLE. (Futrell & Millikan, *Stroke* 1989)

238. The answer is D. Antineutrophilic cytoplasmic antibodies (ANCA) are associated with both Wegener's granulomatosis and polyarteritis nodosa, but mononeuritis multiplex is a classic feature of polyarteritis nodosa that does not occur with Wegener's granulomatosis. Granulomatous angiitis of the CNS is not associated with a positive ANCA. (Kallenberg et al., *Nat Clin Pract Rheumatol* 2006)

239. The answer is A. Ehlers-Danlos syndrome is a congenital, heterogeneous, connective tissue disorder associated with multiple types of collagen anomalies. Patients with Ehlers-Danlos syndrome have abnormal elastic tissue, with joint hypermobility, skin hyperextensibility, and skin hyperelasticity. They are at risk for cerebral aneurysms, carotid-cavernous fistulas, and arterial dissections. They do not have either vasculitis or inflammatory disease, nor do they have any propensity for arterial or venous thrombosis. (Ginsberg & Bogousslavsky, Chapter 122)

240. The answer is A. The sudden onset of severe back pain and evidence of an acute myelopathy in a pregnant woman should lead to emergent evaluation for a spinal epidural hemorrhage and neurosurgical decompression. Although most CNS vascular complications of pregnancy are cerebral, hemorrhage and infarction of the spinal cord can occur. Spinal epidural hemorrhage may occur spontaneously or as a result of vascular malformation leakage with increased vascular volume. Elevated venous pressure in the epidural space, in association with the hemodynamic changes of pregnancy, results in spontaneous hemorrhage from the engorged extradural venous plexus. Prompt surgical decompression and evacuation predicts a generally good recovery. The onset of a myelopathy associated with multiple sclerosis, transverse myelitis, or a malignancy is unlikely to be apoplectic and painful. A psychiatric etiology for her symptoms is not consistent with her examination. (Cywinski, *J Clin Anesth* 2004; Lavi E, et al., *J Neurol Neurosurg Psychiatry* 1986; Szkup et al., *Br J Rad* 2004)

241. The answer is B. According to the North American Symptomatic Carotid Endarterectomy Trial (NASCET) results, ipsilateral CEA is recommended for patients with symptomatic severe carotid artery stenosis. The study found a 17% risk reduction (95% confidence interval, 10–24) at 2 years. The benefit of surgery persisted through the 8 years of follow-up in NASCET. (Barnett et al., *N Engl J Med* 1998)

242. The answer is C. The Warfarin-Aspirin Symptomatic Intracranial Disease (WASID) Trial randomly assigned patients with TIA or stroke associated with angiographically verified intracranial stenosis to receive either warfarin (INR 2–3) or aspirin 1,300 mg daily in a double-blind multicenter trial. The planned mean duration of follow-up was 36 months, but the trial was prematurely terminated because of safety concerns about the use of warfarin. The actual mean duration of follow-up was less than 2 years. Warfarin was associated with significantly higher rates of adverse events and provided no benefit in prevention of the primary end-point (ischemic stroke, brain hemorrhage, or nonstroke vascular death) or the secondary end-points. The rate of vascular death and myocardial infarction was increased on warfarin as compared with aspirin. The investigators concluded that aspirin should be used in preference to warfarin for patients with intracranial stenosis. However, the optimal dose of aspirin for these patients is still unclear. (Chimowitz et al., *N Engl J Med* 2005)

243. The answer is A. In the European Carotid Surgery Trial (ECST), poststenotic narrowing of the internal carotid artery due to reduced distal intra-arterial perfusion pressure was associated with lower risk of ipsilateral stroke with medical treatment. This reduction may be due to the presence of collateral vessels. Plaque ulceration and contralateral internal carotid artery occlusion increase risk of stroke in symptomatic stenosis. Men are more likely to suffer a stroke associated with carotid stenosis than are women. Transient hemispheric symptoms presage an ischemic stroke more frequently than does amaurosis fugax. (Rothwell, *Int J Stroke* 2006)

244. The answer is B. Among medically treated patients, the risk of ipsilateral stroke decreased to an annual level similar to surgically treated patients within 2 to 3 years. Within the 2 to 3 years after surgery, the ipsilateral stroke risk dropped to 2% per year in the surgically treated group and to about 3% per year in the medically treated group. Benefit did not change across the deciles in the moderately stenotic group. The distribution of death did not differ by cause. Left-sided carotid artery disease increased perioperative stroke or death, as did contralateral carotid occlusion. (Barnett et al., *N Engl J Med* 1998)

245. The answers are A 1, B 3, C 5, D 4, E 2. Kawasaki syndrome involves the skin, especially a generalized peeling exanthema in the trunk. Sneddon syndrome involves livedo racemosa (a reddish purple network found on the trunk or extremities), whereas diffuse meningocerebral angiomatosis and leukoencephalopathy presents with livedo reticularis. Malignant atrophic papulosis—Kohlmeier-Degos disease—causes erythematous papules with central atrophy. Epidermal nevus syndrome associates cerebral infarcts and nevi. (Kasner & Gorelick, Chapter 8)

246. The answer is E. The listed disorders all cause transient spells with MRI abnormalities that may be temporary or permanent. However, this presentation is most consistent with stroke-like migraine attacks after radiation therapy (SMART), a newly recognized syndrome that occurs as a delayed consequence of cerebral irradiation. Patients with SMART have prolonged, reversible neurologic signs and symptoms including confusion, visual changes, hemimotor and sensory deficits, aphasia, seizures, and headaches. Transient, diffuse, unilateral cortical enhancement of cerebral gyri in the area of irradiation is seen on MRI. (Black et al., *Cephalgia* 2006)

247. The answer is B. Cerebral vasospasm is an uncommon cause of cerebral infarction. Vasospasm after SAH appears at 3 to 4 days, reaches its maximum at 6 to 8 days, and generally resolves by 12 to 14 days, although it can persist longer. Increased blood on CT scan as measured by the Fisher Scale increases the risk of vasospasm. Nimodipine does not actually decrease cerebral vasospasm, but may improve outcome after SAH-associated vasospasm through neuroprotective mechanisms. (Mohr et al., Chapter 73)

248. The answer is A. The cause of cerebral infarction associated with intranasal, smoked, or parenteral cocaine is variable but most infarctions, both cerebral and coronary, are due to vasoconstriction. (Mohr et al., Chapter 35)

249. The answer is C. Chagas disease, which is endemic in Latin America, is caused by infection with the protozoan parasite, *Trypanosoma cruzi*. Chronic Chagas disease affects the heart, causing congestive heart failure, heart block, arrhythmias or sudden death. The degree of cardiac involvement correlates with the risk of ischemic stroke due to cardiac embolization. Most ischemic strokes in Chagas disease occur in the MCA territory. (Camargo et al., *Neuroimag Clin N Am* 2005)

250. The answer is A. According to the International Study of Unruptured Intracranial Aneurysms (ISUIA), age, size, and location matter in the outcome after surgical treatment of unruptured aneurysms. Anterior circulation aneurysms are more likely to have a favorable surgical outcome than are posterior circulation aneurysms. Age of the patient has a major effect on operative outcome, as compared to the effect of age on the natural history (rupture rate) of the intracranial aneurysm. The deleterious effect of age on outcome is most marked for surgical patients older than 50 years and for endovascular patients older than 70 years. The lowest aneurysmal rupture risk was seen in patients with unruptured intracranial aneurysms smaller than 7 mm in the anterior circulation. Patients with an unruptured aneurysm, who did not have any prior aneurysm causing an SAH, were at a lower risk than those who had a prior ruptured aneurysm in addition to their unruptured aneurysm. Risk is increased in patients who have had a prior ruptured intracranial aneurysm, in addition to an unruptured intracranial aneurysm. (Wiebers, *Neuroimag Clin N Am* 2006)

251. The answer is B. Computed tomography angiography is preferable to MRA in assessing intracranial vasculature in a patient with an acute subarachnoid hemorrhage. Spatial resolution is better with CTA than with MRA, and CTA sensitivity and specificity is reasonable when compared to digital subtraction angiography. Computed tomography angiography is faster and easier to perform in an unstable patient without renal disease; the study can be performed in the intensive care unit using portable scanners. The International Subarachnoid Aneurysm Trial (ISAT) compared the 1-year death and disability outcome with surgical versus endovascular strategies. At 1 year, there was an absolute risk reduction in death and dependency of 7.4% in the coiled group as compared with the surgically treated group. The rebleeding risk in the coiled group after 1 year was approximately 0.2% per patient year. However, the ISAT enrolled patients for whom good surgical outcome would have been expected, with uncertainty persisting about the relative merits of the two treatments. The applicability of this trial to a wider range of ruptured aneurysms and the relative durability of the two treatments are some of the as-yet-unanswered concerns. (Molyneux, *Neuroimag Clin N Am* 2006)

252. The answer is D. This patient has classic isolated angiitis of the CNS. Clinical fluctuations can occur in the disease course, including improvements, but this disease does not remit spontaneously and should be treated aggressively. Prednisone alone may produce temporary improvements, but the combination of prednisone and Cytoxan, or another steroid-sparing immunosuppressive agent, is generally necessary to control this disease. (Moore, *Neurology* 1989)

253. The answer is A. The author of such romantic fiction as *Treasure Island* and *Kidnapped*, as well as *Strange Case of Dr. Jekyll and Mr. Hyde*, was suspected of having hereditary hemorrhagic telangiectasia (HHT), based on a long history of illness including recurrent pulmonary hemorrhage. Because HHT is an autosomal dominant condition with cerebral and pulmonary arteriovenous malformations, his mother's history appears consistent with the diagnosis as well. The diagnosis of HHT is based on the presence of epistaxis, telangiectasias, visceral vascular lesions, and an affected first-degree relative. Von Hippel-Lindau disease is also a genetic disease with hemangioblastomas in the brain, but it is not associated with pulmonary hemorrhage. Sturge-Weber syndrome (encephalotrigeminal angiomatosis) is a congenital, nonfamilial disorder characterized by a facial birthmark and cerebral angiomas. Moyamoya syndrome may present with cerebral hemorrhage in an adult, but is not generally hereditary and does not have lung lesions. Cerebral amyloid angiopathy may rarely occur in families, presenting with intracerebral hemorrhage at a young age, but there is no association with lung lesions. (Guttmacher & Callahan, *Am J Med Genet* 2000)

254. The answer is D. Fewer than 20% of patients with ICH undergo clot removal. Surgery may benefit patients with a cerebellar or subcortical hemorrhage of greater than 3 cm in diameter and impaired consciousness. Comatose patients with ICH in the basal ganglia or thalamus are very unlikely to benefit from clot removal. The STICH study randomized the patients after a spontaneous supratentorial ICH without clear therapeutic choice (clinical equipoise) to either early surgical therapy or conservative management. No definite beneficial effect was seen from early surgery on outcome after supratentorial spontaneous ICH. (Juvela & Kase, *Stroke* 2006)

255. The answer is B. Osler-Weber-Rendu disease (hereditary hemorrhagic telangiectasia [HHT]) is an autosomal dominant disease with skin, nasal, and visceral telangiectasia. Some of these patients also have intracranial AVMs. Neurofibromatosis is associated with occlusive arterial disease. Cerebrovascular disease in Marfan syndrome usually leads to large-artery dissection, as does Ehlers-Danlos syndrome. Sturge-Weber syndrome is characterized pathologically by leptomeningeal vessel calcification and arteriovenous angiomas. (Kasner & Gorelick, Chapter 8)

256. The answer is A. Women in the United States have relatively more strokes than myocardial infarctions, as compared to men. According to the 2006 report of the American Heart Association, each year, about 46,000 more women than men have a stroke. Women have their greatest risk of stroke in their later decades of life. More boys than girls have strokes. Incidence of stroke is greater in men in their 60s and 70s, but stroke is more common in women after age 80 years. Because women live longer than men, more women than men die of stroke each year. Women accounted for 61% of all stroke deaths in 2003. (Thom et al., *Circulation* 2006)

257. The answer is D. Bilateral necrosis of the globus pallidus is the classic finding in carbon monoxide poisoning. Cocaine would show up in the toxicology screen and does not fit the clinical pattern. Bilateral pallidal necrosis does not occur with ischemic stroke or venous sinus thrombus. Schizophrenia would not have this CT finding. The story of this patient was that his girlfriend jilted him. He drove his car to his rented storage garage. He closed the door, left the motor on, and penned a suicide note. He lost consciousness, but the car ran out of gas before the dirty deed was completed. When he woke up, he left the garage. He was wandering around confused. Later, when his family found his car missing, someone thought to look in the storage garage and the pieces of the puzzle fell together. It should be noted that carbon monoxide poisoning is more common in cold weather. Furnace malfunctions contribute, as do people sitting in their cars with the motor running so they can leave the heater on. (Ernst et al., *N Engl J Med* 1999; Osborn)

258. The answer is A. The Quality Standards Subcommittee of the American Academy of Neurology reviewed literature on outcome after cardiac arrest and determined that elevated serum neuron-specific enolase (NSE), a γ-isomer of enolase located in neurons and neuroectodermal cells, was a marker for poor outcome. Neuron-specific enolase levels of more than 33μg/L at days 1 to 3 accurately predicted poor outcome. However, measurement of NSE is not readily available and is not standardized. The prognostic value of other serum and CSF biochemical markers has not been adequately evaluated. (Wijdicks et al., *Neurology* 2006)

259. The answer is B. The Quality Standards Subcommittee of the American Academy of Neurology reviewed literature on outcome after cardiac arrest and determined that bilateral absence of the N20 component of the somatosensory evoked potential with median nerve stimulation on days 1 to 3 after cardiopulmonary resuscitation predicted a poor outcome. Somatosensory evoked potentials are less influenced by drugs and metabolic derangements than is the EEG and are therefore more accurate in their prognostic value. Other evoked potential tests have not been as thoroughly investigated. The predictive value of CT scanning is not clear. (Wijdicks et al., *Neurology* 2006)

260. The answer is E. In patients with a perimesencephalic pattern of hemorrhage on CT scanning, an aneurysm of the vertebrobasilar circulation is rarely found on angiography, and a negative initial four-vessel catheter angiogram study obviates the need for a follow-up study with this specific imaging presentation. Catheter angiography in SAH is associated with a 1.8% rate of ischemic events and 1% to 2% rate of aneurysmal rerupture, thus it is not an innocuous procedure. The sensitivity of MRA is improving, but it is cumbersome in an unstable, ventilated patient and has yet to supplant four-vessel catheter angiography. Computed tomography angiography is easier to perform than an MRA, with sensitivity approaching catheter angiography. (Van Gijn et al., *Lancet* 2007)

261. The answer is B. Anosmia has been reported to occur in almost 30% of patients after SAH. The most common complaints in patients with good neurologic recovery from SAH are cognitive and psychosocial dysfunction. Epilepsy may develop as a function of cortical damage and manipulation. Hydrocephalus is a complication of the acute stage of SAH, and loss of hearing and low back pain are not commonly associated with long-term recovery from SAH. Patients may note continuing headaches after aneurysm resection, especially with posterior fossa surgery. Low back pain may occasionally occur subacutely after a hemorrhage as the blood settles in the thecal sac in the lumbar region. (Van Gijn, *Lancet* 2007)

262. The answer is B. Acute posterior multifocal placoid pigment epitheliopathy (APMPPE) is a chorioretinal disease of unknown etiology that should be considered in young people with strokes or aseptic meningitis of unknown etiology, especially associated with scotomas or visual blurring. There may be radiographic or pathologic evidence of vasculitis. Acute posterior multifocal placoid pigment epitheliopathy is treated with 6 to 12 months of immunosuppressive agents, because strokes generally occur within the first 5 months of disease. It does not have a known genetic pattern. (Comu et al., *Stroke* 1996)

263. The answer is C. High blood levels of digoxin produces both bradycardia and hallucinations. This is the most likely diagnosis in this setting. As individuals age, digoxin metabolism decreases. Failure to decrease the dose in elderly patients may result in digoxin overdose, as can dosage errors and suicide attempts. Although seizures, meningitis, or systemic infections can all produce hallucinations in elderly patients, even when blood counts and temperature are normal, the bradycardia is the key to the correct answer of digoxin toxicity. This is an actual case from the author's practice. (Brunton, Chapter 35; *Physician's Desk Reference*)

264. The answer is D. The antemortem diagnosis of PACNS is difficult to make, and the biopsy can be negative for PACNS; however, the biopsy serves a second function of ruling out other diseases that can mimic vasculitis clinically (diffuse intracranial atherosclerosis, malignancy, infection). Laboratory evaluation for systemic inflammatory diseases is generally negative, although ANA is occasionally positive. When serology is positive, a systemic collagen vascular disease should be considered as an alternate diagnosis. Spinal fluid typically may have pleocytosis and may have elevated protein, but it may be normal. In general, treatment should not be given based on angiography alone because of the low specificity of angiography and the toxicity of the treatments. Because a histologically similar vasculitis occurs in some cases of herpes zoster, an underlying viral process has been suggested. Patients with PACNS do not reactivate a viral disease with immunosuppression, because no clinical evidence of viral infection has been found in these patients. (Moore, *Neurology* 1989)

265. The answer is B. The patient has a Horner's syndrome (ptosis, miosis), and the most likely diagnosis is a traumatic internal carotid artery dissection with his history of neck injury and pain. Both MRA and CTA are noninvasive tests that are useful in the evaluation of potential internal carotid artery dissection. Carotid duplex is an alternative noninvasive screening test, but it will miss distal internal carotid artery dissections. If these noninvasive tests are not diagnostic, then a carotid angiogram would be the next step. Cocaine use is not particularly associated with Horner's syndrome. An apical lordotic chest radiograph or a chest CT is part of the evaluation of an idiopathic Horner's syndrome, to rule out a lung neoplasm, which is unlikely in this man. (Ginsberg & Bogousslavsky, Chapter 76)

266. The answer is C. An internuclear ophthalmoplegia (INO) is characterized by adduction impairment with contralateral abduction nystagmus. Adduction may be preserved during convergence. A skew deviation with a hyperopia may be seen on the side of the medial longitudinal fasciculus (MLF) lesion. An INO can present as an isolated or predominant stroke symptom, with lesions in the pons (rostral or caudal), the pontomesencephalic junction, or mid-brain. Associated vascular lesions can be seen in the basilar artery, the superior cerebellar artery, or the PCA. A gaze paresis accompanying the INO (a one-and-a-half syndrome) indicates paramedian pontine reticular formation, as well as MLF, involvement. The associated gaze paresis usually resolves within days. In a study of patients with an INO as an isolated or predominant stroke symptom, functional recovery was excellent. (Kim, *Neurology* 2004)

267. The answer is A. Mycotic aneurysms form as a result of septic embolization from infective endocarditis. They are found in multiple arterial beds, including the extremities, in addition to the brain. Because the emboli lodge more frequently at distal arterial bifurcations in the brain, the aneurysms are found in this location. These aneurysms can produce SAH. They can become smaller or larger over time, with some completely resolving. Often, surgical or endovascular treatment is not recommended because of their distal location, and they may be treated with a prolonged course of antibiotics. (Brust, *Ann Neurol* 1990; Mylonakis et al., *N Engl J Med* 2001)

268. The answer is C. Tacrolimus is an immunosuppressive agent used after solid-organ and hematopoietic stem cell transplantation. The overall incidence of tacrolimus-associated posterior reversible encephalopathy syndrome (PRES) is variable, up to 8%. This syndrome presents with subacute change in mental status, seizures, and headache, with changes seen on CT or MRI in the subcortical white matter, particularly posteriorly. Hyperintensity of the white matter on T-2 weighted images and FLAIR sequences is characteristically seen on MRI. Hypertension, which has been associated with PRES, is not felt to be a significant contribution to tacrolimus-associated PRES. Most cases are reversible with discontinuation or decreased dosage of the medication. There is nothing specific to indicate tuberculous meningitis or disseminated intravascular coagulopathy (DIC). Herpetic lesions are more commonly seen in the temporal lobes. Bilateral PCA infarcts, involving white and gray matter on imaging, can be distinguished from PRES, which is generally confined to the white matter in a nonvascular distribution. (Wong, *Br J Haemat* 2003)

269. The answers are A 5, B 2, C 4, D 1, E 3. Marfan syndrome, Ehlers-Danlos syndrome type IV and, to a lesser extent, osteogenesis imperfecta, are associated with large-vessel dissections. Marfan syndrome and Ehlers-Danlos syndrome type IV are also associated with cerebral aneurysm formation. Neurofibromatosis type I may result in stenosis of the supraclinoid internal carotid artery with development of moyamoya syndrome. Cerebral autosomal dominant arteriopathy with subcortical infarcts and leukoencephalopathy (CADASIL) is a small-vessel disease of the brain associated with recurrent strokes, headaches, and dementia. (Flossman, *Int J Stroke* 2006)

270. The answers are A 2, B 1, C 3, D 5, E 4. Although Fabry disease may manifest itself in heterozygous women, men are more severely affected. Mitochondrial encephalomyopathy, lactic acidosis, and stroke-like episodes (MELAS) is usually associated with a heteroplasmic A3243G mutation in the mitochondrial gene *MTTL1,* affecting complex 1 of the respiratory chain. Mitochondria are maternally inherited. Pseudoxanthoma elasticum is inherited as an autosomal recessive, or occasionally autosomal dominant disorder, predisposing to occlusive disease of carotid and vertebral arteries. Familial hypertrophic cardiomyopathies are generally transmitted as autosomal dominant disorders with incomplete penetrance. Cerebral amyloid angiopathy is sporadic in the elderly, although rare autosomal dominant forms may lead to cerebral hemorrhage in young Europeans. (Flossman, *Int J Stroke* 2006)

271. The answer is C. According to recently published guidelines for screening of carotid artery disease, mass screening for high-grade asymptomatic extracranial carotid artery stenosis is not cost effective, even with selection for age, gender, or vascular risk factors. Renal artery stenosis, abdominal aortic aneurysms, and need for cardiac surgery (vascular or valvular) are not indications for screening, based on prevalence of coincident disease. However, over 20% of patients with symptomatic peripheral vascular disease have carotid artery stenosis of greater than 60%. This high prevalence of disease led to the recommendation that all patients with symptomatic, but not asymptomatic, peripheral vascular disease be screened for carotid stenosis. Screening for carotid stenosis is not recommended for patients with isolated syncope, dizziness, vertigo, or tinnitus based on the low incidence of associated carotid stenosis. (Qureshi et al., *J Neuroimaging* 2007)

272. The answer is D. Based on increasing rates of ipsilateral and contralateral stenosis with time after radiotherapy, patients surviving head and neck malignancy should be screened 10 years after unilateral or bilateral irradiation. Preliminary studies indicate lower perioperative complications with carotid stenting than with endarterectomy for patients who develop stenosis as a result of head and neck radiation. Screening of these patients prior to radiotherapy should be based on their coincident vascular risk factors. (Qureshi et al., *J Neuroimaging* 2007)

273. The answer is D. Studies of restenosis rates after carotid stenting indicate varying stenosis thresholds and timing criteria to define restenosis. The rates of restenosis quoted in the medical literature are highly variable. No carotid revascularization technique is clearly associated with a lower risk of restenosis. Not all patients who restenose are symptomatic. Most studies reviewing restenosis rates in patients who have undergone angioplasty and stent placement do not examine rate of restenosis as a function of stent type. (Qureshi et al., *J Neuroimaging* 2007)

274. The answer is D. Men, older patients, and patients randomized to surgery within 2 weeks of diagnosis of a TIA or minor stroke did best with CEA. Women had a lower ischemic stroke risk on medical therapy than did men. Women also had a higher operative stroke risk than men. The risk of stroke on medical therapy after a TIA or stroke is highest during the first few weeks after the event. The risk then declines over the subsequent year. Benefit from surgery appears to be greatest in patients with an ischemic stroke, intermediate with a cerebral TIA, and lowest with retinal ischemia. (Rothwell, *Int J Stroke* 2006)

275. The answer is C. The presence of cerebral microbleeds (CMB) on an acute MRI is not a contraindication to intravenous thrombolysis, which appears to be appropriate for this man. Cerebral microbleeds are found on MRI in up to 5% of elderly subjects without symptomatic cerebrovascular disease. The prevalence of CMB increases in patients with hemorrhagic or ischemic cerebrovascular disease. They are also associated with Alzheimer's disease, cerebral microangiopathy, and cerebral amyloid angiopathy. Paroxysmal atrial fibrillation with a thromboembolic event dictates long-term anticoagulation. Without suspicion of cerebral amyloid angiopathy, CMBs are not a contraindication for anticoagulant or antiplatelet therapy. (Fiehler, *Int J Stroke* 2006; Koenneck, *Neurology* 2006)

276. The answer is B. The two major predictors of hemorrhage of an untreated AVM are increasing age and hemorrhagic presentation (as opposed to headaches, seizures, or other nonhemorrhagic presentation at the time of diagnosis). Other independent predictors of hemorrhage are deep brain location and exclusive deep venous drainage. Gender, AVM size, and aneurysms on intranidal or feeding arteries are not associated with increased hemorrhage risk. (Stapf et al., *Neurology* 2006)

277. The answer is C. The lateral medullary (Wallenberg) syndrome results from damage to the anterior lateral system fibers (contralateral loss of pain and thermal sense on the body), the spinal trigeminal tract and nucleus (ipsilateral loss of pain and thermal sense on the face), the nucleus ambiguous and roots of cranial nerves 9 and 10 (bulbar dysfunction), descending hypothalamic fibers (ipsilateral Horner's syndrome), vestibular nuclei (nausea, gait imbalance), and spinocerebellar fibers (ipsilateral ataxia). Contralateral hemiplegia (cortical spinal tract fibers), contralateral loss of position and vibration sense (medial lemniscus), ipsilateral deviation of the tongue (hypoglossal nucleus), and nystagmus (medial longitudinal fasciculus) are symptoms found with infarction of the medial medulla. (Haines, 2004)

278. The answer is D. Central nervous system injury after cardiac surgery includes embolic or hemodynamic ischemic stroke, encephalopathy, delirium, and neurocognitive decline. Magnetic resonance imaging scanning with DWI sequences is more sensitive than CT scanning for evaluation of the neurologically impaired patients after cardiac surgery. This patient had bilateral watershed infarcts in the overlap between the anterior and MCA territories. The MRI showed the characteristic border zone infarct pattern, with small linear lesions affecting the shoulder area of the motor strip ("man in a barrel") bilaterally. This patient had bilateral high-grade carotid artery stenosis discovered postoperatively. The neurologic risk of cardiac surgery is still not well characterized but severe carotid disease increases vascular risk. A decrease in intraoperative blood pressure and increased cardiopulmonary bypass time may result in watershed infarcts in patients with stenotic extracranial disease. (Gottesman et al., *Stroke* 2006)

279. The answer is E. The known involvement of Lp(a) in multiple mechanisms of atherosclerosis should point toward its designation as a significant risk factor for ischemic stroke. No association has been found with hemorrhagic stroke risk. Analysis of Lp(a)'s risk must take into account the increased levels seen in women and African Americans and its correlation with LDL cholesterol (LDL-C) levels. The prospective studies of its clinical relevance in ischemic stroke show variable populations at risk. An elevated level of Lp(a) was an independent predictor of stroke and vascular death in older men, but not in older women. However, an analysis of the Women's Health Study data found that very high levels of Lp(a) in initially healthy older women were predictive of future cardiovascular events, especially when associated with elevated levels of LDL-C. Older men and women who participated in the Atherosclerosis Risk in Communities (ARIC) Study found that a high level of Lp(a) was associated with an increased incidence of ischemic stroke in blacks and white women, but not in white men. At this point, with the uncertainty about its relevance and the difficulty with its assay, routine screening for elevated Lp(a) levels is not advocated. Intervention to decrease elevated levels of Lp(a) is no more specific than management of elevated LDL-C levels. Further studies are needed to show how elevated Lp(a) levels should explicitly dictate patient management. (Ariyo & Thach, *N Engl J Med* 2003; Ohira et al., *Stroke* 2006)

280. The answer is D. This man has a dominant-hemisphere lesion involving motor and visual function, without the additional speech or cortical sensory deficits that would be found with left MCA occlusion. He has an occlusion of the anterior choroidal artery—the distal branch of the internal carotid artery—that interrupts blood supply to the optic tract and the inferior portion of the posterior limb of the internal capsule. The anterior choroidal artery, which can also branch off the M1 portion of the MCA, supplies the choroid plexus of the lateral ventricles, the hippocampus, and globus pallidus, and the posterior limb of the internal capsule. (Haines, 2004; Gilman & Newman, 2003)

281. The answer is E. Hypertension, the most common primary diagnosis in the United States, affects approximately 50 million Americans. According to the JNC 7 Report, using data from the Framingham Heart Study, individuals who are normotensive at 55 years of age have a 90% lifetime risk for developing hypertension. For individuals aged 40 to 70 years, each increment of 20 mm Hg in systolic blood pressure or 10 mm Hg in diastolic blood pressure doubles the risk of cardiovascular disease across the entire blood pressure range from 115/75 to 185/115. (Chobanian et al., *JAMA* 2003)

282. The answer is B. Two episodes of paroxysmal atrial fibrillation in a man younger than 60 years, without heart disease, can be treated with aspirin, rather than warfarin. However, older women with paroxysmal atrial fibrillation who also have evidence of left ventricular dysfunction should be anticoagulated. Warfarin is teratogenic and should not be given during pregnancy. Subcutaneous unfractionated heparin or low-molecular-weight heparin may be given in pregnant patients with high thrombotic risk. A recurrent ischemic event on aspirin is not necessarily an indication for anticoagulation, unless there is a specific indication for anticoagulation, such as newly discovered atrial fibrillation. The woman with lung and brain lesions after orthopedic surgery may have fat embolus syndrome due to the long-bone fracture, not a cardiac source of embolization that warrants anticoagulation. (Hirsch et al., *J Am Coll Cardiol* 2003)

283. The answer is C. Most perioperative strokes are embolic in origin (62%), including strokes that occur related to vascular procedures. Hemorrhagic stroke associated with surgery is exceedingly rare. Perioperative strokes due to cerebral hypoperfusion are rare, and may be related to postoperative volume loss or dehydration. The incidence of stroke after valve replacement alone is in the range of 5% to 9%. The addition of cardiac bypass surgery does not confer additional risk, with approximately 7.5% incidence for the two procedures combined. Aortic atherosclerosis increases the risk of perioperative stroke with cardiac bypass surgery, especially with revascularization of the left mainstem artery. Atrial fibrillation occurs in 30% to 50% of patients after cardiac surgery and is a major cause of stroke in these patients. (Selim, *N Engl J Med* 2007)

284. The answer is B. According to a study of a Finnish population with intracranial aneurysms with or without SAH, there was a fourfold increased risk of having an aneurysm in a close relative as compared to someone in the general population. People with polycystic kidney disease (PCKD) have an increased risk of having an intracranial aneurysm but, according to this study, only 9% of first-degree relatives of a patient with an intracranial aneurysm and PCKD have an intracranial aneurysm, a prevalence that approximated familial risk without PCKD. The prevalence of intracranial aneurysms, especially in men, appears higher in Finns than in other populations. (Ronkainen et al., *Lancet* 1997)

285. The answer is C. Although a migraine can be triggered by exercise and relief from stress, the sudden onset of a severe headache in a young woman without a headache history should raise concern about a SAH. Rarely, the CT scan may not reveal blood in a patient with a SAH, and further testing is recommended. Both a lumbar puncture and an MRI scan may be considered in the hyperacute evaluation of a patient with sudden onset of a severe headache, but the lumbar puncture is generally more available and immediately interpreted. A contrast-enhanced CT scan would not help to differentiate between hemorrhage and migraine. Both headache types may respond to triptans, but sumatriptan should not be given unless a migraine headache is diagnosed. (Suarez et al., *N Engl J Med* 2006)

286. The answer is C. Pituitary apoplexy results from infarction or hemorrhage in a pituitary adenoma. This syndrome is less common now than in previous years, because pituitary adenomas are more frequently diagnosed and treated before this complication occurs. The most devastating cause of pituitary apoplexy is hemorrhage with sudden mass effect from the expansion of the pituitary. This can be catastrophic, causing severe headache, impairment of consciousness, and death. Because the pituitary is near the optic chiasm, visual field defects are frequent with pituitary lesions. Diplopia is another common manifestation. A SAH would be unlikely to produce a bitemporal hemianopia, and an occipital hemorrhage would produce a unilateral hemianopia. Cluster headache is not associated with visual loss. (Keane, *Arch Neurol* 2007; Levy, *J Neurol Psychiatry* 2004)

287. The answer is E. Myoclonic jerks, which are irregular, synchronous, shock-like limb movements, may follow acutely after severe hypoxic–ischemic cerebral injury. Myoclonic activity is generally most prominent in the first 24 to 48 hours after global hypoxic injury. Only an inconsistent relationship exists with paroxysmal EEG activity, and traditional anticonvulsants are generally ineffective. High doses of benzodiazepines may suppress the myoclonic activity. Severe and protracted myoclonus heralds poor prognosis and a high mortality. An action myoclonus syndrome described by Lance and Adams occurs after recovery from coma secondary to cerebral ischemia. The intention myoclonus of the Lance-Adams syndrome is seen in awake patients and may be stimulus-activated. (Ropper, 2004)

288. The answer is B. For explanation, see Answer 289.

289. The answer is C. Although it is a rare disease, this woman has the classic triad of Susac syndrome: subacute encephalopathy, branch retinal artery occlusions, and sensorineural hearing loss. Susac syndrome, a microangiopathy, involves arterioles of the brain, retina, and cochlea. Early in its presentation, it can be confused with other disorders producing multifocal neurologic symptoms. The lack of systemic symptoms in this woman makes syphilis and lupus less likely, and her retinal findings are not seen in multiple sclerosis. Although Cogan syndrome may present with a Ménière syndrome–like symptoms, overlapping the vestibular symptoms of Susac syndrome, the visual symptoms of Cogan syndrome are due to interstitial keratitis or less commonly uveitis. The MRI picture of Susac syndrome reflects the pathology of a microangiopathy involving both gray and white matter. Lesions are seen in the cerebrum, cerebellum, and brainstem. Acute or subacute lesions may enhance during the attack and, rarely, leptomeningeal enhancement is noted. The disease may be monophasic or fluctuating with changes in the MRI lesions over time. (Do et al., *Am J Neuroradiol* 2004)

290. The answer is C. The patient has Cogan syndrome with interstitial keratitis (granular corneal infiltration) and a Ménière-like syndrome with vertigo, nausea, vomiting, tinnitus, and gait instability. Patients with Cogan syndrome develop sensorineural hearing loss. Aortitis with aortic insufficiency is the most characteristic cardiovascular manifestation of Cogan syndrome, with lesions in the aortic wall leading to aneurysmal dilatation. Aortic valve replacement is needed in some patients. (Grasland, *Rheumatology* 2004)

291. The answer is B. Chronic untreated hypertension is the major risk factor for spontaneous ICH, and even young adults with ICH should be evaluated for hypertension. Trauma, vascular malformations, cerebral vasculitis, and anticoagulation may be risk factors in young adults. Alcohol and drug abuse, especially cocaine, are associated with increased vascular risk. Reperfusion injury with ICH is a rare occurrence after revascularization of internal carotid stenosis. Eclampsia is rarely associated with ICH. Nonfamilial forms of cerebral amyloid angiopathy are generally found in elderly individuals. (Qureshi, *N Engl J Med* 2001)

292. The answer is C. Brott et al. performed a prospective observational study of patients with ICH imaged within 3 hours of onset of symptoms. At least 38% of patients had greater than 33% growth in the volume of hemorrhage in the first 24 hours after symptom onset. Early hemorrhage growth was significantly associated with clinical deterioration. No clinical or CT predictor of hemorrhage growth was found, although a trend toward more frequent hemorrhage growth was seen in patients with thalamic hemorrhage. (Brott et al., *Stroke* 1997)

293. The answer is C. Treatment of chronic hypertension, the most important risk factor for spontaneous ICH, results in a substantial decrease in hemorrhage risk. The hypertension-related annual risk of recurrent hemorrhage is around 2% and can be reduced by almost a half with aggressive treatment of chronic hypertension. Cerebral amyloid angiopathy presents as lobar hemorrhages in elderly persons, due to rupture of small- and medium-sized arteries infiltrated by β-amyloid protein. The annual risk of recurrent hemorrhage with amyloid angiopathy is about 10%. The recurrent hemorrhage risk associated with cerebral amyloid angiopathy is tripled by the presence of ε2 and ε4 alleles of the apolipoprotein E gene. These alleles are associated with increased deposition of β-amyloid protein and arterial degenerative changes. Excessive alcohol use and serum cholesterol levels of less than 160 mg/dL are associated with increased spontaneous ICH risk. (Qureshi et al., *N Engl J Med* 2001)

294. The answer is A. The history indicates that this woman has an internal carotid artery dissection, which is not a contraindication to thrombolytic therapy. Heparin is rarely indicated as an acute treatment of ischemic stroke. It may be considered after an acute extracranial arterial dissection, to decrease embolization risk, especially in the setting of a TIA or minor stroke. No data exists to guide the use of heparin in a patient who has had an acute ischemic stroke due to an arterial dissection, although the treatment may occasionally be given. In this case, the acute use of intravenous heparin would preclude thrombolysis. A loading dose of intravenous heparin is generally avoided in a patient with a large acute stroke. Thrombolytic therapy can be considered in pregnant women with acute ischemic stroke, assuming that all the inclusion and exclusion criteria have been considered. The hemorrhagic risk of treatment should be considered if delivery appears imminent during the time of thrombolysis. Intra-arterial treatment of documented arterial thrombosis may confer decreased systemic risk. Because it is a large molecule (7,200 kd), rt-PA does not cross the placenta and has no known teratogenicity. Anecdotal reports of success with rt-PA given either by intravenous or intra-arterial injection in all trimesters indicate that thrombolysis may be an option when the neurologic deficit warrants the risk to the mother and the fetus. (Johnson et al., *Stroke* 2005; Murugappan et al., *Neurology* 2006)

295. The answer is D. Primary postpartum cerebral angiopathy (Call-Fleming syndrome) is a rare, reversible, cerebral vasoconstriction syndrome that presents with headaches, seizures, and focal neurologic deficits. The MRI scan may be initially normal or show cortical lesions. Imaging shows reversible multifocal brain ischemia due to segmental narrowing of large and medium-sized cerebral arteries. Spinal fluid is normal. These patients generally recover without immunosuppressive treatment. The lack of peripheral edema, proteinuria, and hypertension distinguish Call-Fleming syndrome from eclampsia and preeclampsia. Posterior reversible encephalopathy syndrome (PRES), a syndrome of headaches, seizures, visual changes, and accelerated hypertension, can be associated with pregnancy. The MRI shows characteristic changes in the posterior white matter. A progressive headache is generally not due to a SAH. Another potential diagnosis in this case would be cerebral venous thrombosis. (Call et al., *Stroke* 1988)

296. The answer is A. Kittner et al. reviewed data from the Baltimore-Washington Cooperative Young Stroke Study, and found that, for ICH, the adjusted relative risk was 2.5 (95% CI, 1.0–6.4) during pregnancy but 28.3 (95% CI, 13.0–61.4) for the postpartum period. Bateman et al. found a rate of 7.1 pregnancy related ICH per 100,000 at-risk person years compared to 5.0 per 100,000 person-years for nonpregnant women in the same age range. The increased risk was largely associated with ICH in the postpartum period. Intracerebral hemorrhage accounted for 7.1% of all pregnancy-related mortality in the database. Significant independent risk factors included advanced maternal age, African American race, pre-existing or gestational hypertension, preeclampsia/eclampsia, coagulopathy, and tobacco use. (Bateman et al., *Neurology* 2006; Kittner et al., *N Engl J Med* 1996)

297. The answer is C. This woman presented for medical evaluation within 2 hours of the onset of an acute ischemic stroke. Although the precise onset of her stroke is unknown, she was last noted to be neurologically normal within the 3-hour intravenous t-PA treatment window. Her degree of neurologic deficit as measured by the NIHSS is appropriate for treatment with intravenous tissue plasminogen activator. Although her blood pressure was initially elevated, it decreased to levels at which she could receive t-PA. Although aspirin is not given prior to t-PA treatment, it is not a contraindication to t-PA treatment. However, the woman has idiopathic thrombocytopenia purpura (ITP) with a platelet count of less than 100,000, the threshold for treatment with t-PA. (National Institutes of Neurologic Disorders and Stroke rt-TPA Study Group, *N Engl J Med* 1995)

298. The answer is B. This man presents with symptoms possibly suggestive of an acute cerebellar infarct. Although his symptoms could be due to an acute vestibular disorder, his age and medical history make vertebrobasilar disease of primary concern. An MRI with DWI to look for an acute ischemic lesion and an MRA of the posterior circulation could establish the diagnosis in the face of a negative CT scan. An ultrasound study of the neck would not give adequate visualization of the vertebrobasilar system from arch to intracranial vessels. This patient has a risk of edema formation around the area of cerebellar infarction. With acute hydrocephalus, the CT scan would show obliteration of basal cisterns and the fourth ventricle. If the hydrocephalus progresses unrecognized and untreated, transtentorial herniation can cause brainstem compression. Close monitoring by the nursing staff, more frequently than every 6 hours, should pick up changes in mental status from evolving obstructive hydrocephalus. Ventricular drainage or suboccipital decompression of the posterior fossa may avoid life-threatening brainstem compression. This man does not have symptoms suggestive of SAH, and a lumbar puncture in the face of possible posterior fossa obstruction increases herniation risk. (Jensen, *Arch Neurol* 2005)

299. The answer is A. Lowered intravascular volume with dehydration, sepsis, or malnutrition may predispose to cerebral venous thrombosis (CVT). Genetically determined thrombophilias predisposing to CVT include activated protein C resistance, protein S and protein C deficiencies, antithrombin III deficiency, prothrombin gene mutation, and hyperhomocysteinemia. Pregnancy, puerperium, oral contraceptives, and hormone replacement therapy may be associated with CVT. A cardiac evaluation will not yield specific results in this woman. (Ehtisham & Stem, *The Neurologist* 2006; Olesen et al., Chapter 112)

300. The answer is D. Familial hemiplegic migraine (FMH) is a genetically heterogeneous, autosomal dominant migraine subtype. The most common gene associated with FHM is the *CACNA1A*, FHM1 gene, which encodes the pore-forming α1A subunit of P/Q-type voltage-dependent neuronal calcium channels. Fully reversible motor weakness plus fully reversible visual, sensory, or speech deficits are necessary for the diagnosis of FHM. This migraine subtype affects men and women equally. The degree of motor deficit ranges from mild clumsiness to hemiplegia. Permanent cerebellar symptoms, found in up to 20% of patients, include nystagmus and ataxia. (Black, *Semin Neurol* 2006; Olesen et al., 2006)

301. The answer is B. This woman has a headache, neck pain, scalp tenderness, and jaw claudication, suspicious for giant-cell arteritis (GCA). All the listed tests may be used in the evaluation of GCA. Both ESR and CRP are generally elevated in GCA, although the ESR may be lower than expected or even normal in some patients. The ESR is more than 50 mm/hr in 89% and over 100 in 41% of patients with GCA. The C-RP, an acute phase plasma protein, may be more specific for detecting inflammation, and it is not elevated by anemia. The C-RP may be elevated when the ESR is normal in GCA. The elevation of von Willebrand factor, an acute phase reactant, is a nonspecific test. Dampening of the amplitude of the wave form on oculoplethysmography (OPG) may be seen with involvement of the ophthalmic artery in GCA but OPG is rarely used in the diagnosis of GCA. (Olesen et al., Chapter 110)

302. The answer is A. Over a third of patients with ischemic stroke or TIA present with a headache. A headache is more commonly associated with a posterior circulation infarct. Although the size of the infarct does not correlate with the severity of the headache, headaches are less commonly associated with lacunar syndromes. Studies have found no difference in headache frequency between cardioembolic and atherothrombotic strokes. (Olesen et al., Chapter 108)

303. The answer is D. For explanation, see Answer 304.

304. The answer is C. This woman had a venous infarct due to sagittal sinus thrombosis. Cerebral venous thrombosis (CVT) has been associated with pregnancy and the postpartum period, especially in association with congenital or acquired coagulation disorders. Acute treatment with intravenous unfractionated heparin, although concerning in the setting of venous infarction and ICH, appears to improve outcome. Because of the teratogenic effects of warfarin, body weight–adjusted subcutaneous low-molecular-weight heparin should be used for chronic anticoagulation in pregnancy. Local venous thrombolysis has been attempted in pregnant women; however, there is not enough experience to predict outcome. In general, pregnancy-related CVT has a good prognosis for survival. Risk of recurrence of CVT with subsequent pregnancies is unclear, with a suggestion that risk is greatest when the next pregnancy occurs within the next 2 years. (Brown et al., *Stroke* 2006; Ehtisham & Stern, *The Neurologist* 2006)

305. The answer is E. Kurth et al. used data from the Women's Health Study (WHS) of almost 38,000 healthy female health professionals aged 45 years and older to look at lifestyle and weight as risk factors for stroke. A composite healthy lifestyle was associated with a significantly reduced total and ischemic stroke risk, but not hemorrhagic stroke risk. The association was apparent even after controlling for hypertension, diabetes, and elevated cholesterol. Analysis of the individual components of the healthy lifestyle showed substantial reduction of stroke risk in nonsmokers and women with lower body mass indices (BMIs). The associations with alcohol consumption and physical activity were weaker. The healthier diet paradoxically increased risk of ischemic and hemorrhagic stroke, but the overall risk outcomes were unchanged with removal of diet data. (Kurth et al., *Arch Int Med* 2006)

306. The answer is E. Approximately 21 million American women have migraine headaches, a female-predominant disorder. Migraine with aura is less common than migraine without aura, but confers increased risk of cerebral and cardiac ischemic events. The Women's Health Study (WHS) analyzed the correlation between migraine of different types and vascular events. Migraine with aura was found to increase the risk of ischemic stroke, as well as myocardial infarction, coronary revascularization, and angina. Migraine without aura and nonmigraine headaches were not associated with increased vascular risk. (Kurth et al., *JAMA* 2006)

307. The answer is E. Von Hippel-Lindau syndrome is an autosomal dominant disorder caused by deletions or mutations in a tumor-suppressor gene mapped to human chromosome 3p25. Patients develop retinal and CNS hemangioblastomas (cerebellar, spinal, and brainstem), as well as cysts of the kidneys, liver, and pancreas. Clear-cell renal cell carcinoma occurs in up to 70% of patients with von Hippel-Lindau syndrome and is a major cause of death in these patients. Pheochromocytomas may account for elevated blood pressure, and endolymphatic sac tumors can cause tinnitus or deafness. Clear-cell carcinoma of the vagina has been associated with intrauterine exposure to diethylstilbestrol. (Friedrich, *Cancer* 1999)

308. The answer is D. Thrombosis involves cerebral veins, with local effects caused by venous obstruction, and the major sinuses, which causes intracranial hypertension. In the majority of cases, thrombosis involves both veins and sinuses. Transverse sinuses are involved in 86% of cases. The superior sagittal sinus is involved in 62% of cases. The other structures listed are involved in less than 20% of cases. (Stam, *N Engl J Med* 2005)

309. The answer is A. In a review of 13,440 patients in Los Angeles, 31 patients had complete ophthalmoplegia. Miller-Fisher syndrome was diagnosed in 13 patients, and Guillain-Barré syndrome in five. There were four cases of midbrain-thalamic infarcts, one case of pituitary apoplexy, and one case of cranio-facial trauma. (Keane, *Arch Neurol* 2007)

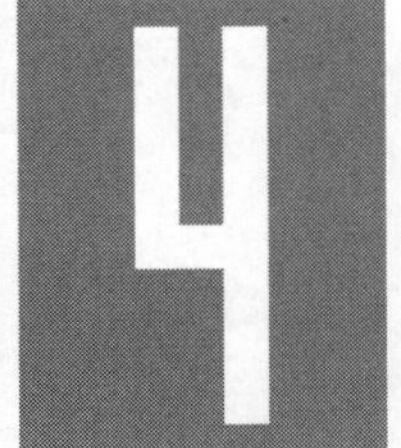

Clinical Cardiology Questions

310. The most sensitive test for a right to left intracardiac shunt with POTENTIAL embolization to the brain is:

A. Transcranial Doppler (TCD) with agitated saline contrast injection.
B. Transthoracic echocardiogram (TTE) with agitated saline contrast injection.
C. Transesophageal echocardiogram (TEE) with agitated saline contrast injection.
D. Computed tomography angiography of the chest

311. The most frequent cardiac cause of cerebral embolism is:

A. Atrial fibrillation.
B. Left ventricular thrombus.
C. Mitral stenosis.
D. Mechanical aortic valve.
E. Left atrial myxoma.

312. Which of the following is in the recommended INR range for stroke prevention in atrial fibrillation?

A. 1.8.
B. 2.2–2.8.
C. 3.0–3.5.
D. 4.0–4.5.

313. What is the approximate prevalence of patent foramen ovale (PFO) in patients with migraine with aura?

A. <10%.
B. 10%–20%.
C. 20%–40%.
D. 40%–60%.
E. 60%–70%.

314. Echocardiography laboratories are certified by the:

A. American College of Radiology (ACR).
B. Intersocietal Accreditation Commission (IAC).
C. Both the ACR and the IAC.
D. Neither the ACR nor the IAC.

315. Mitral stenosis:

A. Is almost always accompanied by atrial fibrillation.
B. Is almost always caused by rheumatic carditis.
C. Generally needs to be followed by TEE.
D. Is not a risk for infective endocarditis.

316. Before the development of the defibrillator and of coronary care units, mortality from acute myocardial infarction was:

A. 3–5%.
B. 10–12%.
C. 25–30%.
D. Above 50%.

317. Thrombolytic therapy for acute myocardial infarction was first used in:

A. 1958.
B. 1969.
D. 1988.
D. 1996.

318. Contrast used in echocardiography is composed in part of:

A. Iodine-containing substances, which cannot be given in patients with iodine allergy.
B. Xenon.
C. Gadolinium.
D. Microbubbles.

319. A 66-year-old man with a history of chronic untreated hypertension came to the emergency room with the sudden onset of severe, stabbing chest pain. His wife reported that he had fallen, with loss of consciousness for about 10 minutes, earlier that day. His blood pressure was 178/96, and he had a left ptosis with a constricted pupil. What bedside test should be performed to diagnose his condition?

A. Carotid ultrasound.
B. Electrocardiogram (ECG).
C. Transesophageal echocardiogram (TEE).
D. Transthoracic echocardiogram (TTE).
E. Chest radiograph.

320. The percentage of acute myocardial infarctions that are unrecognized is approximately:

A. 5%.
B. 15%.
C. 35%.
D. 55%.

321. According to the Framingham study, atrial fibrillation:

A. Has an age-specific prevalence higher in women than in men.
B. Is more common in African Americans than in Caucasians.
C. Is decreasing in prevalence with control of cardiovascular risk factors.
D. Is present in 9% of individuals over the age of 80.

322. The Cox-Maze III surgical protocol for prevention of atrial fibrillation:

A. Eliminates atrial fibrillation in approximately 50% of patients.
B. May eliminate the need for long-term anticoagulation.
C. Carries an operative mortality of approximately 5%.
D. Does not require the cardiopulmonary bypass pump.

323. Catheter ablation for atrial fibrillation:

A. Is most effective in chronic rather than paroxysmal atrial fibrillation.
B. Prevents atrial fibrillation in 70% and improves the response to antiarrhythmic medications in another 15% to 20%.
C. May produce pulmonary artery stenosis.
D. May produce vagal nerve injury.

324. Patients with atrial flutter:

A. Are not at risk for systemic embolization, so anticoagulation is not needed unless the patient also has atrial fibrillation.
B. Should be treated with anticoagulation both before and after cardioversion.
C. Most often have no cardiac disease or other predisposing conditions.
D. Require higher energy with electrical cardioversion than that used with atrial fibrillation.

325. Patients with Wolff-Parkinson-White (WPW) syndrome:

A. Have a shortened P-R interval.
B. Have a 3% risk of sudden death.
C. Should be treated with catheter ablation of the accessory conduction pathway.
D. Should be medically treated with β-blockers and calcium-channel blockers.

326. A long-term patient presented to the vascular neurology clinic for anticoagulation follow-up. She is in and out of atrial fibrillation and was placed on amiodarone (Pacerone) 2 months previously. A finger stick was done, and the INR was found to be 2.6. The medical assistant had her sit on the examination table and began to take her blood pressure; the patient reported feeling light-headed. She began to slump over, and the medical assistant was able to lie her down on the table with no injury. No seizure activity was seen. The physician was called immediately. By the time the physician entered the room (within 2 minutes), the patient was awake and able to speak with no problems. There was no sign of a postictal state. Neurologic exam was normal. Blood pressure was 136/72, pulse was 82 and irregularly irregular. There were no ischemic changes on the EKG, but a long QT interval was found. The most likely etiology of the syncopal event is:

A. Torsades de pointes.
B. Orthostatic hypotension
C. Sick sinus syndrome.
D. Vasovagal syncope.

327. Neurocardiogenic syncope:

A. Is caused primarily by bradycardia.
B. Is most often treated with a cardiac pacemaker.
C. Can be treated by beta blockers.
D. Can be treated with diuretics.

328. Which statement is true about precardioversion care in patients with atrial fibrillation:

A. Three to four weeks of Coumadin therapy is the only proven way to reduce the risk of embolic events during cardioversion.
B. Transesophageal echocardiography to rule out atrial thrombi can be used to avoid the need for anticoagulation.
C. Immediate cardioversion can be done if the TEE rules out atrial thrombi, but therapeutic anticoagulation should be started at the time of the TEE and maintained for 1 month.
D. Transesophageal echocardiography to rule out atrial thrombi should be reserved for patients with contraindications to anticoagulation, because patients screened with TEE have more embolic events than do those treated with anticoagulation.

329. Approximately what percentage of left atrial thrombi originate in the left atrial appendage?

A. 10%.
B. 25%.
C. 50%.
D. 75%.
E. 95%.

330. Patients with no history of atrial fibrillation who have onset of atrial fibrillation following cardiac surgery or catheter PFO closure:

A. Do not need anticoagulation, because they are not at risk for stroke.
B. Can be treated with rate control by calcium-channel blockers to avoid the need for anticoagulation.
C. Require long-term anticoagulation.
D. Generally require only short-term anticoagulation.

331. Spontaneous echo contrast ("smoke") in the left atrium:

A. Is caused by tobacco abuse.
B. Is a normal finding that is not associated with embolic events.
C. Is easily detected by TTE.
D. Is thought do be produced by stagnant blood flow.
E. Disappears with anticoagulant treatment.

332. A patient with acute onset of atrial fibrillation with a resting heart rate of 130 and shortness of breath with minor exercise (such as walking to the bathroom) should be treated with:

A. Intravenous digoxin (Lanoxin).
B. Intravenous diltiazem (Cardizem).
C. Oral verapamil (Calan).
D. Oral metoprolol (Lopressor).

333. Ablation of the atrioventricular (AV) node and permanent ventricular pacing in patients with atrial fibrillation:

A. Is associated with increased mortality when compared with patients treated medically.
B. Is associated with decreased quality of life compared with patients treated medically.
C. Reduces the need for anticoagulation.
D. Reduces the need for antiarrhythmic medications.

334. Which one of the following patients should be best treated with long-term warfarin anticoagulation?

A. A healthy 55-year-old man with two episodes of paroxysmal atrial fibrillation and a normal TEE.
B. A 66-year-old woman with two episodes of symptomatic paroxysmal atrial fibrillation and a TEE that shows mild left ventricular hypokinesis.
C. A 32-year-old woman, who is pregnant, with a past history of cerebral venous thrombosis and activated protein C resistance.
D. A 78-year-old man who had a second stroke on aspirin, with middle cerebral artery stenosis on magnetic resonance angiography (MRA).
E. An 81-year-old woman, who awoke from surgery to replace a broken femoral head, with pulmonary infiltrates and a magnetic resonance image (MRI) of the brain that showed multifocal acute infarcts.

335. Patients with atrial septal defect (ASD):

A. Generally do not need closure of the defect.
B. Should have antibiotic prophylaxis prior to dental work.
C. Are at risk for brain abscess.
D. Are generally asymptomatic.

336. Coarctation of the aorta:

A. Is not a risk for ischemic stroke.
B. May produce stroke because it is a risk factor for aortic dissection.
C. May produce stroke because it is a source of embolism.
D. Requires medical rather than surgical therapy.

337. According to the practice parameter of the American Academy of Neurology, which of the following is the preferred treatment for the prevention of recurrent stroke in patients with PFO and atrial septal aneurysm?

A. Antiplatelet medication.
B. Warfarin.
C. Surgical PFO closure.
D. Percutaneous PFO closure.
E. No preferred treatment.

338. Aortic stenosis is:

A. A major risk factor for ischemic stroke.
B. Not a risk factor for sudden death.
C. Often hereditary.
D. Most often seen in individuals with a tricuspid aortic valve.

339. Which of the following groups of potential cardiac sources of emboli contain lesions that are all considered major stroke risks?

A. Calcific aortic stenosis, mechanical mitral valve, atrial myxoma.
B. Dilated cardiomyopathy, inferior wall hypokinesis, infective endocarditis.
C. Mitral stenosis, recent anterior wall myocardial infarction, Libman-Sacks endocarditis.
D. Atrial fibrillation, mitral valve prolapse, mobile left ventricular thrombus.

340. Which of the following causes of aortic dissection is found most commonly as a cause of dissection in patients under age 40 years?

A. Marfan syndrome.
B. Turner syndrome.
C. Noonan's syndrome.
D. Ehlers-Danlos syndrome.
E. Cocaine use.

341. The ductus arteriosus is:

A. A congenital heart abnormality.
B. A connection between the pulmonary artery and the ascending aorta.
C. Also known as the foramen ovale.
D. Responsible for shunting poorly oxygenated blood to the placenta.

342. The fossa ovalis:

A. Can be seen from the right atrium.
B. Can be seen from the left atrium.
C. Is part of the interventricular septum.
D. Has a central protruding segment.

343. The left atrial appendage:

A. Is smaller than the right atrial appendage.
B. Is generally a bilobed structure.
C. Is generally a single lobed structure.
D. Is visualized adequately on transthoracic echo.

344. The most common type of ASD is:

A. An ostium primum defect.
B. An ostium secundum defect.
C. A coronary sinus defect.
D. A sinus venosus defect.

345. Lambl's excrescences are:

A. Platelet aggregates on the chordae.
B. Not a risk factor for stroke.
C. Fine fibrous strands on the nodule of Arantius or on the mitral valve.
D. Congenital.
E. An indication for chronic anticoagulation therapy.

346. Which statement is true about transthoracic (TTE) and transesophageal (TEE) echocardiography in the detection of infective endocarditis?

A. Transthoracic echocardiography and TEE have equivalent sensitivity in the detection of vegetations caused by endocarditis.
B. With clinically suspected endocarditis, TEE should be performed.
C. If TTE is normal TEE is not necessary.
D. Even with both TTE and TEE, cases of active infective endocarditis can be missed.

347. Stress echocardiography:

A. Provides useful information in the quantitation of aortic stenosis.
B. Produces adequate data on valvular heart disease and cardiac wall motion, so that TTE does not need to be performed on stroke patients who have had a recent stress echo.
C. Is always performed on a treadmill.
D. Is associated with a high risk of cardiac ischemia or arrhythmia during the test.

348. Which statement is true about ASD and echocardiography?

A. Transthoracic echocardiography will detect most ASDs.
B. Transesophageal echocardiography is needed to verify the diagnosis in just over half of patients with ASD.
C. Bidirectional shunting following contrast injection is rarely seen with ASD.
D. Long tunnels are frequently seen in connection with ASD.

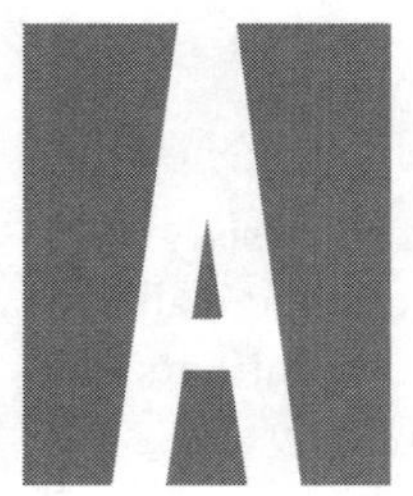

Clinical Cardiology Answers

310. The answer is A. Transcranial Doppler (TCD) with agitated saline is the most sensitive test for detecting a right-to-left shunt with potential embolization to the brain. The sensitivity of a transthoracic echocardiogram (TTE) is low for patent foramen ovale (PFO) detection. A transesophageal echocardiogram (TEE) is not quite as sensitive as TCD for the shunt, but is able to determine whether a patent foramen ovale (PFO) or an atrial septal defect (ASD) is present. Transesophageal echo also demonstrates anatomic features that may be important, such as atrial septal aneurysms, presence and size of a tunnel, and presence or absence of a Eustachian valve. Computed tomography angiography of the chest can determine if a pulmonary arteriovenous malformation is present in a patient with a right-to-left shunt on TCD, but not intracardiac shunt on TEE. (Belvis et al., *J Neuroimaging* 2006)

311. The answer is A. All the listed items can lead to cerebral embolization from the heart, but approximately half of all cardioembolic strokes are caused by atrial fibrillation. This is because of the high prevalence of atrial fibrillation, which is increasing with increased life expectancy in the population. The overall risk of ischemic stroke associated with atrial fibrillation is about 5% a year, but subpopulations, including those with prior thromboembolic event, hypertension, diabetes, and left ventricular dysfunction, have a significantly higher rate. Ventricular thrombi and rheumatic heart disease each account for approximately 10% of cardioembolic strokes, with 5% due to mechanical prosthetic mitral and aortic valves. Atrial myxomas are rare. (Ginsberg & Bogousslavsky, Chapter 103)

312. The answer is B. The recommended ranges of anticoagulation are related to the optimal intensity to prevent stroke, combined with the need to reduce risk of bleeding complications. An INR near 2.5 is recommended for patients with atrial fibrillation. An INR of 1.8 is appropriate for prevention of venous thrombus in many patients. An INR of 3 to 3.5 is recommended for patients with mechanical heart valves. An INR of 4.0 or more is associated with high bleeding complications and would rarely be appropriate for stroke prevention. (Ginsberg & Bogousslavsky, Chapter 103)

313. The answer is D. Studies on patients with migraine headaches, as defined by the International Headache Society criteria, have used TEE or TCD to diagnose PFO. Correlation depends on headache type. Patent foramen ovale has been demonstrated to be present in 40% to 60% of migraineurs with aura, compared to a prevalence of 20% to 30% in migraineurs without aura and in the general population. An association between PFO and migraine without aura has not been found in studies that examined the relationship between PFO and migraine types. Likewise migraine without aura is present in 10% of patients with PFO, a proportion similar to that expected in the general population. Migraine with aura is present in 15% to 50% of patients with PFO of any size, and is present in 45% to 60% of patients with large PFOs. The two conditions may share genetic colocalization, or a PFO may play a role in the triggering of migraine with aura. With preliminary data indicating a possible relationship between PFO closure and improvement in migraine with aura, multiple clinical trials of devices to close PFOs in migraine patients are under way. (Schwedt & Dodick, *Headache* 2006)

314. The answer is B. The Intersocietal Accreditation Commission (IAC) was initially founded to certify vascular laboratories. The Intrasocietal Commission for the Accreditation of Vascular Laboratories (ICAVL) was a cooperative effort between neurology, neurosurgery, cardiology and vascular surgery to monitor quality and certify laboratories as an alternate to the American College of Radiology (ACR). This was, in large part, politically necessary to protect nonradiology specialties involved in vascular imaging. When echocardiography was a new technique the IAC incorporated ICEAL. Cardiology maintained control of that technique, which was not certified by the ACR. Subsequently the IAC founded ICANL (Nuclear Cardiology, Nuclear Imaging, and PET Imaging), ICAMRL (MRI), and ICACTL (CT). The IAC certifies qualified neurologists who direct vascular laboratories, CT, or MRI facilities. Neurologists who own carotid duplex equipment can add a cardiac echo probe and/or a TEE probe to this equipment in order to perform echocardiography. If certified technologists are used and board certified cardiologists interpret the studies (and perform the studies in the case of TEE) ICEAL certification can be obtained for studies performed in a neurology clinic. This is convenient for patients, saves scheduling, saves clinic personnel time, and adds technical revenue for the clinic. TTE and TEE are performed at the Intermountain Stroke Center. (Intersocietal Accrediation Commission, website)

315. The answer is B. Congenital mitral stenosis and mitral stenosis from a severely calcified mitral annulus is rare. Left atrial myxomas can obstruct mitral outflow. Fifty percent of patients with severe mitral stenosis also have atrial fibrillation. Transthoracic echo with Doppler is the recommended test for evaluating the anatomy of the mitral valve and to rule out mitral valve thrombi. In cases where the TTE is not adequate, TEE is an alternative. Mitral stenosis is a significant risk for infective endocarditis. (Fuster, Chapter 67)

316. The answer is C. Close monitoring of the cardiac patient by nurses skilled in cardiac disease was initiated in 1961. The defibrillator was the first major technology to treat the potentially fatal ventricular arrhythmias that are the most dangerous complication of acute myocardial infarction. The first medical therapy for angina was amyl nitrate, followed by nitroglycerine. Both therapies were initially used in the late 19th century. (Fuster, Chapter 1)

317. The answer is A. Streptokinase administered intravenously was first used by Fletcher and Sherry in 1958. The first intracoronary infusion was in 1960. The current usage profile did not begin until the late 1970s, when intracoronary infusion and extension with IV infusion became commonplace. Intravenous tissue plasminogen activator (t-PA) for myocardial infarction was introduced in 1987. The most devastating complication was cerebral hemorrhage, leading to a delay in applying this therapy to acute stroke patients. The sentinel paper on t-PA and stroke was published in the *New England Journal of Medicine* in 1995, and the U.S. Food and Drug Administration (FDA) approved t-PA for acute stroke in 1996. (Fuster, Chapter 1)

318. The answer is D. The standard echo contrast is produced by filling 10% of a syringe with air and then adding sterile saline. With the help of a three-way stopcock, the contents of the syringe are moved back and forth between two syringes. This breaks up the air into microbubbles, which are then injected intravenously. This contrast has proven safe and effective. It is used in both echocardiography and in TCD, to detect intracardiac shunts. Iodine-containing substances are used in CT contrast. Xenon has been used in the past in some CT perfusion studies, but is no longer available because of a recent Food and Drug Administration (FDA) ruling. Iodine-based contrasts are most often used presently. Gadolinium is the standard MRI contrast. (Fuster, Chapter 15)

319. The answer is C. This man with chronic hypertension has chest pain, syncope, and a Horner syndrome, consistent with a dissection originating in the ascending aorta and propagating to the arch (type A). Up to a third of cases of aortic dissection lead to neurologic deficits, including syncope, cerebral ischemia, spinal cord ischemia, and peripheral nerve injuries. The sensitivity and specificity of TEE is much greater than that of TTE, making it preferable for the bedside diagnosis of an aortic dissection. The findings on electrocardiogram (ECG) and chest radiograph in aortic dissection are nonspecific. An MRI scan can diagnose the dissection but may not be appropriate in medically unstable patients. (Khan & Nair, *Chest* 2002)

320. The answer is C. Approximately 35% of MIs go unrecognized. Half of the unrecognized myocardial infarctions are clinically silent; the other half present with atypical symptoms that go unrecognized by patients and physicians. More than half of these patients eventually develop clinically recognizable symptoms of coronary artery disease. (Fuster, Chapter 2)

321. The answer is D. The age-specific prevalence of atrial fibrillation is higher in men than in women. The prevalence of atrial fibrillation increases with advanced age. Because women have a longer life expectancy than men, atrial fibrillation prevalence is approximately equal in men and women. African Americans have a lower incidence of atrial fibrillation, for reasons that are not understood. Although modifiable risk factors for atrial fibrillation include hypertension and diabetes, age is a very strong risk factor. The impact of the aging of the population far outweighs control of other risk factors, and the prevalence of atrial fibrillation is increasing in the United States. Currently 390 million individuals over age 65 are alive worldwide. This is projected to increase to 800 million by 2015. (Fuster, Chapter 2)

322. The answer is B. This surgical procedure includes electrical isolation of the pulmonary veins and linear ablation in the left or right atria. (There is a high prevalence of foci that trigger atrial fibrillation in pulmonary veins.) The left atrial appendage is also treated (oversewing, amputation, or ligation) to decrease the risk of future embolization. This eliminates the need for long-term anticoagulation. Atrial fibrillation is eliminated in 75% to 99% of patients undergoing this surgery. The operative mortality is less than 1%. One of the main indications for this surgery in patients who need to undergo open heart surgery for other reasons. Recurrent emboli, despite anticoagulation, is another indication for the surgery. Even though the surgical thoracic incision is relatively small, cardiopulmonary bypass is required. (Fuster, Chapter 29,)

323. The answer is B. Catheter ablation is more effective in patients with paroxysmal atrial fibrillation. Complications of the procedure include pulmonary vein stenosis, phrenic nerve injury, stroke, and pericardial tamponade. (Fuster, Chapter 29)

324. The answer is B. Anticoagulation is recommended before and after cardioversion. Although atrial fibrillation caries a much higher rate of embolization than does atrial flutter, anticoagulation is advised in atrial flutter patients who have other risk factors such as left atrial enlargement, diabetes, hypertension, or history of embolic events. Most atrial flutter patients do have predisposing medical conditions or underlying heart disease, particularly heart failure. Coexisting atrial fibrillation and atrial flutter is not uncommon. Calcium-channel blockers and β-blockers can be used to slow the rate of atrial flutter. Cardioversion of atrial flutter requires lower electrical energy than that needed for atrial fibrillation. (Fuster, Chapter 29)

325. The answer is A. Wolff-Parkinson-White (WPW) is a syndrome including atrial tachycardia and an accessory electrical pathway between the atrium and the ventricle. The hallmark of this pathway is early ventricular depolarization (pre-excitation), which shortens the P-R interval. The other electrocardiographic (EKG) change is the δ wave, which appears as a curved, gradual upstroke on the QRS complex. Palpitations are common, and syncope occurs in about a third of patients. Sudden death occurs in 0.15% to 0.39% of patients. Because 40% to 50% of these patients are asymptomatic, not all need to be treated. Catheter ablation is the treatment of choice for symptomatic patients. β-Blockers and calcium-channel blockers are generally not recommended for patients with pre-excitation. (Fuster, Chapter 30)

326. The answer is A. A long QT interval can be an inherited disorder associated with sudden death, but the most common cause of long QT syndrome is iatrogenic. Torsade de pointes is the classic arrhythmia associated with the long QT interval. It is a rapid ventricular tachycardia that oscillates above and below the line on the EKG. It can be brief, causing only presyncope, or it can cause syncope or sudden cardiac death. Several cardiac antiarrhythmic drugs can cause torsades de pointes, including amiodarone (Pacerone), disopyramide (Norpace), procainamide, quinidine, and sotalol (Betapace). Other relatively commonly noncardiac drugs, including haloperidol (Haldol), droperidol (Inapsine), methadone, and erythromycin can cause torsades. Answers B, C, and D are all common causes of syncope, but the long Q-T interval is the key in this situation. (As an interesting aside, there was a question about torsades de pointes in the first Vascular Neurology board exam. Many of us chuckled together about this "obscure" topic of which we knew nothing. In the process of writing this book and reviewing the

Hurst cardiac textbook, it becomes clear that many of our patients are on medications that precipitate this syndrome, and it behooves us to be aware of this!) (Fuster, Chapter 31)

327. The answer is C. Neurocardiogenic syncope is a common syndrome and is an abnormality of maintaining perfusion (particularly cerebral) in the upright posture. Adrenergic stimulation may be the beginning of a cascade of events that results in neurocardiogenic syncope, thus it may be potentially preventable with β-blockade. Abnormal tilt testing with isoproterenol infusion may identify those patients most likely to respond to β-blockers. Some patients have incidental bradycardia during neurocardiogenic syncope, but it is not the major cause. Pacemakers are indicated in neurocardiac syncope in those unusual cases with prolonged asystole Other potential treatments include volume expansion, anticholinergic agents (scopolamine), serotonin reuptake inhibitors, α-antagonists (midodrine), and methylxanthines (theophylline). Diuretics would likely worsen neurocardiogenic syncope. (Fuster, Chapter 40)

328. The answer is C. The Analysis of Coronary Ultrasound Thrombolysis Endpoints in Acute Myocardial Infarction (ACUTE) study looked at 1,222 patients, randomized to 2 to 3 weeks of anticoagulation versus TEE screening for atrial thrombi prior to cardioversion. There was a lower risk of bleeding in the TEE group, and there was no increase of embolic events when atrial thrombi were not seen on TEE. The standard protocol is heparin and, at the time of the TEE, switching to warfarin and maintaining therapeutic anticoagulation for 1 month. (Rosenschein et al., *Circulation* 1997)

329. The answer is C. Although the left atrial thrombi may be detected by TTE, TEE is required to reliably detect thrombi in the left atrial appendage. Thus, a normal TTE does not completely rule out a cardiac source of emboli in patients with stroke. (Fuster, Chapter 15)

330. The answer is D. Atrial fibrillation following cardiac procedures is generally transient, not requiring long-term anticoagulation. These patients are at risk for stroke, so anticoagulation is indicated temporarily. Calcium-channel blockers will control rate but, as in other patients with atrial fibrillation, they do not decrease the risk of embolization. (Fuster, Chapter 29)

331. The answer is D. The descriptive term "smoke" has been used to describe a visual phenomenon in the left atrium, which may be produced by an aggregation of red blood cells and plasma proteins. It is a risk for emboli but the appropriate therapeutic intervention is not clear. Spontaneous echo contrast is essentially unseen on TTE, requiring TEE for detection. It can still be missed if gain signals are not appropriately high. Spontaneous echo contrast does not disappear with therapeutic anticoagulation. (Fuster, Chapters 15 and 29)

332. The answer is B. In a patient with atrial fibrillation who has severe symptoms due to a rapid ventricular response, immediate rate control is necessary. This can be achieved within 5 minutes using IV verapamil, diltiazem, metoprolol, or osmolal. Intravenous digoxin does not act as quickly, so it is less useful in this setting. Oral medications are appropriate for patients with mild or moderate symptoms from rapid ventricular response. (Fuster, Chapter 29)

333. The answer is D. Atrioventricular (AV) node ablation and permanent ventricular pacing is an appropriate therapy for selected patients in atrial fibrillation following the failure of medications to control symptoms associated with a rapid ventricular rhythm. Because a prolonged ventricular rate (over 120) can lead to a tachycardia-induced cardiomyopathy, this treatment should be considered when medications are not effective. It is *not* associated with increased mortality when compared to medical therapy. In patients with low left ventricular ejection fraction, it improves the quality of life, improves exercise tolerance, and decreases the symptoms of congestive heart failure. The indication for anticoagulation remains unchanged. (Fuster, Chapter 29)

334. The answer is B. Two episodes of paroxysmal atrial fibrillation in a man younger than 60 years old without heart disease can be treated with aspirin, rather than warfarin. However, older women with paroxysmal atrial fibrillation who also have evidence of left ventricular dysfunction should be anticoagulated. Warfarin is teratogenic and should not be given during pregnancy, at least in the first trimester. Subcutaneous unfractionated heparin or low-molecular-weight heparin may be given in pregnant patients with high thrombotic risk. A recurrent ischemic event on aspirin is not an indication for anticoagulation, unless a specific indication for anticoagulation exists, such as newly discovered atrial fibrillation or a hypercoagulable state. The woman with lung and brain lesions after orthopedic surgery may have fat embolus syndrome because of the long-bone fracture, rather than a cardiac source of embolization that warrants anticoagulation. (Hirsch, *J Am Coll Cardiol* 2003)

335. The answer is C. Patients with ASD develop multiple complications, including pulmonary hypertension, pulmonary emboli, paradoxical emboli, and brain abscess. The most common cause of death is congestive heart failure. These defects should be closed, and transcatheter closure (which is approved by the

FDA) is an acceptable alternative in many patients. These patients are not symptomatic during the first 1 to 2 years of life, but become symptomatic in their teens and twenties. By the fourth decade, severe symptoms are present. Atrial septal defect is not a risk for infective endocarditis, so antibiotic treatment is not recommended prior to dental work. (Fuster, Chapter 73)

336. The answer is B. Coarctation of the aorta is a relatively common heart defect, with an aneurysmal dilatation distal to a congenital narrowing of the aorta at the level of the obliterated ductus arteriosis. Complications of coarctation of the aorta include aortic dissection and fusiform aneurysm formation in the descending thoracic aorta. Dissection is less common now that early surgical intervention is undertaken to repair the defect. (Asher, Chapter 56)

337. The answer is E. The review of the literature on the prevention of secondary stroke in patients with PFO and/or atrial septal aneurysm found that PFO alone was not associated with an increased risk, whereas the combination did seem to increase risk in young adults. Insufficient evidence was available to determine if warfarin or aspirin was preferable for medical therapy or to evaluate the different closure techniques. (Messe et al., *Neurology* 2004)

338. The answer is C. A bicuspid aortic valve, which is frequently hereditary, is a risk for development of aortic stenosis. Aortic stenosis, unlike mitral stenosis, is not a major risk factor for stroke. Aortic stenosis is associated with cardiac arrhythmias and is a risk for sudden death. (Fuster, Chapter 73)

339. The answer is C. High-risk embolic sources include mechanical aortic and mitral valves, both infective and Libman-Sacks endocarditis, mitral stenosis, atrial fibrillation, atrial myxoma, recent anterior wall myocardial infarction, dilated cardiomyopathy, and left ventricular thrombus. Minor risk sources include mitral valve prolapse, severe mitral annular calcification, calcified aortic stenosis, and focal hypokinesis without thrombus. The degree of stroke risk in young adults with PFO, with or without atrial septal aneurysm, is still unclear. (Ginsberg & Bogousslavsky, Chapter 103)

340. The answer is A. Most aortic dissections occur in men older than age 50 years and are related to chronic hypertension. However, Marfan syndrome accounts for the majority of causes of aortic dissection in patients younger than 40 years of age. Pregnancy, which may be associated with elevated blood pressure, is the most common association in women younger than 40 years old. (Khan & Nair, *Chest* 2002)

341. The answer is B. The nature of the fetal circulation is essential to the understanding of various congenital cardiac defects and intracardiac shunts, which may increase the risk of stroke. With the interest in PFO among medical professionals and the public, this knowledge is important in explaining PFO to patients.

In the fetus, the blood in the inferior vena cava (IVC), some of which has passed through the placenta and been oxygenated, has a higher oxygen saturation than the blood in the superior vena cava (SVC), which has not been oxygenated. The more highly oxygenated blood in the IVC is diverted by the crista dividends and the Eustachian valve toward the foramen ovale in the right atrium, where the blood pushes the flap of the foramen ovale open and crosses into the left atrium. This blood is then pumped into the left ventricle and to the *ascending* aorta, which perfuses particularly the coronary arteries and the brain, along with portions of the upper body. The less oxygenated blood from the SVC goes preferentially through the right atrium into the right ventricle. When it is pumped from the right ventricle into the pulmonary artery, there is very little flow into the pulmonary circulation because of the extremely high resistance of these vessels. Instead, the majority of the blood passes through the ductus arteriosus, which is a connection between the pulmonary artery and the *descending* aorta. Some of this less-oxygenated blood then goes to the placenta for reoxygenation.

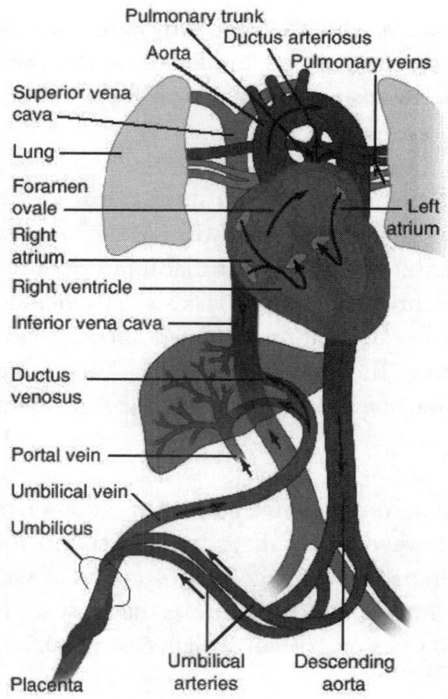

At birth, when spontaneous respirations begin, the lungs expand, and the previously constricted pulmonary arteries dilate. This causes a *decrease* in pulmonary vascular resistance. Then, when the umbilical cord is cut or clamped, fetal circulation is suddenly cut off from the placenta. This produces an *increase* in systemic vascular resistance, so blood is then unable to pass from the lower-pressure pulmonary artery to the now higher-pressure descending aorta. (The subsequent mechanism for the closing of the ductus is not completely understood.) The loss of shunting through the ductus arteriosus increases the pulmonary venous return into the left atrium. This increases left atrial pressure and pushes the flap of the foramen ovale back to the atrial septum, stopping the right-to-left shunt that operates in the fetus. (Fuster, Chapter 73)

342. The answer is A. The fossa ovalis of the interatrial septum is the anatomic hallmark of the right atrium. The limbus of the fossa ovalis is the muscular, horseshoe-shaped outer portion, with a central depressed area that is the valve of the fossa ovalis. The limbus is thick walled, and the valve is thin. The foramen ovale is the potential space between the limbus and the valve. (Chan, *Br Heart J* 1993)

343. The answer is A. At least 80% of left atrial appendages are multilobed, with up to four 4 lobes. The anatomic variants of the left atrial appendage were not appreciated until the advent of TEE. It is important that all lobes of the left atrial appendage be examined by TEE, to avoid overlooking a thrombus as a potential source of cardiogenic emboli. (Pollick and Taylor, *Circulation* 1991)

344. The answer is B. During fetal development, the two atria of the heart are separated by the septum primum, which has an opening, the ostium primum, connecting the two atria. The septum primum develops a second opening, the ostium secundum, which forms before the ostium primum closes. When the septum secundum grows over the ostium secundum, the foramen ovale is the only residual connection between the two atria. The most common ASD is the ostium secundum defect. The coronary sinus defect and the venous sinus defect are much less common. (Fuster, Chapter 73)

345. The answer is C. Lambl's excrescences are fibrous strands, not related to the chordae or to platelet aggregates. They may be a risk factor for stroke but the appropriate therapy is unclear. They are not congenital, but are age-related changes. (Magerey, *J Pathol Bacteriol* 2005)

346. The answer is D. Transesophageal echocardiography is more sensitive than TTE in the diagnosis of endocarditis. Many cases will be detected by TTE, so the less invasive and less expensive test is the preferred initial test. If TTE is negative, TEE should be performed, because additional cases may be detected. Even when both TTE and TEE are done, some vegetations may be missed, particularly in association with valvular abnormalities, such as calcification, which can obscure small vegetations. This remains a clinical diagnosis, with blood cultures remaining an integral part of the diagnostic investigation. Occasionally, multiple blood cultures must be obtained. (Fuster, Chapter 15)

347. The answer is A. Stress echo is performed with either exercise or pharmacologic stress. Under either stress, areas of decreased cardiac wall motion are predictive of coronary artery insufficiency. Stress echocardiography is useful in assessing mitral and aortic stenosis, but TTE is preferable in evaluating most valvular disease, because it is not subject to the patient movement and time constraints inherent in stress echocardiography The risk of cardiac ischemia and arrhythmia during the test is fortunately quite low. (Fuster, Chapter 15)

348. The answer is A. Most ASDs are easily detected on TTE. The exception is the sinus venous defects, which often require TEE. The ASD is frequently associated with bidirectional shunting. Tunnels are a feature associated with PFO rather than ASD. (Fuster, Chapter 40)

5 Clinical Hematology Questions

349. Lupus anticoagulant (LA):

A. Is associated with a decrease in the partial thromboplastin time (PTT).
B. Is associated with an increase in the PTT, which corrects with the addition of fresh frozen plasma.
C. Occurs only in patients with discoid or systemic lupus erythematosus (SLE).
D. Is frequently accompanied by elevations of immunoglobulin (Ig)-G anticardiolipin antibodies.
E. None of the above.

350. Antiphospholipid syndrome (APS):

A. Can be diagnosed based on laboratory criteria alone.
B. Can be associated with elevated levels of anti-β_2 glycoprotein-1.
C. Requires only one positive assay of an elevated antiphospholipid level for diagnosis.
D. Causes fetal loss only prior to the 10th week of gestation.
E. All of the above.

351. Which of the following treatments is most often indicated in the primary prevention of stroke in children with sickle cell disease (SCD)?

A. Antiplatelet medications.
B. Warfarin.
C. Chronic transfusions.
D. Bone marrow transplantation.
E. Hydroxyurea.

352. Which statement best describes antiphospholipid syndrome (APS)?

A. Antiphospholipid syndrome is associated with a reduced incidence of cardiac valvular disease in SLE patients.
B. Ischemic arterial stroke is the most common clinical manifestation of primary APS.
C. Antiphospholipid syndrome is rarely associated with ischemic stroke in patients without SLE.
D. Patients with APS are at increased risk of cerebral venous thrombosis (CVT).
E. Chorea is more frequent in patients with SLE than in patients with APS.

353. Which of the following statements applies to LA?

A. Lupus anticoagulant correlates better with thrombosis in SLE than does anticardiolipin antibody.
B. Testing for LA includes activated partial thromboplastin time (aPTT)-based assays and dilute Russell's viper venom time (dRVVT).
C. Either aPTT or dRVVT with correction suffices for LA positivity.
D. Testing can be run on a blood sample with an INR <3.5.
E. All of the above.

354. Ristocetin induces platelet activity and is useful for the diagnosis of:

A. Elevated platelet counts.
B. Von Willebrand's disease.
C. Hemophilia.
D. Therapeutic blood levels of aspirin.

355. The PTT:

A. Is elevated only in patients with LA or on heparin therapy.
B. Is strongly influenced by the levels of tissue factor and factor VII.
C. Is a test of the intrinsic and common pathways of clotting.
D. Is not a predictor of a hypercoagulable state when the value is low.

356. The prothrombin time (PT):

A. Measures only the extrinsic coagulation pathway.
B. Requires contact or chemical activation.
C. Is affected by platelet levels.
D. Is very sensitive to low levels of factor VII and X.
E. Is most sensitive to low levels of prothrombin.

357. Vitamin K–dependent clotting factors include:

A. Prothrombin and factors VII and X.
B. Prothrombin and factors VIII, XI, and XII.
C. Fibrinogen and factors VIII, XI, and XII.
D. Prothrombin, fibrinogen, and factor VIII.

358. Thrombotic thrombocytopenic purpura (TTP):

A. Presents with thrombocytopenia, hemolytic anemia, and hemorrhage.
B. Presents with thrombocytopenia, hemolytic anemia, and small-vessel occlusions.
C. Does not produce neurologic signs and symptoms.
D. Occurs with increased frequency in patients with SLE.

359. Thrombotic thrombocytopenic purpura is treated with:

A. Platelet inhibition.
B. Platelet transfusion.
C. Corticosteroids.
D. Exchange plasmapheresis.

360. Essential thrombocytosis:

A. May cause both arterial and venous occlusions in the brain.
B. Cannot be treated with platelet inhibition because of the risk of increased bleeding time and hemorrhage.
C. Is associated with the Philadelphia chromosome.
D. Is generally accompanied by polycythemia.

361. Which of the following is most often a cause of hypercoagulability?

A. Protein C deficiency.
B. Von Willebrand's disease.
C. Factor V Leiden mutation.
D. Prothrombin G20210A gene mutation.
E. Antithrombin III deficiency.

362. Protein C deficiency:

A. Produces a clinical hypercoagulable state in almost all individuals with this trait.
B. Is an indication for lifetime anticoagulation in patients presenting with deep venous thrombosis (DVT).
C. Is a risk for acute tissue necrosis in patients beginning Coumadin (warfarin) therapy.
D. Can be diagnosed in patients taking warfarin.

363. Activated protein C resistance (APC-R) is:

A. Diagnostic of factor V Leiden mutation.
B. Associated with protein C deficiency.
C. May be caused by antiphospholipid antibodies.
D. Associated with antithrombin III deficiency.

364. Factor V Leiden mutation:

A. Is inherited in an autosomal recessive fashion.
B. Is most common in individuals of Asian or African descent.
C. Is an indication for lifetime anticoagulation in individuals presenting with any thrombotic event.
D. Is associated with cerebral venous thrombosis.
E. Is not a risk factor for arterial thrombosis.

365. When initiating warfarin therapy in patients on heparin:

A. Therapeutic anticoagulation will not be achieved sooner by giving loading doses.
B. Heparin can be discontinued when the INR reaches 2.5.
C. Patients should be counseled to avoid vitamin K–containing food.
D. Warfarin loads cannot be administered.

366. A 67-year-old man presented to the neurology clinic with a complaint of severe headache and a rushing sound in his ears for 2 weeks He had the acute onset of imbalance noted an hour ago. His face was ruddy, and he was bald. On funduscopic examination, his retinal veins were engorged and mild papilledema was present. His gait was wide-based with a tendency to veer to the left. The most important test to diagnose this patient's underlying disorder is:

A. Complete blood counts with differential and platelet count.
B. Metabolic panel.
C. Antinuclear antibody (ANA) titer.
D. Fibrinogen level.

367. The most effective immediate treatment to prevent stroke in the patient described in Question 366 is:

A. Corticosteroids.
B. Platelet inhibition.
C. Hydroxyurea.
D. Interferon-α.
E. Phlebotomy.

368. Heparin-induced thrombocytopenia (HIT):

A. Is an immune mediated drug reaction initiated by antibodies directed against the platelet glycoprotein IIb/IIIa receptor.
B. Does not warrant discontinuation of clinically indicated heparin.
C. Is associated with both arterial and venous thrombosis.
D. Is more common with low-molecular-weight heparin than with unfractionated heparin.
E. Requires the use of warfarin for anticoagulation.

369. Argatroban, dabigatran, and hirudin:

A. Inhibit the tissue factor–factor VIIa complex.
B. Inactivate cofactors Va and VIIIa.
C. Target factor Xa and thrombin.
D. Inactivate fibrin-bound thrombin.
E. Inhibit the platelet glycoprotein IIb/IIIa receptor.

370. The most appropriate anticoagulation treatment for patients with a history of HIT is:

A. Intravenous unfractionated heparin.
B. Subcutaneous unfractionated heparin.
C. Subcutaneous enoxaparin (Lovenox).
D. Intravenous argatroban (Novastatin).
E. Oral anticoagulation with dabigatran.

371. Aspirin resistance:

A. Is defined as the failure of aspirin to inhibit platelet thromboxane A_2 production.
B. Is determined by reproducible laboratory testing with defined sensitivity and specificity.
C. Has a single etiologic mechanism, which explains aspirin treatment failure.
D. Is defined by a clear cut-off in platelet responsiveness.
E. Is easily recognized and treated.

372. What is the most common inherited bleeding disorder?

A. Von Willebrand's disease.
B. Bernard-Soulier's syndrome.
C. Hemophilia A.
D. Hemophilia B.
E. Christmas' disease.

373. Factor V Leiden and prothrombin G20210A gene mutations:

A. Are strong risk factors for ischemic arterial stroke in young people.
B. Increase the risk of ischemic stroke in patients with atrial fibrillation.
C. May increase the risk of venous thrombosis in women on oral contraceptives.
D. In combination do not increase the risk of venous thrombosis.
E. All of the above.

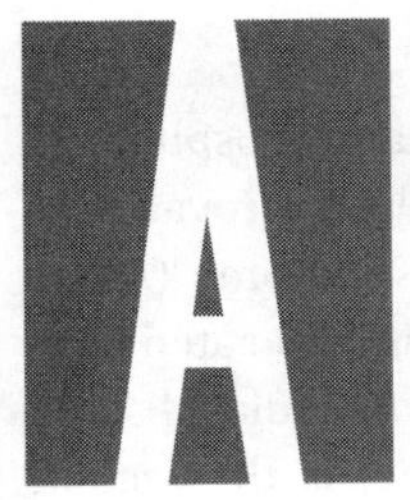

Clinical Hematology
Answers

349. The answer is D. Lupus anticoagulant (LA) and anticardiolipin antibodies are overlapping groups of antiphospholipid antibodies. They were first identified in patients with systemic lupus erythematosus (SLE), but occur frequently in patients with no evidence of lupus. The diagnosis of LA is made when the PTT is elevated and fails to correct with the addition of fresh frozen plasma. Because this is exactly the laboratory picture seen in patients on heparin, LA was initially called a "circulating anticoagulant." Lupus anticoagulant is now known to be associated with risk of thrombus formation. (Bertolaccini & Hughes, *Rheum Dis Clin North Am* 2006)

350. The answer is B. Published classification criteria for APS dictate at least one clinical and one laboratory criteria. The clinical criteria are either objective evidence of arterial or venous thrombosis and/or fetal loss or prematurity due to vascular disease. The fetal loss can be one fetal death beyond 10 weeks or three sequential spontaneous abortions before the 10th week. The laboratory criteria are based on the presence of LA, or elevated levels of anticardiolipin antibody, or anti-β_2 glycoprotein-1. There should be two positive assays of elevated titers or presence of LA, separated by 6 to 12 weeks, to avoid misclassification of an ephemeral laboratory finding. (Miyakis et al., *J Thromb Haemost* 2006)

351. The answer is C. In the Stroke Prevention Trial in Sickle Cell Anemia (STOP) study, children with mean blood flow velocities of ≥200 cm/sec on transcranial Doppler were randomized to either regular blood transfusions or to no transfusions. Transfusion lowered hemoglobin S levels to less than 30%. There was a 90% reduction in first stroke with transfusions. Hydroxyurea is being studied in children with SCD. No specific recommendations exist on the use of anticoagulants and antiplatelet medications. Data is limited on the use of bone marrow transplantation in stroke prevention in children with SCD. (Mehta & Adams, *Curr Treat Opt Neurol* 2006)

352. The answer is D. Anticardiolipin antibodies and LA are antiphospholipid antibodies (aPL) that are associated with venous thrombosis and cerebrovascular disease. Elevated levels of aPLs are found in antiphospholipid syndrome (APS), which is divided into primary or secondary APS. Secondary APS is associated with connective tissue disease, most frequently SLE. Ischemic cerebrovascular disease (strokes, transient ischemic attack [TIA], multi-infarct dementia) is the second most common clinical manifestation of primary APS, after venous thrombosis. Cardiac emboli, especially from left-sided valvular disease, can cause cerebral ischemia in patients with APS. The brain magnetic resonance imaging (MRI) of patients with APS may show evidence of either large- or small-vessel disease, as well as nonspecific white matter changes. Most studies indicate that elevated levels of aPLs are associated with an increased risk of ischemic stroke, independent of SLE. Central venous thrombosis (CVT) is seen infrequently in patients with APS, as well as in other hypercoagulable states. Chorea is more frequent in patients with primary APS than in patients with SLE. Antiphospholipid syndrome associated chorea is bilateral. The acute onset of unilateral chorea in patients with APS is generally due to cerebrovascular disease. (Sanna et al., *Rheumatology* 2003)

353. The answer is E. Lupus anticoagulant correlates better with thrombosis, pregnancy morbidity, and thrombosis in SLE patients than does anticardiolipin antibody. Testing for LA includes activated partial thromboplastin time (aPTT)-based assays and dilute Russell's viper venom time (dRVVT), with one of the two tests positive needed to rule in LA and both tests negative needed to rule out LA. The aPTT used for LA testing should be LA-sensitive, with a heparin neutralizer or measurement of the thrombin time, to exclude the inadvertent presence of heparin. Laboratory testing for APS requires two positive assays for LA or anticardiolipin antibodies separated in time by at least 12 weeks. Also, with APS based on the presence of either LA or anticardiolipin antibodies, both laboratory and clinical criteria must be satisfied. Testing for LA can be run on a blood sample with an INR of <3.5 if it is diluted 1:2 with normal plasma before the test is performed. (Miyakis et al. *J Thromb Haemost* 2006)

354. The answer is B. Ristocetin is an antibiotic that induces platelet aggregation in vitro. Activity of von Willebrand factor (vWF) in plasma is determined by the ability of the patient's plasma to support ristocetin-induced agglutination of normal formalin-fixed platelets. Reduced levels are characteristic of von Willebrand's disease, in which factor VIII levels are usually reduced proportionately. Falsely elevated values may occur with inflammation, pregnancy, or estrogen therapy. The other answers are distractors, because the use of ristocetin is specific for von Willebrand's disease. (Greer et al., Chapter 51)

355. The answer is C. The intrinsic pathway of activation of the coagulation cascade includes factors VIII, IX, XI, and XII, along with prekallikrein, phospholipids, and high-molecular-weight kininogen. The common pathway includes phospholipids, factors V and X, prothrombin, and fibrinogen. Because the intrinsic pathway requires contact activation, various methods of activation are used in performing this assay. Originally, the glass tube provided the contact activation, but now ellagic acid or kaolin produces better and more standard activation. The PTT is elevated in patients with lupus anticoagulant or those who are on heparin therapy, but it can also be elevated in patients with factor deficiencies, particularly factors VIII and IX. Factor VII, along with tissue factor, belongs to the extrinsic pathway and does not influence the PTT. A low PTT is indeed an independent predictor of a hypercoagulable state. (Greer et al., Chapter 51)

356. The answer is D. The prothrombin time (PT) measures the activity of the extrinsic and common pathways of coagulation. The extrinsic pathway includes tissue factor and factor VII. The common pathway includes phospholipids, factors V and X, prothrombin, and fibrinogen. Although the name of the test may incorrectly suggest that the test is most sensitive to prothrombin, the test is actually most sensitive to low levels of factors VII and X. The test is not affected by platelet levels. Unlike the PTT, the PT requires no activation. (Greer et al., Chapter 51)

357. The answer is A. The vitamin K–dependent factors, which are decreased by warfarin (Coumadin) and related agents, include prothrombin and factors VII, and X. Fibrinogen and factors VIII, XI, and XII are not vitamin K–dependent factors. (Greer et al., Chapter 51)

358. The answer is B. Fever is also present in 50% of thrombotic thrombocytopenic purpura (TTP) patients. Many of the clinical manifestations of this disorder are caused by diffuse microangiopathic thrombotic occlusions, which can occur in the brain, kidney, and other organs. Idiopathic thrombocytopenic purpura (ITP) is frequently associated with lupus, but TTP is not. Thrombotic thrombocytopenic purpura has been associated with thienopyridine, generally ticlopidine, use. (Greer et al., Chapter 54)

359. The answer is D. Although platelet inhibition and steroids are often used, their benefit is uncertain. Platelet transfusion is contraindicated, because it is associated with worsening of renal function and neurologic complications. (Greer et al., Chapter 54)

360. The answer is A. Essential thrombocytosis is *not* accompanied by polycythemia or the Philadelphia chromosome, both of which are features of polycythemia vera. Aspirin is useful in reducing the symptoms of cerebral microthrombosis. Aspirin does increase the bleeding time more in patients with essential thrombocytosis than in normal patients, but it is considered the treatment of choice in some patients with essential thrombocytosis, particularly in those with erythromelalgia. (Greer et al., Chapter 57)

361. The answer is C. Factor V Leiden is present in 3% to 7% of the general population, whereas the other hypercoagulable factors are present in 3% or less of the general population. Elevated anticardiolipin antibodies are also common, being present in 2% to 7% of the population, and mild homocystinemia is present in 5% to 10 % of the general population. When evaluating patients presenting with a first venous thromboembolism, factor V Leiden, hyperhomocysteinemia, LA, factor VIII elevation, and elevated anticardiolipin antibodies are each found in excess of 10% of these patients. Similar data are not available related to patients presenting with stroke or TIA. Von Willebrand's disease is not a hypercoagulable state, but produces excess hemorrhage. (Greer et al., Chapter 61)

362. The answer is C. Warfarin-induced skin necrosis occurs rarely in patients who are not on parenteral anticoagulation when started on large doses of warfarin. Protein C levels are reduced by warfarin before the vitamin K–dependent procoagulant factors, resulting in a worsening of the protein C–induced hypercoagulable state. As warfarin reduces protein C levels, protein C deficiency cannot be diagnosed in a patient on warfarin. Many patients with protein C deficiency are asymptomatic and do not require specific treatment. The recommendation for warfarin therapy is 3 to 6 months following a first deep venous thrombosis (DVT). If recurrent DVT or life-threatening thrombosis occurs, lifetime warfarin should be considered. (Greer et al., Chapter 61)

363. The answer is C. Ninety-two percent of individuals with activated protein C resistance (APC-R) have factor V Leiden mutation. Because APC-R testing is less expensive than is polymerase chain reaction (PCR) for factor V Leiden, it is the recommend screening test. Pregnancy, oral contraceptives, cancer, certain antiphospholipid antibodies, and other factors can also cause APC-R, so confirmation by PCR for factor V Leiden mutation is necessary. Activated protein C resistance is sensitive but not specific. Patients with negative APC-R do not require PCR for factor V Leiden. Activated protein C resistance is not associated with protein C deficiency or with antithrombin III deficiency. (Greer et al., Chapter 61)

364. The answer is D. Factor V Leiden mutation is associated with a two- to tenfold lifetime increase in the risk of venous thromboembolism. Although there is a notable absence of association with arterial thrombi, it is a risk factor for myocardial infarction in young women, particularly in smokers. This mutation is most common in individuals of European descent, and it is rare in those of Asian and African descent. The inheritance is autosomal dominant, similar to most other hypercoagulable states. Factor V Leiden is not an indication for lifetime anticoagulation after a thrombotic event, unless multiple events or one severe life-threatening event occurs. (Greer et al., Chapter 61)

365. The answer is A. Factor VII has a half-life of only 4 to 6 hours. Loading doses will produce a more rapid fall in factor VII and an increased PT, but therapeutic anticoagulation is not reached until other factors with longer half-lives are also affected. Although the warfarin-induced tissue necrosis may be prevented by heparin, therapeutic anticoagulation is not reached earlier with loading doses. Even without warfarin load, the PT may increase after only 1 day of warfarin, but therapeutic anticoagulation requires a minimum of 4 to 5 days. Thus, heparin should be continued for 4 to 5 days after the initiation of warfarin therapy, even when the INR reaches standard therapeutic levels within a shorter time frame. (Greer et al., Chapter 54)

366. The answer is A. This patient has the classic clinical presentation for polycythemia vera. The hallmark of this disorder is an elevated hematocrit. Frequently, elevated leukocyte and platelet counts also will be present. Patients have facial rubor, leading to a complexion described as "ruddy." Neurologic symptoms include headache, vertigo, visual disturbances, focal neurologic deficits, and seizures. Retinal vascular engorgement and papilledema may occur because of sludging. A metabolic panel and an ANA will be of no help in making the appropriate diagnosis, although spurious elevation of potassium levels may occur with this disorder. Fibrinogen consumption can occur, with a corresponding decrease of fibrinogen, but a fibrinogen level is not diagnostic for polycythemia vera. (Greer et al., Chapter 85)

367. The answer is E. Phlebotomy has the advantage of immediately lowering the red cell mass. Some patients can be treated with repeated phlebotomy alone. When phlebotomy does not adequately control the disorder, hydroxyurea is the most widely used treatment of polycythemia vera. Interferon-α is another effective agent. Steroids are of no value. Platelet inhibition has been studied, in combination with phlebotomy, to reduce the incidence of thrombotic complications of polycythemia vera, with conflicting results, but there has been no study of platelet inhibition alone. (Greer et al., Chapter 85)

368. The answer is C. Heparin-induced thrombocytopenia (HIT), an immune-mediated drug reaction, is caused by antibodies against complexes of platelet factor 4 (PF4) and heparin. It presents with a low platelet count (<150,000 per cubic millimeter or a relative decrease of >50% of baseline) in patients on parenteral heparin. Heparin-induced thrombocytopenia is about ten times more common with unfractionated heparin than with low-molecular-weight heparin. Arterial or venous thrombotic complications develop in 20% to 50% of patients with HIT. The mortality of HIT related thrombosis is high, and heparin therapy should be discontinued when HIT is diagnosed. When HIT is diagnosed by serologic or functional assays, the patient can be parenterally anticoagulated with direct thrombin inhibitors or heparinoids. (Arepally & Ortel, *N Engl J Med* 2006; Pohl et al., *Neurology* 2005)

369. The answer is D. The coagulation system is triggered by the formation of the tissue factor–factor VIIa complex at the site of vascular injury. Drugs that block this complex are potent anticoagulants, but are still under development. Propagation of the thrombus occurs when factor IXa binds to its cofactor VIIIa, to form a complex that activates factor X. Factor Xa binds to its cofactor Va to form prothrombinase, which converts prothrombin to thrombin. Thrombin generation is blocked by drugs targeting these propagating coagulation factors. Thrombin activates platelet-bound factor XI, promoting factor Xa generation. In the final step of coagulation, thrombin converts fibrinogen to fibrin. Low-molecular-weight heparin and unfractionated heparin are indirect thrombin inhibitors that catalyze natural thrombin inhibitors but do not act against fibrin-bound thrombin. The parenteral direct thrombin inhibitors, hirudin, argatroban, and bivalirudin, inactivate fibrin-bound thrombin directly with a more predictable anticoagulation action than do the indirect inhibitors. The only approved thrombin inhibitors are parenteral (as of 2007), although oral agents are being investigated in clinical trials. Dabigatran is an oral direct thrombin inhibitor being studied for the prevention of stroke in patients with atrial fibrillation. Fibrin interacts with the platelet at the glycoprotein IIb/IIIa receptor to form a cross-linking platelet–fibrin network. (Weitz & Bates, *J Thromb Haemost* 2005)

370. The answer is D. Patients who develop HIT and continue to need anticoagulation should be treated with the intravenous direct thrombin inhibitor argatroban (Novastatin). The oral direct thrombin inhibitor dabigatran is still being tested for safety and efficacy and is not yet approved for clinical use. Unfractionated heparin, low-molecular weight-heparin, and glycoprotein IIb/IIIa inhibitors should not be used in patients with HIT. (DiNiso, *N Engl J Med* 2005)

371. The answer is A. Aspirin resistance is the inability of aspirin to reduce the platelet activation and aggregation initiated by the production of thromboxane A_2. The correlation of the laboratory measure of resistance to the clinical outcome of reduction of vascular events is under investigation, as are the therapeutic options when an aspirin treatment failure occurs. Multiple etiologies for aspirin treatment failure range from medication noncompliance to many causes of platelet alteration. No standard, reproducible laboratory measure of the antiplatelet effects of aspirin exists, although methods exist to measure thromboxane production and thromboxane-dependent platelet function. Resistance to the antiplatelet effects of clopidogrel is also being investigated, but as with aspirin, the clinical relevance is as yet uncertain. (Hankey & Eikelboom, *Lancet* 2006; Helgason et al. *Stroke* 1994)

372. The answer is A. Von Willebrand's disease, the most common inherited bleeding disorder, is caused by a quantitative (type 1 and 3) or qualitative (type 2) defect of vWF. Patients are treated with desmopressin or plasma concentrates containing factor VIII and vWF. Bernard-Soulier's syndrome, along with May-Hegglin's anomaly and gray platelet syndrome, is an inherited giant-platelet disorder characterized by abnormally large platelets, thrombocytopenia, and bleeding tendency. Hemophilia A (a deficiency of factor VIII) is more common than hemophilia B (a deficiency of factor IX), which is also known as Christmas' disease, named after the first patient diagnosed with this deficiency during the 1950s. (Franchini, *Hematology* 2005; Hayward et al., *Haemophilia* 2006; Peyvandi et al., *Haemophilia* 2006)

373. The answer is C. Although different studies show some variability in results, these gene mutations do not appear to be strong risk factors for ischemic arterial stroke, either in young people or in patients with atrial fibrillation. Although some association exists with ischemic stroke in patients with PFO, this may relate to their propensity for venous thrombosis. Although these mutations have differing risk of venous thrombosis, more with factor V Leiden and prothrombin than with methylenetetrahydrofolate reductase, in combination, the risk is additive. (Almawi et al., *J Thromb Thrombolysis* 2005; Berge et al., *Stroke* 2007; Lopaciuk et al., *Clin Appl Thromb Hemost* 2001; Wu et al., *Thromb Haemost* 2005)

6 Clinical Pediatrics Questions

374. Causes of embolic stroke in children include:

A. Atrial fibrillation and atrial myxoma.
B. Infective endocarditis and orbital infections.
C. Patent foramen ovale (PFO) and cavernous sinus thrombosis.
D. Fat emboli and leukemia.

375. Which of the following is the most common cause of arterial (nonvenous) ischemic stroke in children?

A. Sickle cell disease.
B. Moyamoya syndrome.
C. Cardiac disease.
D. Mitochondrial encephalomyopathy lactic acidosis and stroke-like symptoms (MELAS).
E. Homocystinuria.

376. Tangier disease:

A. Is named after a city in northern Morocco where the disorder was initially discovered.
B. Is associated with atrophic tonsils in children.
C. Is caused by mutations in the adenosine triphosphate (ATP)-binding cassette transporter A1 (ABCA1).
D. Confers increased vascular risk due to very high levels of triglycerides.
E. Is rarely associated with peripheral neuropathy.

377. Arterial dissection leading to ischemic stroke in children:

A. Rarely if every occurs.
B. Has a male predominance explained by more head and neck trauma with boys.
C. Is most commonly intracranial when it occurs in the anterior circulation.
D. Occurs most commonly at the origin of the vertebral artery when it occurs in the posterior circulation.
E. Rarely if ever recurs.

378. Arteriovenous malformations (AVMs) in children:

A. Rarely bleed.
B. Are rarely associated with migraine-type headaches.
C. Produce a cranial bruit in 10% of cases.
D. May cause high-output congestive heart failure.
E. Are associated with alternating hemiplegia of childhood.

379. Cerebral aneurysms presenting as subarachnoid hemorrhage (SAH) in childhood:

A. Are responsible for 5% to 10% of all SAHs.
B. Are generally located in the circle of Willis.
C. Have a higher morbidity and mortality than in adults.
D. Can occur in children under 1 year of age.

380. Alternating hemiplegia of childhood:

A. Is inherited in an autosomal recessive pattern.
B. Starts generally at age 5 to 7 years.
C. Is associated with episodes of hemiparesis that last minutes to weeks and resolve spontaneously.
D. Usually has a benign prognosis.
E. Is more common during sleep.

381. What percentage of neonates with ischemic stroke have prothrombotic risk factors, including factor V Leiden mutation, factor II mutation (prothrombin 20210 gene mutation), methylenetetrahydrofolate reductase (MTHFR) mutation, elevated lipoprotein (a) (Lp(a)), decreased antithrombin III, decreased proteins C or S, or elevated anticardiolipin antibodies?

A. Under 5%.
B. 20–30%.
C. 50–60%.
D. 75–85%.

382. Periventricular leukomalacia on magnetic resonance imaging (MRI) in infants and children:

A. Does not occur, because this is a disorder that occurs exclusively with aging.
B. Is associated with prematurity.
C. Is almost always associated with hemorrhage.
D. Is an uncommon finding in children with spastic diplegia.

383. In premature infants:

A. The incidence of intracranial hemorrhage is 60% to 80%.
B. Subependymal hemorrhage is most often related to forceps delivery.
C. Intracranial hemorrhage most often occurs prenatally.
D. Intracranial hemorrhage occurs most often in the first 4 days of life.

384. Subdural hemorrhage in newborns:

A. Occurs in term infants, not in premature infants.
B. May cause hemiparesis.
C. Is most often clinically evident.
D. Is easily differentiated from intracerebellar hemorrhage by computed tomography (CT) scan.

385. Intracerebellar hemorrhage in newborns:

A. Occurs almost always in term infants.
B. Occurs almost always in premature infants.
C. Can be diagnosed by cranial ultrasonography.
D. Is not treated surgically.

386. What is the most common presentation of cerebral venous thrombosis (CVT) in neonates?

A. Lethargy.
B. Seizures.
C. Poor feeding.
D. Weight loss.
E. Respiratory distress.

387. A 10-year-old boy presented with an ischemic stroke and fever. He had an erythematous rash on his trunk and multiple enlarged lymph nodes. His MRI showed small old hemorrhages as well as a new MCA infarct. What diagnosis should be considered?

A. Malignant atrophic papulosis.
B. Sneddon syndrome.
C. Kawasaki syndrome.
D. Epidermal nevus syndrome.
E. Diffuse meningocerebral angiomatosis and leukoencephalopathy.

388. The most common hemorrhagic cerebrovascular disorder in infants is:

A. Periventricular hemorrhage.
B. Subarachnoid hemorrhage.
C. Subdural hematoma.
D. Lobar hemorrhage.

389. Perinatal ischemic stroke:

A. Most commonly occurs in the left MCA territory.
B. Rarely presents with neonatal seizures.
C. Is always symptomatic at birth.
D. Is rarely associated with thrombophilias.
E. Almost always has an unfavorable outcome.

390. In the United States, which stroke type most commonly causes death in children?

A. Intracerebral hemorrhage.
B. Subarachnoid hemorrhage.
C. Ischemic stroke (arterial).
D. Cerebral venous thrombosis.

391. Which statement is true about stroke mortality in individuals under age 20?

A. Although stroke mortality has been decreasing in adults over the last few decades, it is increasing in children.
B. More boys than girls die from SAH and ICH, but mortality from ischemic stroke is equivalent in boys and girls.
C. More deaths occur from stroke in white children as compared with black children.
D. Sickle cell disease is the main cause of fatal stroke in black children.

392. Which one of the following children is most likely to develop Moyamoya syndrome after treatment of the underlying disease?

A. A 7-year-old girl with neurofibromatosis type 1 (NF1) and an optic nerve glioma with progressive tumor following chemotherapy.
B. A 16-year-old boy with a pineal teratoma.
C. A 4-year-old girl with acute lymphocytic leukemia and malignant cells in the spinal fluid.
D. A 2-year-old girl with enucleation for a left eye retinoblastoma who has developed tumors in the right eye.

393. Which statement about Varicella zoster virus (VZV) infection and stroke in children under age 12 is true?

A. Varicella predisposes to stroke by producing a hypercoagulable state.
B. Varicella can produce a vasculopathy, probably from varicella zoster virus in the arterial wall.
C. Varicella predisposes to stroke by causing a severe cardiomyopathy.
D. Varicella causes Moyamoya syndrome.

394. Which of the following is the most common risk factor for venous and arterial thrombosis in children?

A. Congenital heart disease.
B. Hyperhomocysteinemia.
C. Dehydration.
D. Catheterization.
E. Factor V Leiden mutation.

395. Which test is essential in the evaluation of a child with suspected primary central nervous system (CNS) vasculitis?

A. Computed tomography scan of the brain with contrast.
B. Electroencephalography (EEG).
C. C-reactive protein (C-RP).
D. Cerebrospinal fluid (CSF) varicella zoster virus immunoglobulin (Ig)-M titer.
E. Brain biopsy.

396. Which is the most common cause of intraparenchymal hemorrhage in children?

A. Arteriovenous malformation.
B. Cavernous malformation.
C. Hematologic disease.
D. Aneurysm.
E. Intracranial tumor.

397. Which organism is associated with Lemierre syndrome, a rare cause of cavernous sinus thrombosis and internal carotid artery stenosis in children?

A. *Fusobacterium necrophorum.*
B. *Mycobacterium massiliense.*
C. *Enterobacter sakazakii.*
D. *Cunninghamella bertholletiae.*
E. *Nocardia brasiliensis.*

398. Which of the following is the most common CNS abnormality associated with posterior fossa malformations, hemangiomas, arterial anomalies, coarctation of the aorta and other cardiac defects, and eye abnormalities (PHACE syndrome)?

A. Arachnoid cyst.
B. Cerebellar hypoplasia.
C. Dandy-Walker malformation.
D. Absent cerebellar vermis.
E. Optic nerve hypoplasia.

399. Which congenital cutaneovascular syndrome is characterized by multiple intracranial arterial and venous CNS malformations?

A. Neurofibromatosis.
B. Osler-Weber-Rendu disease.
C. Ehlers Danlos syndrome.
D. Sturge-Weber syndrome.
E. Marfan syndrome.

400. Which statement is true about the use of thrombolysis in children?

A. Streptokinase is the agent of choice.
B. The recommended dose for children is the same per body weight as in adults.
C. Thrombolysis should not be used in children due to the high risk of hemorrhage.
D. Urokinase is the agent of choice.
E. Effective in both arterial and venous thrombi at doses of 0.1 mg/kg.

401. Alagille syndrome:

A. Is associated with an increased risk of aneurysmal SAH.
B. Has an autosomal recessive inheritance pattern.
C. Has an unknown genetic defect.
D. Causes death in infancy.
E. Is found only in girls.

402. Which of the following best describes hemiplegic migraine?

A. Motor deficit is the only manifestation of the aura.
B. Hemiplegic migraine always has an autosomal dominant inheritance.
C. Hemiplegic migraine is rarely confused with ischemic stroke.
D. Attacks of hemiplegic migraine may occur in children as young as 5 years old.
E. β-Blockers are routinely used for prevention of hemiplegic migraine.

403. Which of the following is associated with increased risk of primary hemorrhagic stroke in children with sickle cell disease?

A. Recent blood transfusion.
B. Previous ischemic stroke.
C. Aneurysms.
D. Anemia.
E. Elevated leukocyte count.

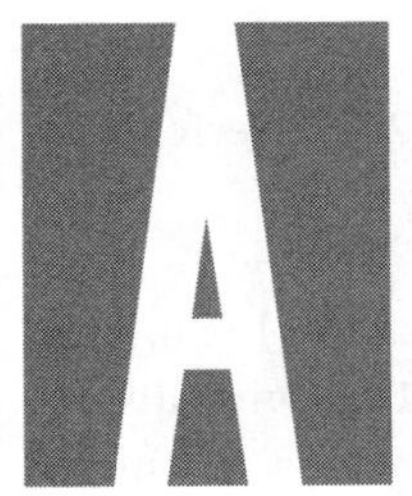

Clinical Pediatrics
Answers

374. The answer is A. Atrial fibrillation and atrial myxoma are potential causes of embolic stroke in children. Infective endocarditis, patent foramen ovale (PFO) and fat emboli from long-bone fractures are also related to cerebral embolization in children. The other choices, including orbital infections, cavernous sinus thrombosis, and leukemia, are not sources of emboli and are mainly related to cerebral venous thrombus. (Behrman, Chapter 593)

375. The answer is C. Arterial ischemic stroke occurs in approximately 3 per 100,000 children per year. The most common cause of ischemic stroke in children overall is heart disease, including congenital and acquired. Sickle cell disease is the most common cause of ischemic stroke in African American children, occurring in approximately 11% of patients with SCD by age 20. Moyamoya syndrome is a rare noninflammatory vasculopathy presenting as ischemic strokes in children and intracerebral hemorrhages (ICH) in adults. Homocystinuria and mitochondrial encephalomyopathy lactic acidosis and stroke-like symptoms (MELAS) are rare causes of stroke in children. (Jordan, *Neurologist* 2006)

376. The answer is C. Tangier disease is an autosomal codominant disorder in which homozygotes have very low levels of high-density lipoprotein (HDL) cholesterol and apolipoprotein (apo) A-I (both <10 mg/dL), decreased low-density lipoprotein (LDL) cholesterol levels (about 40% of normal), and mild hypertriglyceridemia. It is caused by mutations in the adenosine triphosphate (ATP)-binding cassette transporter A1 (ABCA1). Tangier disease was initially discovered almost half a century ago in families inhabiting Tangier Island in the Chesapeake Bay, but has since been found in other individuals. Abnormalities in reverse cholesterol transport leading to storage of cholesterol esters in reticuloendothelial tissues produce the characteristic large orange tonsils as well as infiltration of other organs. The major neurologic manifestation is peripheral neuropathy, but the affected individuals also may have cardiovascular and cerebrovascular disease occurring prematurely or late in life. (Maxfield & Tabas, *Nature* 2005; Serfaty-Lacrosniere et al., *Atherosclerosis* 1994)

377. The answer is C. Arterial dissection leading to ischemic stroke in children occurs spontaneously or related to trauma. In a study of children with dissections, a marked male predominance was not explained by increased trauma in boys. Unlike in adults, 60% of anterior circulation dissections in children are intracranial, as opposed to occurring in extracranial internal carotid arteries. When the dissections occur in the posterior circulation, over half are at the level of the C1 to C2 vertebral bodies in the vertebral artery. None of the children with posterior circulation dissections but 10% of the children with anterior circulation dissections had recurrent dissections. (Fullerton et al., *Neurology* 2001)

378. The answer is D. An arteriovenous malformation (AVM) of the vein of Galen can produce high-output heart failure due to shunting of blood. It can also cause hydrocephalus if the cerebrospinal fluid drainage is blocked. Arteriovenous malformations can bleed at any age, but are the most common cause of intraparenchymal hemorrhage in children. They may be associated with migraine-like headaches in children with hemicranial pain that does not alternate sides. Cranial bruits are audible by auscultation over the skull in 50% of children. Arteriovenous malformations do not produce symptoms that alternate sides. Hemiplegia caused by a hemorrhagic AVM is unilateral, with a longer duration than occurs with alternating hemiplegia episodes in children. (Garcia-Monaco et al, *Childs Nerv Syst* 1991)

379. The answer is D. Aneurysms in babies are unusual, with approximately 131 reported in the literature, accounting for less than 1% of all subarachnoid hemorrhages (SAHs). The majority of cerebral aneurysms diagnosed in childhood (73%) present with SAH. Aneurysms in childhood are significantly different in anatomic localization and outcome from cerebral aneurysms in adults. Aneurysms of the middle cerebral artery (MCA) are by far the most common; nearly three times higher than in any other vessel. Giant aneurysms, on the other hand, are more common in the posterior circulation, which is different from adults. Aneurysms in childhood are less likely to occur at bifurcations in the circle of Willis, the most common areas for aneurysm formation in adults. Outcome after SAH is better for children than for adults. (Buis, *Childs Nervous Syst* 2006; Pasquilin, *Child Nervous Syst* 1986)

380. The answer is C. The etiology of alternating hemiplegia of childhood is usually unknown, although it may be occasionally related to migraine. It is generally sporadic. It most frequently starts in infancy, between 2 and 18 months. The prognosis is poor, often leading to progressive mental retardation and eventual development of choreoathetosis. The symptoms may spontaneously regress with sleep and worsen on awakening. A benign form, which has an older onset and may be inherited, has recently been reported. (Chaves-Vischer, *Neurology* 2001)

381. The answer is C. Of 215 neonates with ischemic stroke, 125 (59.1%) had at least one of the listed prothrombotic risk factors. Most common was elevated lipoprotein (a) (Lp(a)) titers in 45 patients, followed by the factor V Leiden mutation found in 32 patients. Only one patient each had protein S deficiency or antithrombin III deficiency. (Kurnik, *Stroke* 2003)

382. The answer is B. Periventricular leukomalacia occurs in infants. It is associated with prematurity and occurs in approximately 32% of infants with cerebral palsy born weighing under 1,000 g. Secondary hemorrhage (which may be relatively minor) is reported in 25% of infants by autopsy. Approximately 44% of patients who develop spastic diplegia have periventricular leukomalacia. (Tangwai, *Pediatr Neurol* 2006; Bodensteiner, *J Child Neurol* 2006)

383. The answer is D. The most common intracranial hemorrhage in premature infants is associated with rupture of fragile subependymal vessels in the germinal matrix. Despite a decreased incidence with improved perinatal intensive care, it still occurs in 20% to 40% of premature infants. Half the hemorrhages occur in the first day of life. Up to 90% of the hemorrhages occur in the first 4 days of life. Forceps delivery may cause a subdural hematoma, but not subependymal hemorrhage. (MacDonald, Chapter 50)

384. The answer is B. Subdural hemorrhage occurs in both premature and term infants. Clinical symptoms include motor asymmetry, seizures, and altered consciousness. Mild subdural hemorrhages are not associated with symptoms and may go unrecognized. Thus, the true incidence of subdural hemorrhage is unknown. Differentiating a subdural from an intracerebellar hemorrhage on CT scan can be difficult if the blood is in the posterior fossa. (MacDonald, Chapter 50)

385. The answer is C. Intracerebellar hemorrhage occurs in both premature and term infants. It can be seen on intracranial ultrasound. It may be treated surgically or conservatively, depending on the size and the clinical situation. (Avery, Chapter 50)

386. The answer is B. All the listed choices are symptoms of cerebral venous thrombosis (CVT) in neonates, but about two-thirds of cases in neonates present with seizures. Respiratory distress occurs in about one-third of neonates with CVT. The majority of neonates with CVT have an acute illness at the time of diagnosis. The superior sagittal sinus and the lateral sinuses are most typically involved, but the straight sinus and deep venous system are more often involved in neonates than in adults. Functional outcome is generally worse than in adults. (Bousser & Ferro, *Lancet Neurol* 2007)

387. The answer is C. Kawasaki syndrome—a mucocutaneous lymph node syndrome—involves the skin and mucous membranes of children or young adults. Fever is followed by skin lesions, conjunctivitis, and generalized lymphadenopathy. Vascular involvement includes ischemic stroke, SAH, or myocardial infarction. Sneddon syndrome involves livedo racemosa and ischemic stroke, generally in adult women. Malignant atrophic papulosis occurs in young adults with skin lesions, gastrointestinal symptoms, and multifocal infarctions or hemorrhages. Epidermal nevus syndrome associates cerebral infarcts and nevi. Diffuse meningocerebral angiomatosis and leukoencephalopathy presents as livedo reticularis, progressive dementia, and seizures in the setting of brain infarcts, demyelination, and cerebromeningeal angiomatosis. (Kasner & Gorelick, Chapter 8)

388. The answer is A. Periventricular hemorrhage is common in preterm infants, occurring in 23% to 75% of infants weighing under 1,500 g (3.3 pounds). Subarachnoid hemorrhage is rare in infants. Subdural hematoma occurs infrequently, but can occur perinatally in infants associated with difficult forceps deliveries. Lobar hemorrhage is most commonly associated with amyloid angiopathy, almost invariably associated with advanced age. (Ginsberg & Bogousslavsky, Chapter 60)

389. The answer is A. Symptomatic perinatal stroke occurs in about 1 in 4,000 term neonates. Most perinatal strokes occur in the territory of the MCA. Left-sided predominance may be attributable to the hemodynamic aspects of flow from a patent ductus arteriosus or from the left common carotid artery. Focal seizures are a common presentation for neonates who have had an ischemic stroke, although the diagnosis may be recognized later in life when asymmetry in grasp and reach is noted or when there is a delay in achieving milestones. Thrombophilias may lead to perinatal ischemic stroke due to thrombosis on the maternal side of the placenta (maternal thrombophilia) or on the fetal side of the placenta (maternal or paternal inherited thrombophilias). About half of neonates with ischemic stroke are clinically normal later in infancy. (Nelson & Lynch, *Lancet Neurol* 2004)

390. The answer is A. Databases from the National Center for Health Statistics were searched to examine the demographics of stroke in children. In the United States, from 1979 to 1998 there were 4,881 deaths in stroke patients under 20 years of age. Of these, 2,055 (42%) of these were from ICH, 1,566 (32%) from SAH, and 872 (17%) from ischemic stroke. About 8% of acute cerebrovascular disease cases in children were ill-defined. There were no deaths from nonpyogenic cerebral venous thrombosis. (Fullerton, *Neurology* 2002)

391. The answer is B. Stroke mortality has decreased in the United States in adults and in children in recent decades. The decline in stroke mortality in children is especially marked in ICH and SAH, as compared with ischemic stroke. Stroke mortality is dramatically higher in neonates, accounting for one in three stroke-related deaths under age 20 years, with especially high death rates due to ICH. More stroke-related deaths occur per 100,000 population in black children compared with white children. Sickle cell disease causes ischemic stroke, but most (76%) of the stroke deaths in black children were from ICH or SAH. (Fullerton, *Neurology* 2002)

392. The answer is A. Cranial irradiation is particularly toxic in children. Although it is effective in treating low-grade gliomas, the toxicity is greater in children under 10 years, so it is generally reserved for tumors failing chemotherapy. Moyamoya syndrome is a complication of head and neck irradiation, because irradiation of major arteries can result in accelerated atherosclerosis and stenosis. The risk is increased with neurofibromatosis type 1 (NF1) and with irradiation near the circle of Willis. Pineal teratoma is treated with surgery and, if irradiation is needed, it is not as likely to produce Moyamoya syndrome as does irradiation of an optic nerve glioma. Leukemia is treated with chemotherapy. Treatment for retinoblastoma is not near the circle of Willis, and it is generally treated using laser therapy rather than irradiation. (Ullrich, *Neurology* 2007)

393. The answer is B. Varicella zoster virus (VZV) produces a cerebral vasculopathy with stenosis. On autopsy studies, the virus has been found in diseased cerebral arteries. Patients with VZV-associated vasculopathy may have ischemic strokes or transient ischemic attacks (TIAs). The stenosis can regress, but recurrent TIA or stroke may still occur. The other three options are not causes of stroke due to VZV. (Lanthier, *Neurology* 2005)

394. The answer is D. All the listed choices are thrombotic risk factors in children, but the most common is central venous or arterial catheterization producing venous or arterial thrombosis respectively. Central venous catheterization is the cause of 80% of deep venous thrombosis (DVT) in the upper venous system in newborns and of 60% of DVT in older children. Noncatheter-related arterial thrombosis is relatively rare in children. (Tormene et al., *Semin Thromb Hemost* 2006)

395. The answer is D. Primary central nervous system (CNS) vasculitis is an inflammatory disease of the brain and spine that can occur in children as well as adults. In immunocompetent children, VZV is associated with two overlapping CNS vasculidities in children, post-varicella arteriopathy and transient cerebral arteriopathy. The VZV to IgM ratio in the cerebrospinal fluid (CSF) or serum should be assayed to evaluate an underlying infectious etiology. A CT scan and an electroencephalogram (EEG) are not specific enough to be helpful in the diagnosis. A normal C-reactive protein (C-RP) does not rule out vasculitis. Brain biopsies may be considered in the child with a newly acquired, progressive neurologic deficit associated with CSF and MRI abnormalities. (Benseler, *Curr Rheumatol Rep* 2006)

396. The answer is A. All the listed conditions are associated with intraparenchymal hemorrhage, but about 50% of childhood intraparenchymal hemorrhages are due to an AVM. A cavernous malformation may be difficult to diagnose immediately after the hemorrhage. Hematologic causes include liver failure, hemophilia, disseminated intravascular coagulation, thrombocytopenia, sickle cell disease, and anticoagulant medications. Brain tumors in children rarely hemorrhage but, when they do, the hemorrhage-associated mortality rate may be as high as 50%. (Jordan & Hillis, *Pediatr Neurol* 2007)

397. The answer is A. Lemierre syndrome (also called postanginal sepsis) is an extremely rare complication of a pharyngeal infection due to *Fusobacterium necrophorum* (a gram-negative anaerobic rod) that can occur in immunocompetent children or adults. Septicemia may result in remote infection characteristically involving the lungs. Rare neurologic complications include meningitis, vasculitis, ischemic stroke, subdural empyema, cerebral venous thrombosis, and internal carotid artery stenosis. Patients treated with surgery and antibiotics generally survive. The other organisms are distracters. (Westhout et al., *J Neurosurg* 2007)

398. The answer is C. All the listed disorders are associated with posterior fossa malformations, hemangiomas, arterial anomalies, coarctation of the aorta and other cardiac defects, and eye abnormalities (PHACE syndrome), a neurocutaneous syndrome of infancy, but Dandy-Walker malformation is most commonly reported with this increasingly recognized disorder. The hallmark of PHACE, which is more common in girls than boys, is a massive facial hemangioma, and all infants with prominent facial hemangiomas should have brain imaging to rule out an associated CNS abnormality. Ischemic stroke is common, related to congenital or progressive anomalies in the cervical and cerebral vasculature, or to cardiac defects. Moyamoya syndrome may result from a progressive arterial vasculopathy with large artery stenosis. Sternal clefting or a supraumbilical abdominal raphe may also occur. The cause of this syndrome is unknown, with speculation that it develops in the first trimester of gestation. (Coates et al., *Ophthalmology* 1999; Drolet et al., *Pediatrics* 2006)

399. The answer is B. Osler-Weber-Rendu disease (hereditary hemorrhagic telangiectasia) is an autosomal dominant disease with skin, nasal, and visceral telangiectasia. Neurofibromatosis is associated with occlusive arterial disease. Cerebrovascular disease in Marfan syndrome usually leads to large-artery dissection, as does Ehlers-Danlos syndrome. Sturge-Weber syndrome is characterized pathologically by leptomeningeal vessel calcification and arteriovenous angiomas. (Kasner & Gorelick, Chapter 8)

400. The answer is E. Although thrombolysis has not formally been studied in children, and its usage should be limited to clinical trials as much as possible until formal criteria are established, low dose therapy of 0.1 mg/kg has been shown to be effective. In children, "high dose" therapy is defined as 0.5 mg/kg. Urokinase is no longer approved by the FDA. Streptokinase should not be used due to the high prevalence of anti-streptococcal neutralizing antibody. (Manco-Johnson et al., *Thromb Haemost* 2002)

401. The answer is A. Alagille syndrome is an autosomal dominant arteriodysplastic syndrome with multiorgan symptoms resulting from a mutation in the *Jagged1* gene, which encodes a ligand for the Notch receptor. Although renal, gastrointestinal, cardiovascular, and pulmonary abnormalities are most often described, cerebrovascular involvement has also been reported. The risk of intracranial hemorrhage is increased (reported to be as high as 16%), because of aneurysmal SAH. Moyamoya syndrome may also be seen in these boys or girls, who have typical peculiar facies, chronic cholestasis, butterfly-like vertebral arch defects, polycystic kidneys, posterior embryotoxon, and other developmental abnormalities. (Turnialan et al., *Pediatr Neurosurg* 2006)

402. The answer is D. Hemiplegic migraine attacks may present with acute neurologic signs and symptoms indistinguishable from ischemic stroke, and the focal neurologic manifestations may persist for hours to days. Sensory, visual, or aphasic symptoms occur along with the motor aura. Although the mean age of onset is in the teens, some children may begin to have auras followed by headaches as toddlers. Hemiplegic migraine can be sporadic or inherited in an autosomal dominant pattern. Familial hemiplegic migraine has been mapped to specific genes, including a mutation of a P/Q voltage-gated Ca^{2+} channel (CACNA1A) gene on chromosome 19p13. Although triptans, ergotamines, and β-blockers are generally proscribed in hemiplegic migraine, the risk with their use is poorly characterized. (Black, *Semin Neurol* 2006)

403. The answer is A. Primary hemorrhagic stroke is an uncommon complication of SCD. Stroke is found in adults more often than in children. The mortality of primary hemorrhagic stroke associated with SCD ranges from 24% to 65%. In a retrospective study of children with SCD, an increased risk of hemorrhagic stroke was associated with a history of hypertension, transfusion within the last 14 days, treatment with corticosteroids, and possibly with the use of nonsteroidal anti-inflammatory drugs. (Strouse et al., *Pediatrics* 2006)

7 Imaging Questions

404. This magnetic resonance image (MRI) was obtained in a 67-year-old woman who was seen at the Intermountain Stroke Center for a 5-minute episode of mild right-sided hemiparesis and word-finding difficulty. Her family also reported memory problems and decreased energy. Given the findings on this MRI, of the following choices, which test should be done on the most urgent basis?

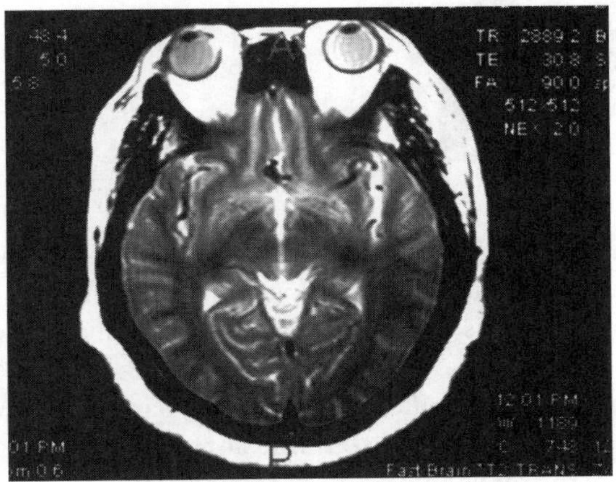

A. Carotid duplex.
B. Echocardiography.
C. Computed tomography angiography (CTA) or MR angiography (MRA).
D. Transcranial Doppler (TCD).

405. A 52-year-old man presented to the emergency room with a moderately severe right-sided hemiparesis and aphasia. His wife stated that his symptoms had started 2 hours prior to his arrival. His past medical history was remarkable for hypertension. His blood pressure was 160/72, and his electrocardiogram (EKG) revealed atrial fibrillation with a rate of 138. Blood counts, chemistries, and coagulation studies were all normal. This was the patient's CT, taken 135 minutes following the reported onset of his stroke.

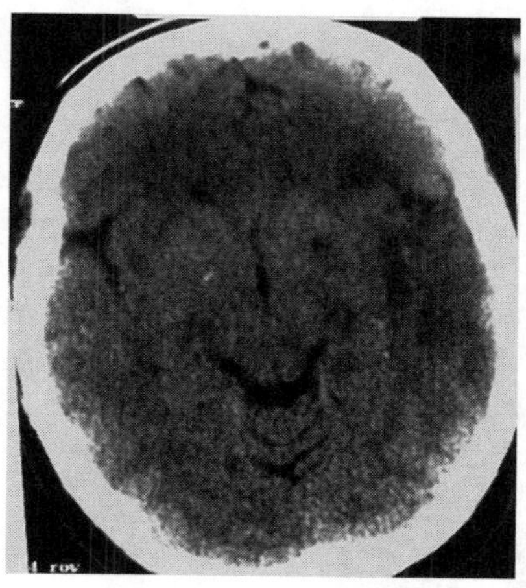

Which statement is true?

A. Tissue plasminogen activator (t-PA) should be given immediately because his symptoms started well within the 3 hour window.
B. Tissue plasminogen activator is risky in this patient and unlikely to result in appreciable improvement.
C. Tissue plasminogen activator should be given immediately, and cardioversion should be performed after the t-PA infusion is completed.
D. Tissue plasminogen activator should be given immediately, along with IV mediations to control his heart rate.

406. A 74-year-old male presented for evaluation of "amyloid angiopathy." He had a seizure disorder and was on both phenytoin (Dilantin) and gabapentin (Neurontin). His wife noted that he had "slowed down," had memory problems, and that his mood seemed less stable. This MRI was obtained, and the patient was referred to a vascular neurologist. This disorder:

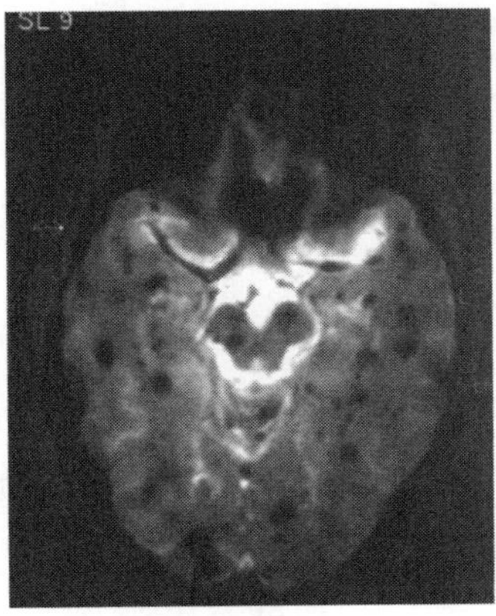

A. Has an autosomal dominant inheritance pattern.
B. Affects only the brain.
C. Has normal findings on CT angiography of the brain.
D. Presents most often with focal neurologic deficits.

407. The patient described in question 406 has three children. The recommended advice to the children is:

A. No testing unless symptoms develop.
B. Magnetic resonance imaging of the brain with and without contrast.
C. Cerebral angiography.
D. Computed tomography of the brain with and without contrast.
E. Computed tomography angiography (CTA) or MRA of the brain.

408. This MRI is most compatible with:

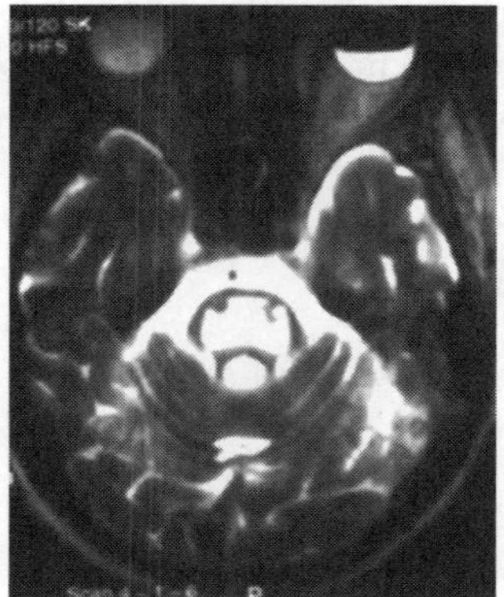

A. Occlusion of the basilar artery.
B. Aortic atherosclerosis.
C. Fetal origin of the posterior cerebral artery.
D. Cardiogenic embolus.
E. Alcoholism.

409. The structure indicated by the arrow is the:

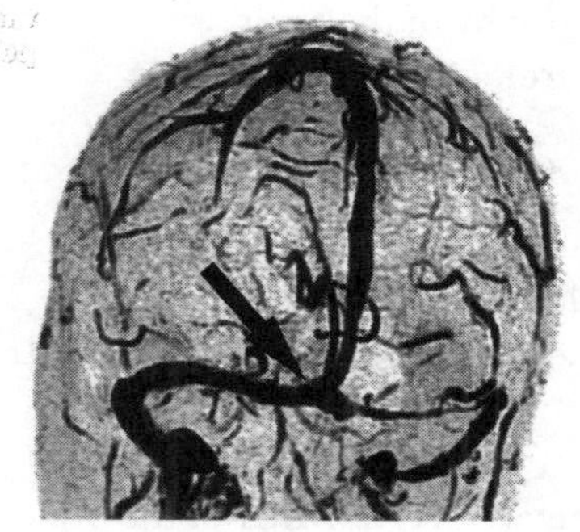

A. Superior sagittal sinus.
B. Transverse sinus.
C. Torcular Herophili.
D. Inferior anastomotic vein.

410. A 46-year-old man presented with a huge nondominant stroke, with left hemiplegia and neglect. The MRI revealed an infarct of essentially the entire right MCA territory. A TCD was done and four of the tracings are shown here. Which of the following is the most likely clinical implication of the TCD?

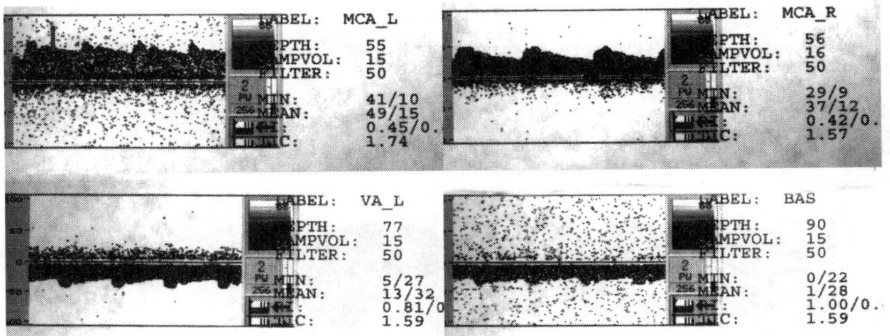

A. Middle cerebral artery stenosis.
B. Chronic hypertension.
C. Increased cerebrovascular resistance.
D. Cardiomyopathy.
E. Alcohol abuse.

411. The most important immediate intervention for the patient described in Question 410 is:

A. Administration of Lanoxin (digoxin).
B. Heart transplant.
C. Placement of an intracardiac defibrillator (ICD).
D. Placement of a demand pacemaker.
E. Diuresis.

412. Compared to gray matter, fresh (hyperacute) blood in the brain can be:

A. Hyperintense on T1 and hyperintense on T2.
B. Hyperintense on T1 and isointense on T2.
C. Isointense on T1 and hyperintense on T2.
D. Isointense on T1 and hypointense on T2.

413. On MRI, intraparenchymal hemosiderin can be:

A. Hyperintense on T1 and hyperintense on T2.
B. Hyperintense on T1 and hypointense on T2.
C. Hypointense on T1 and hyperintense on T2.
D. Hypointense on T1 and hypointense on T2.

414. The timing of a hemorrhage seen on MRI:

A. Is highly accurate.
B. Is based on the imaging properties of oxygen bound to hemoglobin.
C. Is frequently inaccurate because of overlapping signal characteristics of hemoglobin breakdown products.
D. Is only understood by neuroradiologists.

415. Match the arrows with the structures. Each answer can be used only once, but some answers will not be used. Match arrows 1 through 5 with the following answers:

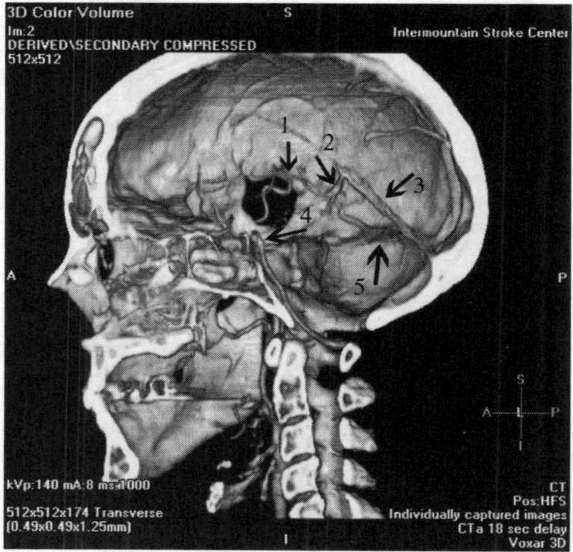

See color section following page 282.

A. Middle cerebral artery.
B. Vein of Galen.
C. Jugular vein.
D. Sigmoid sinus.
E. Superior sagittal sinus.
F. Transverse sinus.
G. Straight sinus.
H. Internal cerebral vein.
I. Vertebral artery.
J. Basilar artery.

416. The "duplex" in carotid duplex stands for:

A. The combination of color-flow and grayscale imaging.
B. The imaging of both the internal and the external carotid arteries.
C. B-mode imaging with simultaneous measurement of flow velocity.
D. The use of a two-channel pulsed wave Doppler system.

417. "B-mode" refers to:

A. Grayscale imaging.
B. Measurement of velocity.
C. Biologic imaging.
D. Spectral analysis.

418. At the bifurcation, the position of the internal carotid artery (ICA) in relationship to the external carotid artery (ECA) is most often:

A. Medial.
B. Lateral.
C. Dorsal.
D. Dorsolateral.
E. Dorsomedial.

419. Low-resistance arteries include:

A. External carotid artery, superficial temporal artery, maxillary artery.
B. Internal carotid, vertebral artery, basilar artery.
C. Subclavian artery, iliac artery, radial artery, aorta.
D. Facial artery, occipital artery, superior thyroid artery.

420. Which statement is true about the Doppler sounds produced by normal ICAs and ECAs?

A. The ICA makes a soft sound, whereas the ECA makes a whip-like sound.
B. The ECA makes a soft sound, whereas the ICA makes a whip-like sound.
C. There is no difference in the sound of the Doppler signal between the ICA and ECA.
D. The sounds produced by the ICA and the ECA are not useful in identifying the vessels.

421. A 72-year-old woman with treated hypertension and hypercholesterolemia had a TIA with left-sided face, arm, and leg numbness with mild weakness lasting 10 minutes. Her MRI showed nine bilateral hyperintense lesions on T2 images, 4 to 8 mm in size, randomly distributed. Below is the grayscale image of her right carotid artery and her Doppler waveform with velocities. What degree of stenosis is represented?

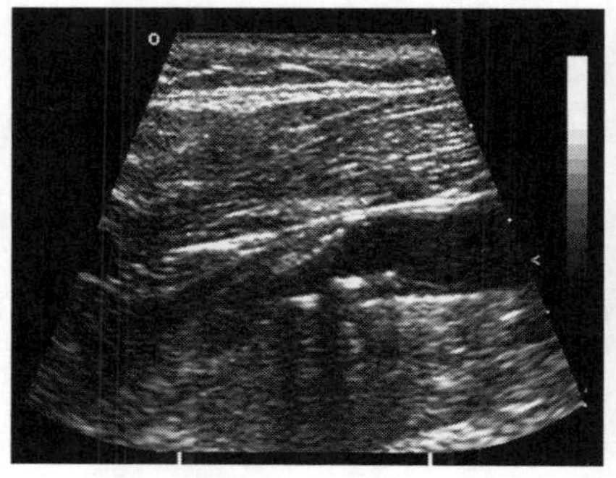

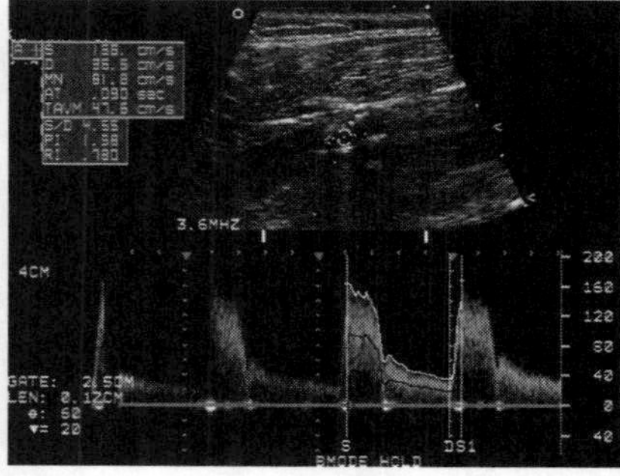

A. Less than 40%.
B. 40–59%.
C. 60–89%.
D. 90–95%.
E. Subtotal or total occlusion.

422. This TCD is most compatible with:

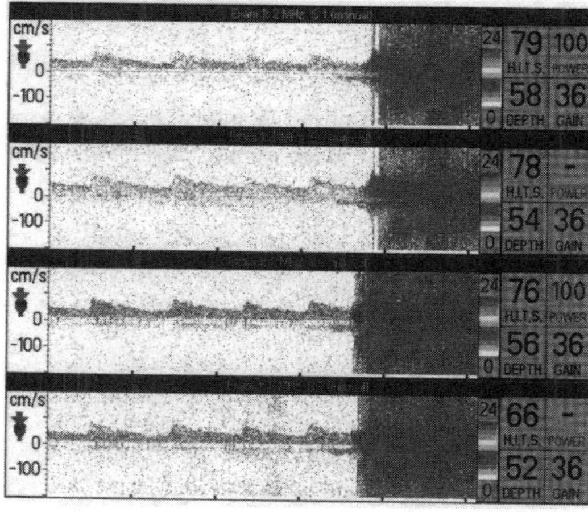

See color section following page 282.

A. Carotid occlusion.
B. Left-to-right intracardiac shunt.
C. Right-to-left intracardiac shunt.
D. Pulmonary AVM.

423. Which window or access point is used to insonate the carotid siphon using TCD?

A. Transorbital.
B. Anterior temporal.
C. Posterior temporal.
D. Nuchal or transforaminal.

424. Using a transtemporal window, an artery insonated at 50 mm, with the direction of flow being toward the probe, is most likely the:

A. Anterior cerebral artery (ACA).
B. Middle cerebral artery (MCA).
C. Posterior cerebral artery (PCA).
D. Vertebral artery.

425. Which statement is true about normal intracranial arterial velocities as recorded by TCD?

A. The normal velocities of the arteries in the anterior and posterior circulation are approximately the same.
B. The normal velocities of arteries in the anterior circulation are higher than that of the posterior circulation.
C. The normal velocities of arteries in the anterior circulation are lower than that of the posterior circulation.
D. The highest velocity is generally seen in the ophthalmic arteries.

426. A TCD done in a 68-year-old man revealed peak systolic velocities (PSV) of 78 cm/sec in the right MCA and 220 cm/sec in the left MCA. Which conclusion is most appropriate?

A. There is decreased velocity in the right MCA, consistent with distal stenosis or occlusion.
B. There is a moderate stenosis of the left MCA.
C. There is a severe stenosis of the left MCA.
D. There is a probable right carotid artery occlusion.

427. The TCD tracing from a right temporal window at a depth of 70 mm is most consistent with:

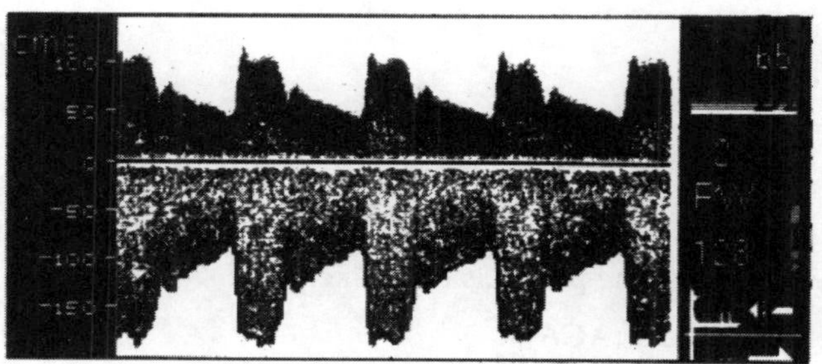

A. Right ACA moderate stenosis.
B. Right MCA moderate stenosis.
C. Left internal carotid occlusion.
D. Normal velocities.

428. Biphasic flow in the left MCA on TCD, with waveforms alternating above and below the line, is most consistent with:

A. Distal MCA occlusion.
B. Brain death.
C. Previous EC-IC bypass surgery.
D. Embolic signals.

429. A 46-year-old man presented with a huge right hemispheric stroke. Echo cardiogram showed a dilated cardiomyopathy with an ejection fraction of 26%. Eighteen months later, the patient had a heart transplant and was placed on immunosuppressive agents. Six months following the transplant, he had a generalized seizure and this MRI was obtained. Findings include a large infarct of the right MCA territory and:

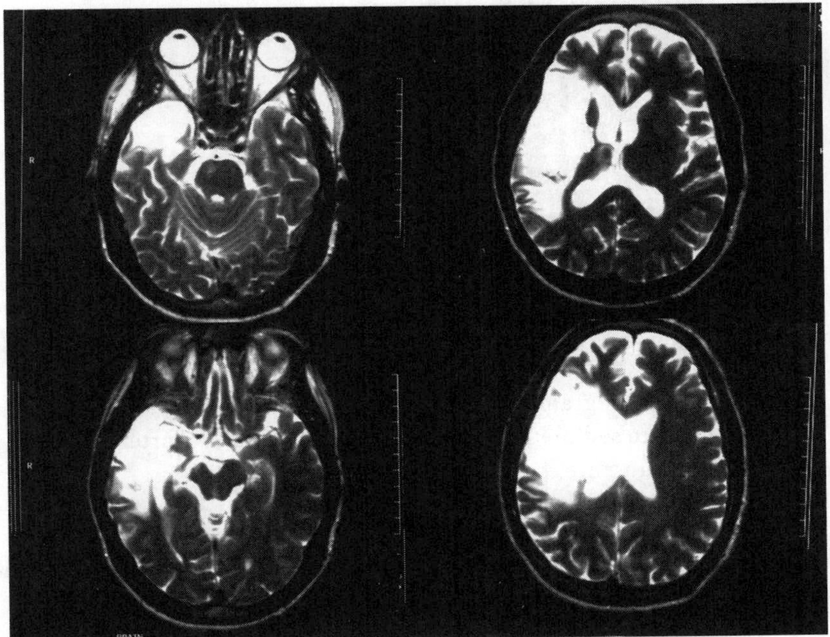

A. Right thalamic abscess.
B. Ischemia of the right basis pontis.
C. Wallerian degeneration.
D. Infective cerebritis most likely due to sepic embolic from an opportunistic pulmonary infection.

430. A 47-year-old woman presented to her primary physician with left temple and jaw pain. He ordered an MRI. When the report was obtained, he sent the patient to the stroke clinic. Based on the MRI picture, the test(s) most likely to confirm this patient's diagnosis to be:

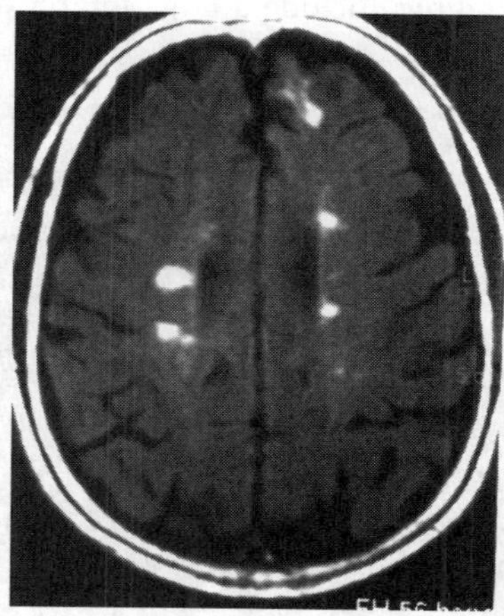

A. Cerebral angiogram.
B. Erythrocyte sedimentation rate (ESR) and temporal artery biopsy.
C. Lumbar puncture.
D. Gene testing for hereditary angiopathy.

431. Which of the following statements regarding MRA, CTA, and carotid duplex is correct?

A. Carotid duplex is technically limited in patients with calcified carotid atheromas.
B. Because of the technical limitations of noninvasive vascular imaging (MRA, CTA, and carotid duplex), catheter angiography is still needed in most stroke patients.
C. Performing a MRA or CTA is less expensive than carotid duplex.
D. The MRA tends to underestimate high-grade arterial stenosis.

432. An epidural hematoma:

A. Appears as a biconvex intra-axial hematoma on CT scan.
B. Occurs most frequently as a “contre-coup” lesion.
C. Is most frequently caused from an arterial hemorrhage.
D. Is most often caused from bleeding from a vascular malformation.
E. Is most commonly located in the posterior fossa.

433. The finding in this image is:

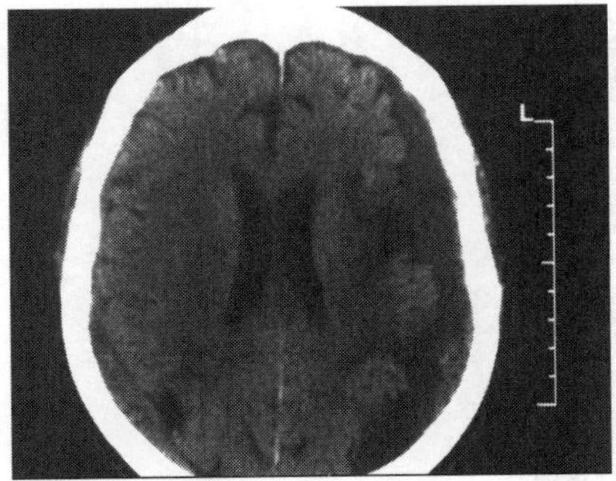

A. Caused by tears of bridging veins.
B. An intra-axial lesion.
C. More common with age, particularly in men.
D. Most often cause by a vascular malformation.

434. A 65-year-old man presented for aneurysm screening. His mother had two aneurysms, one treated surgically and one treated endovascularly. His mother is 96 and independent for activities of daily living. The patient has a long history of migraines and has had short-term memory loss since a mild closed-head injury. He is otherwise healthy and has no vascular risks, although he had not had a lipid panel for 5 years. A CTA was done.

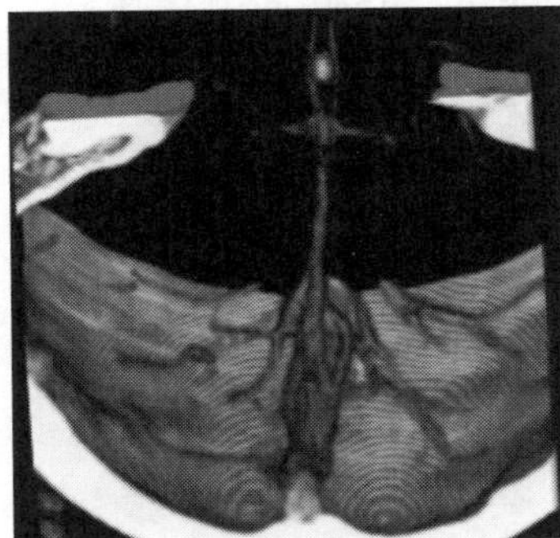

See color section following page 282.

After seeing this image, the next action should be:

A. Digital subtraction angiography.
B. Full cerebral angiography with cut films.
C. Neurosurgical consultation.
D. Lumbar puncture.
E. Lipid panel.

435. This vessel (*arrow*) is the:

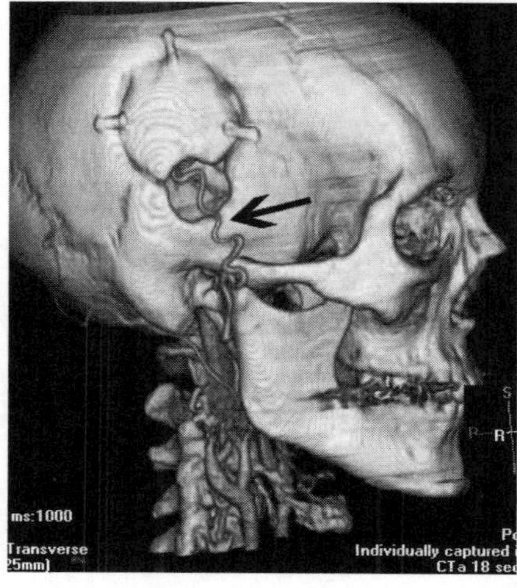

See color section following page 282.

A. Facial artery.
B. Internal jugular vein.
C. Middle cerebral artery.
D. Superficial temporal artery.

436. This TCD tracing was taken at a depth of 56 mm using a right temporal window in a 28-year-old woman. The most likely diagnosis is:

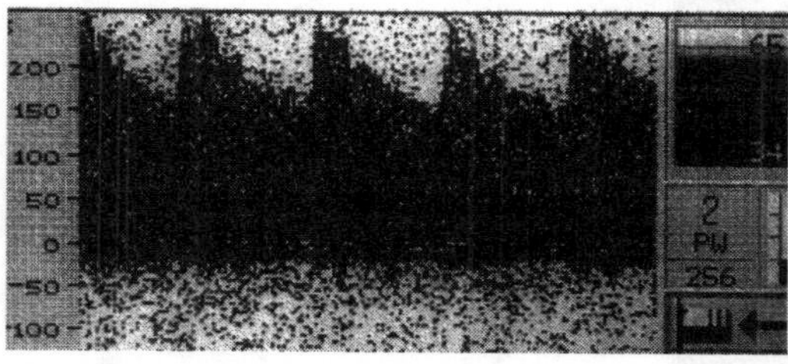

A. Right ACA stenosis.
B. Migraine headache.
C. Left ACA stenosis with collateral flow from the right ACA.
D. Right MCA stenosis.
E. Artifact.

437. The vessel indicated by the arrow is the:

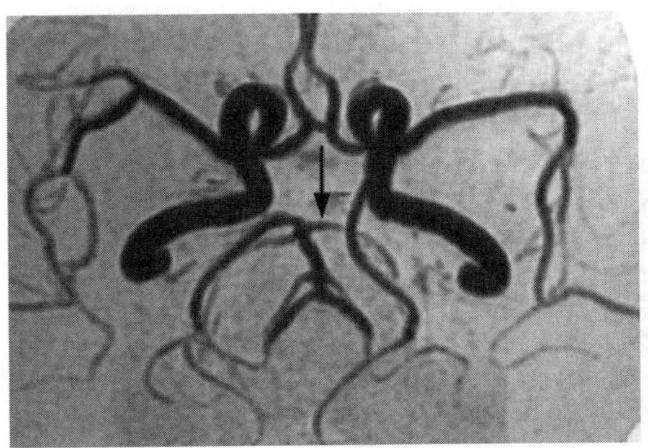

A. Left superior cerebellar artery.
B. Left PCA.
C. Anterior cerebral artery.
D. Anterior spinal artery.

438. The "delta sign" or the "empty delta sign" is most commonly associated with:

A. Airline strikes.
B. Bilateral paramedian hemorrhages.
C. Subdural hematoma.
D. Transverse sinus thrombosis.

439. A 69-year-old woman with hypertension and osteoarthritis was admitted to the hospital with crescendo TIAs consisting of left hemiparesis and hemianesthesia. She had no history of headaches. Noncontrasted MRI was ordered, but when the image on the left was seen, contrast was injected. The findings on this MRI are most consistent with:

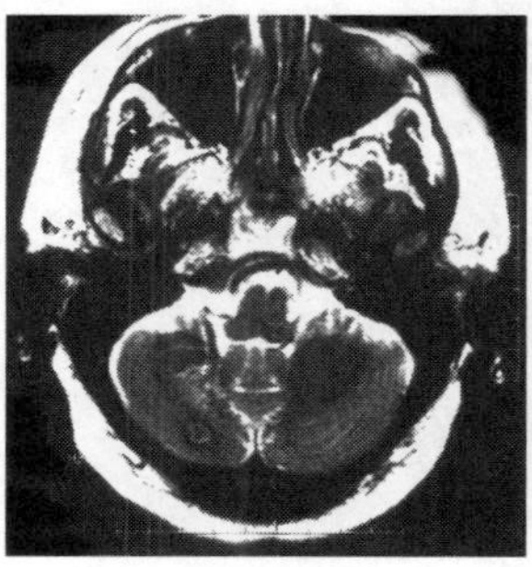

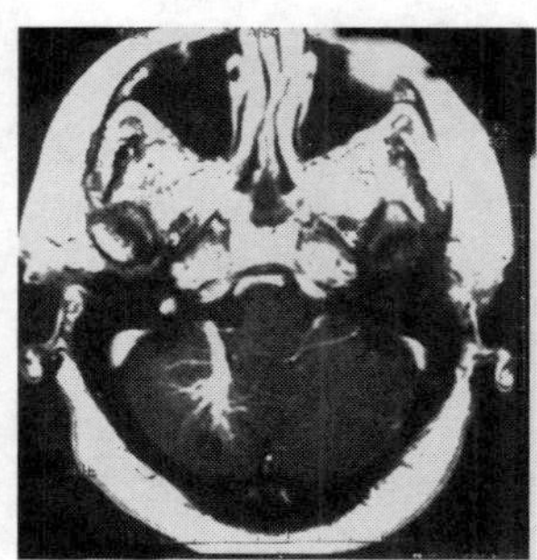

A. Developmental venous anomaly (DVA, previously referred to as venous angioma), along with a cavernous malformation.
B. Cavernous malformation alone.
C. A DVA alone.
D. Sturge-Weber syndrome.
E. Acute right cerebellar hemorrhage.

440. A 39-year-old white woman presented with a history of migraine-type headaches accompanied by numbness in the left arm. An MRI was obtained. The structure indicated by the arrow is most likely:

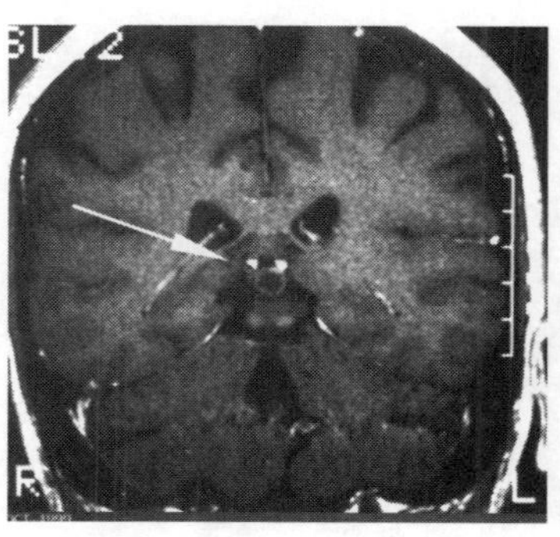

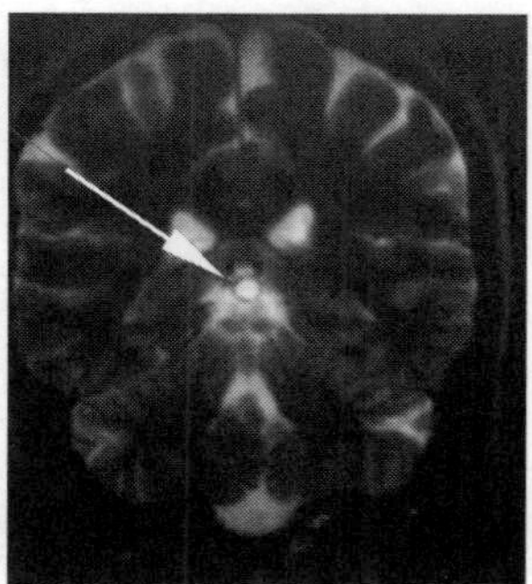

A. Basilar aneurysm.
B. Pineal cyst.
C. Artifact of MRI.
D. Colloid cyst.

441. A 77-year-old man with atrial fibrillation presented with a 30-minute episode of moderate aphasia. He had a past history of trauma years prior that left him blind in the left eye. His medications included aspirin and two antihypertensive medications. His MRI showed multiple small strokes. He was treated with warfarin. Two years later, he went to his eye doctor complaining about his vision in the right eye. No visual fields were done, and new glasses were prescribed. Two weeks later, he presented in the neurology clinic for evaluation of worsening visual loss. The INR was 3.8. The MRI obtained suggests:

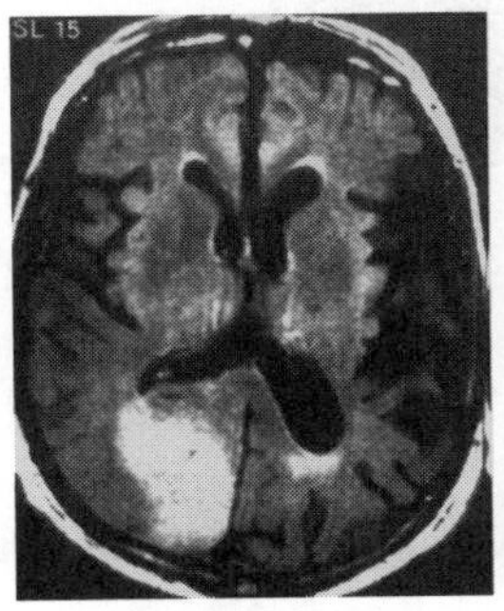

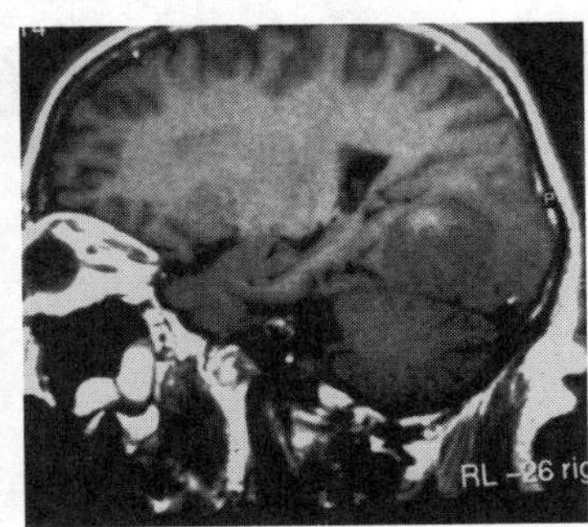

A. Hemorrhagic transformation of a cardioembolic infarct.
B. Abscess.
C. Primary brain tumor.
D. Lobar hemorrhage.

442. This MRA illustrates a:

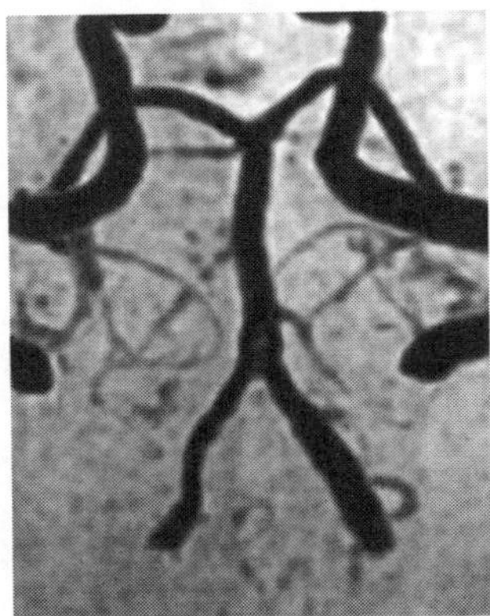

A. Fenestrated basilar artery.
B. Basilar dissection with hematoma in the vessel wall.
C. Dolichoectasia of the basilar artery.
D. Basilar thrombosis.

443. This is a suboccipital TCD tracing at a depth of 96 mm. This is most likely a:

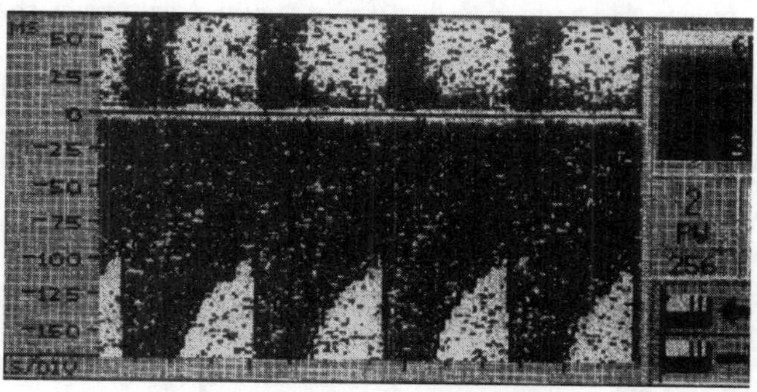

A. Vertebral stenosis.
B. Basilar stenosis.
C. Subclavian steal with reversal of flow.
D. Venous signal.

444. A disorder of which organ may be a contraindication for the use of gadolinium-containing contrast agents?

A. Liver.
B. Kidneys.
C. Pancreas.
D. Thyroid.
E. Skin.

445. An infant of African descent was adopted by a couple in the United States. The birth parents were both healthy, and the birth mother used no alcohol or drugs (prescription or recreational) during the pregnancy. Pregnancy and delivery were normal. In the first 3 to 4 months, the infant met developmental milestones normally, although it was noted that she reached for things preferentially with her left hand. As her motor skills progressed, decreased fine motor skills and posturing in the right upper extremity were noted. At 6 months, she presented to the Intermountain Stroke Center after the CTs were obtained. She was alert and attentive to her environment. Vision seemed intact. She had hypertonia, posturing, and decreased fine motor control in the right hand with mild hypertonia in the right leg. The most likely diagnosis is:

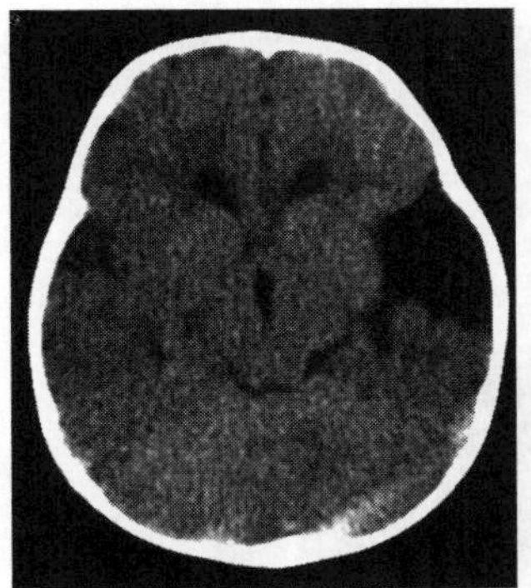

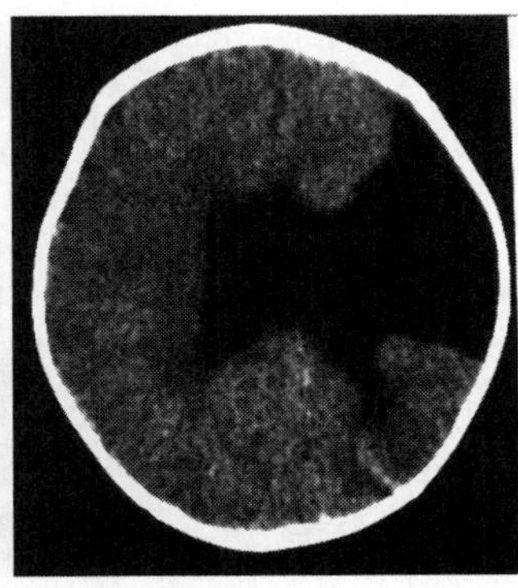

A. Prenatal or perinatal left MCA ischemic stroke.
B. Schizencephaly.
C. Prenatal or perinatal intracranial hemorrhage.
D. Congenital absence of the left MCA.

446. Which of the following statements best describes CT scanning done within 3 hours of an acute ischemic stroke?

A. Attenuation of the lentiform nuclei is a poor prognostic sign.
B. A hyperdense MCA sign is a contraindication for thrombolytic therapy.
C. Attenuation of the lentiform nuclei accurately predicts the side of the acute stroke.
D. Hypodensity of 50% of the MCA territory is a poor prognostic sign.

447. The definitive diagnosis of a developmental venous anomaly (DVA) is best made by:

A. Using catheter angiography.
B. Using either MR or CT angiography.
C. Using MRI with contrast.
D. Using MRI without contrast.
E. Using CT without contrast.

448. A halo sign on duplex evaluation of the superficial temporal artery is most consistent with:

A. Previous EC-IC bypass surgery.
B. Right internal artery occlusion and internalization of the right ECA branches.
C. 90% probability of temporal arteritis.
D. 70% probability of temporal arteritis.

449. This velocity tracing from a carotid duplex study is most compatible with:

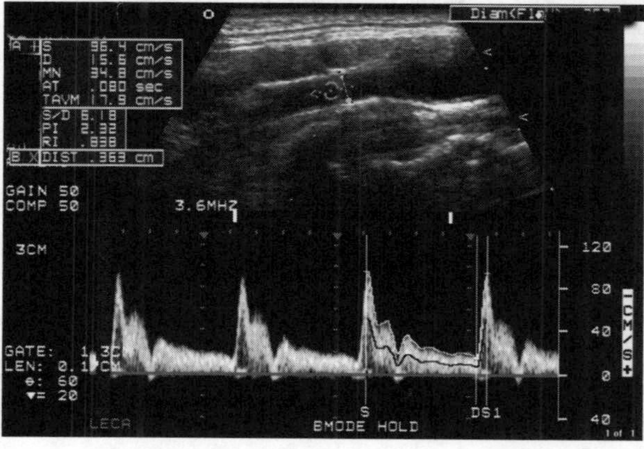

A. Normal common carotid artery.
B. Normal ICA.
C. Normal ECA.
D. Normal vertebral artery.

450. A 48-year-old man presented with a 75% symptomatic right carotid stenosis. Endarterectomy was performed. His elevated cholesterol was controlled, and he was place on medication for platelet inhibition. Six weeks later, the endarterectomy was patent. On his 3-month follow-up, no restenosis was found. Six months, later mild endothelial thickening was seen in the proximal ICA, with what seemed to be a paradoxical elevation of PSV to 131 cm/sec with an end diastolic velocity of 40 cm/sec. Six months, later a peak systolic of 466 cm/sec was obtained in the proximal ICA, with an end diastolic velocity of 275 cm/sec. This CT angiogram was obtained on the CereTOM scanner.

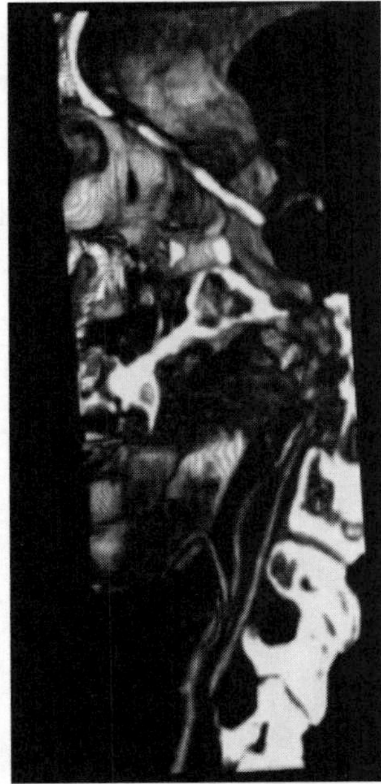

See color section following page 282.

The most appropriate intervention is:

A. Maintain the same regimen and repeat the duplex in 4 weeks.
B. Addition of anticoagulation to the platelet inhibition.
C. Repeat endarterectomy as soon as possible.
D. Angioplasty and stent placement.
E. Perform an EC-IC bypass.

451. This TCD tracing, taken at a depth of 96 mm from a suboccipital approach, peak systolic 41 cm/cm, is most consistent with:

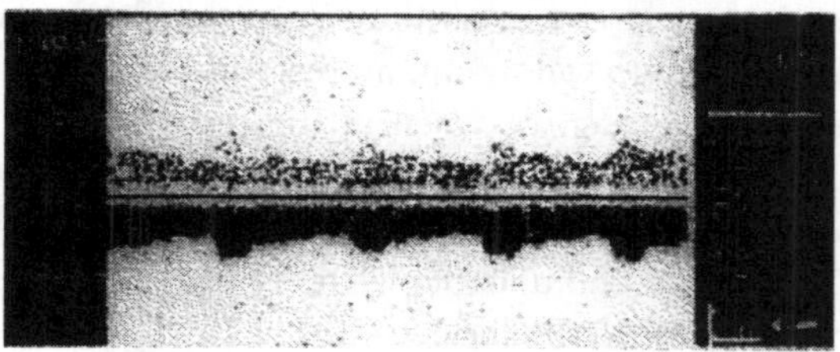

A. Normal basilar artery.
B. Normal vertebral artery.
C. Fetal origin of both posterior cerebral arteries.
D. Subclavian steal.

452. This is the relative blood flow component of a CT perfusion scan. This is most compatible with:

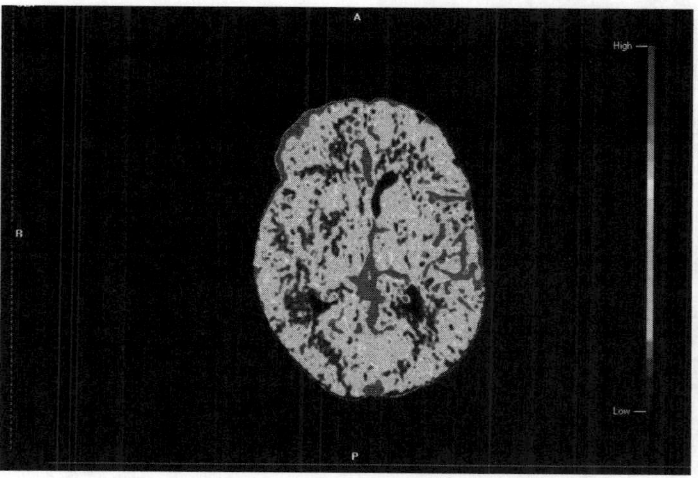

A. Cerebral vasculitis.
B. Normal study.
C. Right carotid occlusion.
D. Postischemic hyperperfusion in the left hemisphere.

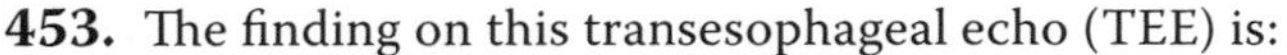

453. The finding on this transesophageal echo (TEE) is:

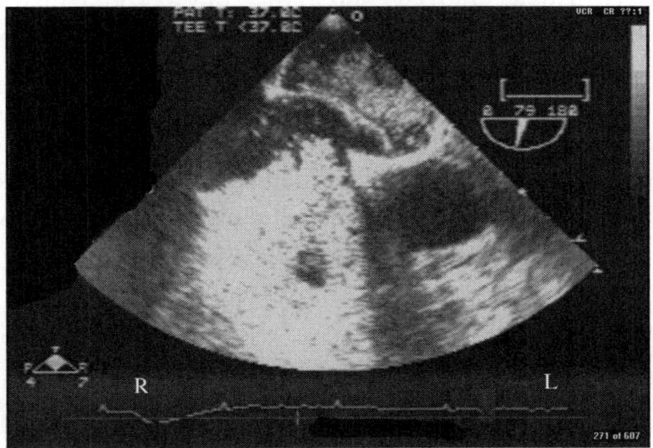

A. A Eustachian valve.
B. A long tunnel defect.
C. A left-to-right shunt.
D. An atrial myxoma.

454. A 60-year-old man, who was taking 81 mg aspirin a day, had five stereotypic episodes of transient numbness in the left arm and leg occurring periodically over a week. With one episode, he had clumsiness of his left hand. When he awakened and had yet another similar episode, his wife brought him to the emergency department. No flow was seen in the right ICA by carotid duplex Doppler examination. What advice should be given to this patient?

A. His ICA is occluded, so there is no point in attempted surgical intervention.
B. An MRA should be preformed, because a focal signal dropout will prove occlusion.
C. Catheter cerebral arteriography or CTA should be performed urgently.
D. He should stop aspirin and take either Plavix or Aggrenox.
E. Cardiac echo should be performed immediately.

455. A 70 -year-old physician presented to the Intermountain Stroke Center for evaluation of dizziness. He usually enjoyed a dip in the hot tub following his daily 60 minute work-out. One day, he noted that he was light headed for 30 to 60 seconds as he stepped out of the hot tub. During his medical training, he was found to have an occluded left carotid artery when residents were practicing carotid Duplex on each other. He assumed this was likely a traumatic occlusion from his high school football escapades, but he was concerned that perhaps decreased cerebral blood flow from this occlusion could be producing his symptoms. A CTA was done. Figure A is the left common carotid with its distal course. Figure B is a source image. What is the diagnosis?

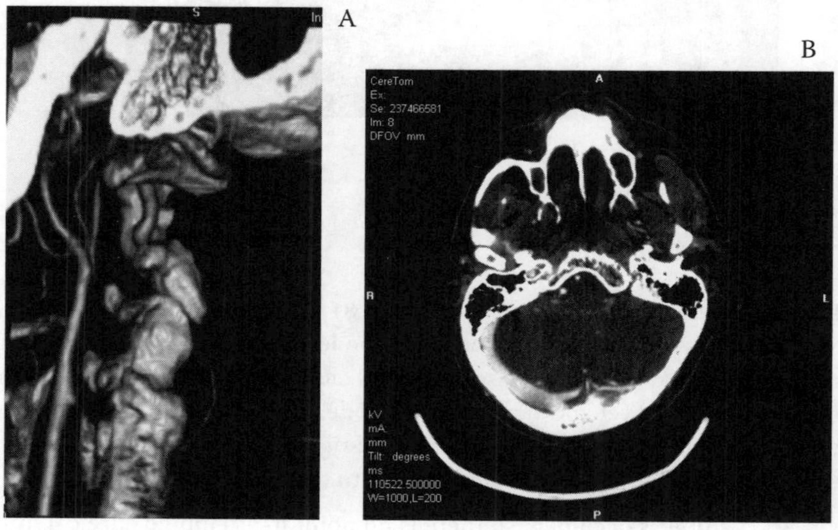

A. Atherosclerotic occlusion of the left ICA.
B. Probable traumatic occlusion of the left ICA, most likely related to old dissection.
C. Congenital absence of the left ICA.
D. Internalization of the left ECA.
E. Occlusion of the ECA with an intact ICA.

456. The most important factor in obtaining accurate velocity measurements when performing carotid duplex is:

A. The use of a large sample volume.
B. The Doppler angle.
C. The use of color Doppler.
D. The use of power Doppler.

457. Which carotid duplex findings are most consistent with this CTA? The PSV is peak diastolic velocity, EDV is end diastolic velocity. All velocities are in cm/sec.

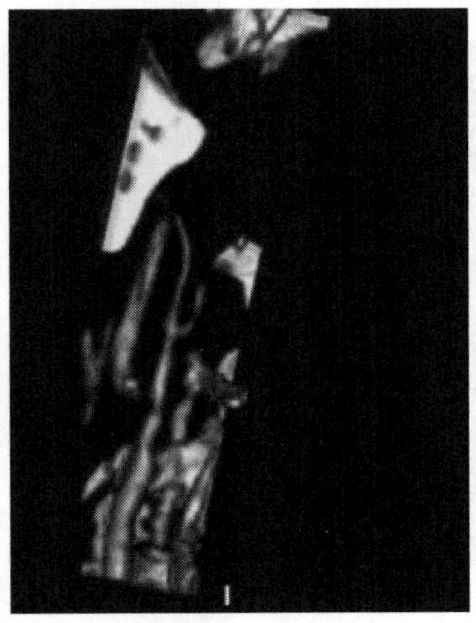

A. PSV 85, EDV 18.
B. PSV 155, EDV 35.
C. PSV 210, EDV 45.
D. PSV 380, EDV 160.

458. These MRIs are from a 55-year-old woman who was having episodic neurologic events with variable combinations of garbled speech, distorted vision, and right-sided arm numbness, arm pain, arm weakness, and/or poor coordination in the right arm. She had 12 events in a 2-week period. She was seen in the emergency department, at which time her neurologic examination was normal. Stress was suspected, because her nephew had recently undergone bilateral leg amputations following a motorcycle accident. She was sent home. The next day, she presented with a moderate right hemiparesis and Wernicke aphasia. Carotid duplex suggested an occluded left ICA. What is the most likely explanation for the patient's strokes?

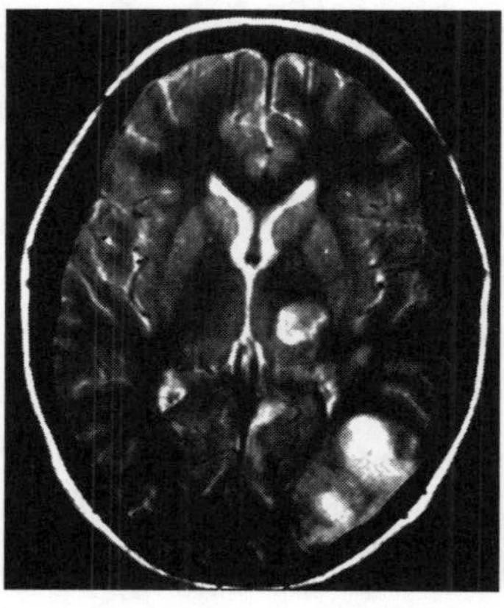

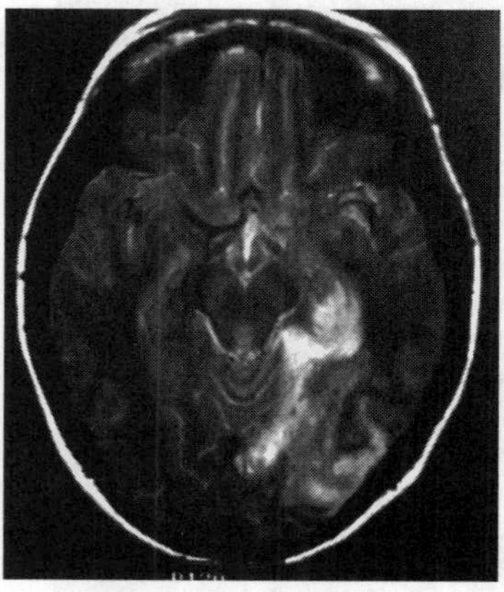

A. Cardiogenic emboli.
B. Emboli from a basilar stenosis entering the left PCA.
C. Fetal origin of the left PCA.
D. Hypotension with watershed infarcts.

459. Which of the following is a definite contraindication to CTA?

A. Shellfish allergy.
B. Claustrophobia.
C. Cardiac pacer.
D. Pregnancy.

460. Match the window for insonation with the detected using TCD.

A. Transtemporal approach.
B. Transorbital approach.
C. Transforaminal approach.
D. Submandibular approach.

1. Ophthalmic artery (OA).
2. Basilar artery.
3. Anterior cerebral artery (ACA).
4. Distal ICA at the skull base.

461. Cerebral microbleeds:

A. Are most easily noted on gradient-echo T2*-weighted MRI sequences.
B. Indicate focal acute hemorrhage.
C. Are independent of increasing age.
D. Are independent of hypertension.
E. Are associated with increased serum cholesterol.

462. Which of the following statements best describes the use of MRI in the diagnosis of TIA?

A. In patients with TIAs, the diffusion-weighted imaging (DWI) lesions consistently evolve into completed infarctions.
B. Use of DWI offers little added information over conventional MRI imaging sequences.
C. Most TIA patients have early DWI lesions but no later imaging evidence of infarction.
D. In a study of TIA patients, a DWI lesion was found in 70% of patients who had symptom duration of 12 to 24 hours.
E. Perfusion-weighted imaging (PWI) appears to show no benefit over DWI in detecting acute ischemic changes in patients with TIA.

463. A 58-year-old man had multiple episodes of transient bilateral blurred vision. The most recent and prolonged one occurred 5 hours prior to arrival in the emergency department. His blood pressure was elevated, but his neurologic examination was normal. The CT scan of the brain and the carotid ultrasound were normal. Because of his recent chemotherapy for lymphoma, you are suspicious of posterior reversible encephalopathy syndrome (PRES) but your colleague thinks that he had posterior embolic ischemia. Which MRI sequence will best resolve this dispute?

A. T1-weighted images.
B. T2-weighted images.
C. Fluid-attenuated inversion recovery (FLAIR).
D. Diffusion-weighted images (DWI).
E. Apparent diffusion coefficient (ADC) map.

464. An acute ischemic stroke characteristically produces a hyperintense signal seen on DWI. Which of the following can also cause a hyperintense signal on DWI?

A. A subacute ischemic stroke.
B. Cerebral abscess.
C. Glioblastoma multiforme.
D. Herpes encephalitis.
E. All of the above.

465. The most characteristic MRI lesion in Susac syndrome is seen in which anatomic location?

A. Basal ganglia.
B. Corpus callosum.
C. Cerebellum.
D. Thalamus.
E. Leptomeninges.

466. Which is true about intracranial and extracranial dissections?

A. The combination of MRI and MRA have specificity for dissection equivalent to conventional angiography.
B. Angioplasty and stenting is of proven value in the treatment of dissection.
C. Angiography is the preferred initial test if dissection is strongly suspected.
D. Intramural hematomas are not seen on MRI.

467. Transcranial Doppler tracings become more difficult to obtain as the the skull thickens with age. Based on the ability to obtain TCD readings, the thickest skulls are in:

A. Men.
B. Women.
C. No gender difference.

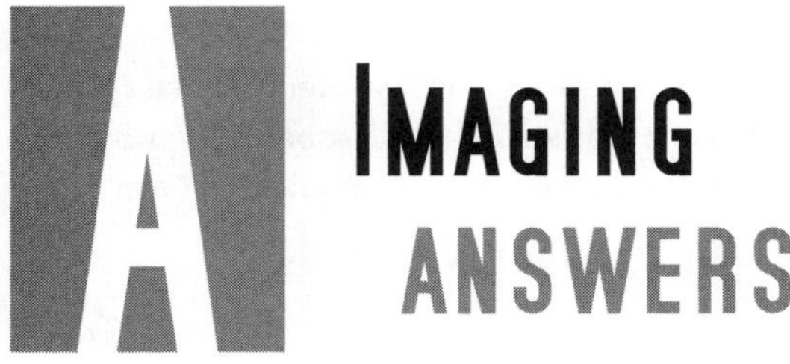

Imaging Answers

404. The answer is C. The pertinent finding on this magnetic resonance imaging (MRI) is a large flow void in the midline in the area of the anterior communicating artery. This computed tomography (CT) angiogram was obtained in the clinic using the CereTOM CT scanner; it reveals a 6 mm anterior communicating aneurysm. This finding was confirmed by digital subtraction angiography, and the aneurysm was clipped without complications. Carotid duplex and echocardiography are part of a full stroke work-up, but they would not explain the MRI finding. Transcranial Doppler (TCD) findings are not diagnostic of cerebral aneurysms. (Osborn, Chapters I, 3, 15)

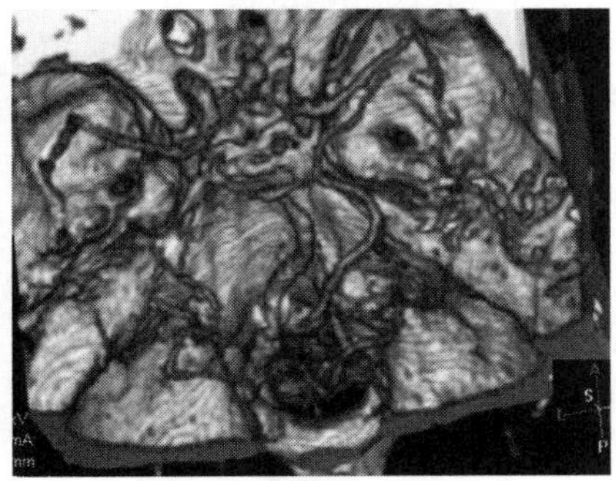

See color section following page 282.

405. The answer is B. The CT scan shows hypodensity of more than one-third of the middle cerebral artery (MCA) territory. The bleeding risk is increased in this patient, and the chances of clinical benefit are very small with so much permanently damaged tissue. Interestingly, after tissue plasminogen activator (t-PA) was appropriately withheld from this patient, additional history became available from other individuals. The patient's wife apparently returned from a rendezvous with a male companion and found her husband on the floor unable to move his right side. Because she did not want her children to know about the "other man," she fabricated the story that she was with him at the time of onset. The actual time of the stroke was in fact unknown. The patient was last seen normal 6 hours earlier. Based on the degree of hypodensity, this stroke was probably over 3 hours old in any case. (The boyfriend bailed out of this relationship quickly.) (von Kummer, *Stroke* 1999)

406. The answer is A. This is an MRI of a patient with HHT—hereditary hemorrhagic telangiectasia, also know as Osler-Weber-Rendu syndrome, who was evaluated at the Intermountain Stroke Center. This disorder is inherited as an autosomal dominant. This patient had a history of epistaxis, which is the most common presentation. He had telangiectasias on his lips. He also had a history of gastrointestinal bleed. When he had a transient ischemic attack (TIA), he was placed on aspirin and clopidogrel with no CT scan of the brain. When neurologic symptoms recurred, this MRI was obtained. Acute and chronic blood was present on MRI and CT. The symptoms and the acute hemorrhagic changes improved when platelet inhibition was discontinued. Computed tomography angiography of the brain may demonstrate high flow arteriovenous malformations (AVMs). (Osborn, Chapters I, 1, 14)

407. The answer is B. Because of the autosomal inheritance pattern of HHT and the potentially devastating consequences in those patients with HHT who do have cerebral AVMs, screening of first-degree relatives is recommended. The test of choice is MRI with and without contrast. Invasive or noninvasive vascular imaging may be appropriate in patients with abnormal MRIs, depending on the findings. This screening should also be done in patients with systemic evidence of HHT, including mucocutaneous and visceral telangiectasias. In this case, the patient's sister had a history of epistaxis and hemorrhagic changes on MRI, as did his daughter. The patient recommended that his daughter come in for evaluation, but she refused. In the 2 years since this MRI, was done the patient's daughter has become disabled by a major hemorrhage from a cerebral AVM. Since the antiplatelet agents have been stopped in this patient, he has improved. (Osborn, Chapters I, 1, 14)

408. The answer is E. This patient was a chronic alcohol abuser with ataxia and confusion. A year previously, he had been seen in the emergency department with an alcohol level of 230. His sodium level was corrected according to established guidelines but, despite this, he became gradually more confused and somnolent. This particular MRI was taken 6 months later, when the patient presented for evaluation of choreoathetotic movements. This represents the outcome of central pontine myelinolysis. The sparing of the rim of tissue at the superficial portion of the basis pontis rules out stroke, because no vessel has such a distribution. (Adams, Victor, & Mancall, *Arch Neurol Psychiatry* 1959)

409. The answer is C. The structure in question is the sinus confluence, also called the torcular Herophili. It forms the confluence of the superior sagittal sinus, the straight sinus, and the transverse sinuses. The superior sagittal sinus, transverse sinus, and the inferior anastomotic vein are also demonstrated in this image. The large arrow shows the superior sagittal sinus. The curved arrow points to the transverse sinus. The small arrow points to the vein of Labbe, also known as the inferior anastomotic vein. (Harnsberger, Part 1, Section 8)

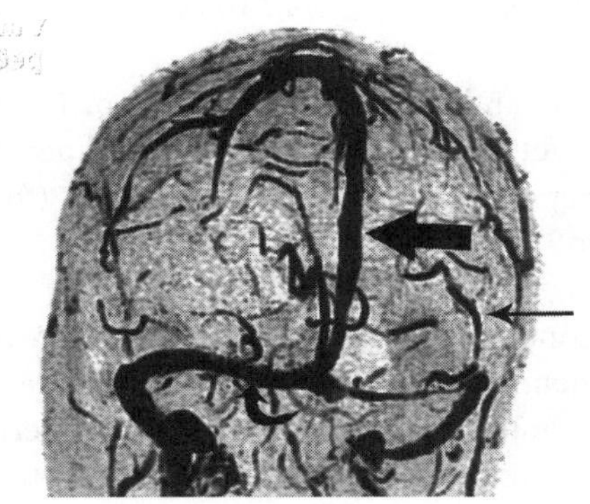

410. The answer is D. This patient had a severe dilated cardiomyopathy with an ejection fraction of 26%. This TCD is typical of low cardiac output with autoregulation producing an extremely low resistance pattern. This tracing shows a very low pulse pressure in all arteries sampled, which improves following heart transplant. Below is the TCD tracing of this patient following his heart transplant.

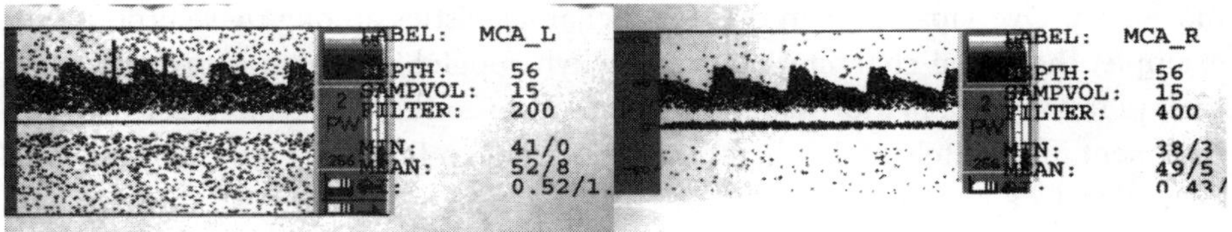

It should be noted that TCD is *not* a measurement of cerebral blood flow, but when blood flow drops maximal decreased resistance occurs, resulting in a lower pulse pressure.

Middle cerebral artery stenosis would show high peak systolic velocities in the MCA, with other waveforms being normal. Increased resistance would produce a lower diastolic flow. Alcohol abuse does not produce particular TCD changes, unless it results in a cardiomyopathy. (Gruhn et al., *Stroke* 2001; Hennerici, Chapter 3)

411. The answer is C. Intracardiac defibrillators (ICDs) were initially developed to prevent sudden death in patients with a history of ventricular fibrillation and ventricular tachycardia (VT). Patients with dilated cardiomyopathy have frequent episodes of nonsustained VT that results in sudden death. Electrophysiologic studies have not been successful in predicting these patients, and medications have not been successful in treating them, so ICD placement is preferred. Heart transplant may be necessary, but cannot be done urgently. A demand pacemaker will be of no value. (Gregoratos et al., *J Am Coll Cardiol* 1998)

412. The answer is C. On T1, fresh blood can be either hypointense or isointense. On T2, fresh blood is hyperintense, but a fresh hematoma will frequently have a surrounding rim of hypointensity representing early deoxygenation (formation of oxyhemoglobin). (Atlas, Chapter 9)

413. The answer is D. Hemosiderin is contained in macrophages and can be present in areas of hemorrhage for an indefinite period, first appearing several days following hemorrhage as macrophages enter the tissue. On T2, hemosiderin is always hypointense, but it can be either hypointense or isointense on T1. (Atlas, Chapter 9)

414. The answer is C. The dating of hemorrhagic changes by MRI is fraught with inaccuracies. The signal characteristics of hemorrhagic tissue is based on the magnetic properties of iron and of the hemoglobin breakdown products, including, deoxyhemoglobin, intracellular and extracellular methemoglobin, and hemosiderin. Overlaps occur in the signal characteristics among these groups. For example, the signal characteristics of deoxyhemoglobin, which is present hours to days following a hemorrhage, can be identical to those of hemosiderin, which is present indefinitely after a hemorrhage. Although D may be true, it should not be! (Atlas, Chapter 9)

415. The answer is 1A, 2B, 3G, 4J, 5F. This is a CTA/CTV of a patient with an extracranial-intracranial (EC-IC) bypass. This was obtained using the CereTOM CT scanner. The CT angiogram has the advantage of imaging arteries and veins simultaneously. In this situation, the superior temporal artery enters the intracranial space via the surgical skull defect and anastomoses with the MCA, representing an EC-IC bypass. The other vessels are standard normal anatomy. (Harnsberger, Part 1, Sections 7 and 8)

416. The answer is C. Duplex systems were developed before the advent of color-flow technology. The standard equipment is now a color-flow duplex system. Both external and internal carotid arteries can be imaged, but this has no relationship to the name of the technique. Continuous-wave Doppler is single channel; pulse-wave Doppler is multichannel. (Hennerici, Chapter 1)

417. The answer is A. When the ultrasound propagation speed is measured by "brightness modulation" (called B-mode), this produces a grayscale image. The velocity measurement is Doppler. Biologic imaging is meaningless; this answer is merely a distractor. Spectral analysis is part of the analysis of the multiple frequencies in the Doppler signal. (Hennerici, Chapter 1)

418. The answer is D. A huge variability exists in the relative locations of the internal carotid arteries (ICA) and external carotid arteries (ECA) in the neck. In 49% of patients, the ICA is dorsolateral to the ECA. It is medial in only 3%. It is dorsal in 21% and dorsomedial in 18%. It is ventromedial in 8%. The important message here is that the relative locations of the two branches of the common carotid artery are not useful in identifying the vessel. Other techniques, including resistance patterning and percussion are more useful. (Hennerici, Chapter 1)

419. The answer is B. Arteries supplying the brain exhibit low resistance. Low-resistance arteries have higher diastolic flow than do high-resistance arteries, thus providing forward systolic and diastolic flow. Arteries to muscle and skin have high resistance, with low diastolic flow. In the aorta, the resistance is so high that backward diastolic flow occurs. The difference in resistance in the ICA and ECA is useful in distinguishing between these arteries on carotid duplex in relatively normal patients. (Hennerici, Chapter 2)

420. The answer is A. This describes the sound of normal arteries. The whip-like sound of the ECA is typical of a high-resistance artery. In stenotic arteries with increased velocities, a higher-pitched sound occurs. The sound of the Doppler signal can be useful in differentiating between arteries and in listening for stenotic "sounding" signals. (Hennerici, Chapter 2)

421. The answer is B. The most reliable measure of stenosis is the peak systolic velocity, which is 166 cm/sec. This fits a 40% to 59% stenosis. The end diastolic velocity is 36.6 cm/sec, also well within the 40% to 59% stenosis range. With stenosis of 60% or more, end diastolic velocity goes above 40 cm/sec. The apparent interruption of color flow is commonly seen whenever frames are isolated. When one views the real-time images, there is no interruption of flow when an entire cardiac cycle is followed. This loss of information from a single frame is one reason most neurologists prefer to read from video or digital real-time images. (Hennerici, Chapter 2)

422. The answer is C. This is a classic right-to-left intracardiac shunt, which in this patient turned out to be a patent foramen ovale (PFO). This TCD was done using agitated saline bubble contrast. The IV injection would have to pass right-to-left to be detected in the brain. Left-to-right intracardiac shunts do occur, but TEE is necessary to detect this shunt. Pulmonary AVM can produce a right-to-left shunt, but these are much less common than intracardiac shunts and will generally produce a lower level of shunting. Carotid occlusion has no relationship to this TCD. This level of shunting can be described as a "curtain" or as a level "5", depending on the classification system being used. (Droste et al., *Stroke* 1999)

423. The answer is A. The temporal windows are used to insonate anterior, middle, and posterior cerebral arteries. The intracranial portion of the ICA can also be seen through this window, but bone obscures the carotid siphon from this approach. The transforaminal approach is used to insonate the vertebral and basilar arteries. (Hennerici, Chapter 3)

424. The answer is B. The MCA starts at a depth of approximately 60 mm, and it and its branches can be traced distally to a depth of 30 to 40 mm. The direction of the MCA is toward the probe. At a depth of 60 mm, a waveform flowing away from the probe can be detected and followed to a depth of 70 mm. This is the anterior cerebral artery (ACA). With an ipsilateral carotid occlusion, the contralateral ICA may provide collateral flow via the ACA. In this case, both the ACA and the MCA will have flow directed toward the probe. The posterior cerebral artery (PCA) is seen at 55 to 80 mm. The PCA has flow both toward and away from the probe, because of the curve of this vessel. The vertebral artery is not seen via the transtemporal approach. (Hennerici, Chapter 3)

425. The answer is B. Normally, the highest velocity is in the MCA, with slightly lower velocity in the ACA. When the ACA is providing collateral flow to the contralateral hemisphere, this relationship will be reversed, and the ACA will have a velocity higher than the ipsilateral ACA. All vessels in the posterior circulation have a lower velocity than the MCA and the ACA in normal subjects. The ophthalmic artery generally has the lowest velocities. (Hennerici, Chapter 3)

426. The answer is B. The normal MCA velocity is under 140 cm/sec. The velocity in the right MCA is normal. Mild stenosis produces a peak systolic velocity of 140 to 209 cm/sec. Moderate stenosis produces a PSV of 210 to 280 cm/sec, with severe stenosis producing a PSV of over 280 cm/sec. In high-grade stenosis, there will also be increases in diastolic velocity. With a critical stenosis, the velocities will eventually decrease with near occlusion. (Hennerici, Chapter 3)

427. The answer is C. In a normal TCD, the MCA peak systolic velocity (PSV) is slightly higher than the ACA. In this tracing, the PSV in the ACA is more than 50% higher than the MCA. This patient has a left carotid occlusion. As the right ACA is providing collateral flow to the left hemisphere, the velocity is elevated because of the increased blood volume coursing through this vessel. Anterior cerebral artery stenosis is less likely. This velocity is not high enough to suggest a moderate stenosis, and the waveform is normal, not resembling a stenotic waveform. The right MCA velocity is normal. (Hennerici, Chapter 3)

428. The answer is B. This is a classic picture of brain death or cerebrocirculatory arrest. The advantage of this confirmatory test for brain death is that it is not influenced by sedatives, as are some other tests for brain death (e.g., the electroencephalogram or EEG). Distal MCA occlusion may have a dampened waveform, but will not have biphasic flow. An EC-IC bypass may produce reversal of flow in the MCA. Embolic signals are single "blips" on the TCD. (Hennerici, Chapter 3)

429. The answer is C. The motor and sensory neurons in the right frontal lobe have been destroyed, leading to demyelination of the nerve fibers (Wallerian degeneration). This will produce atrophy and hyperintensity along the pathways involving these neurons, including diencephalon and brainstem structures. The rounded hyperintensity in the right thalamus and the hyperintensity in the right cerebral peduncle and the right basis pontis is consistent with demyelination of the corticospinal and sensory fibers. Wallerian degeneration also produces atrophy in the brainstem, which is seen here in the right pons and midbrain. With immunosupression, opportunistic infections in the lung can embolize to the brain, but this image does not support this diagnosis. (Osborn, Chapters I, 10, 91)

430. The answer is C. This patient had a lumbar puncture with positive oligoclonal bands, and her visual evoked potentials were consistent with the diagnosis of multiple sclerosis (MS). The characteristic lesions of MS include ovoid lesions that are periventricular and oriented radially. All the lesions on this MRI are periventricular, which is another clue to the correct final diagnosis. These MRI findings are not absolutely diagnostic, but primary demyelinating disease must be considered. Cerebral angiogram would be performed for the possibility of cerebral vasculitis, and a temporal artery biopsy would be indicated to diagnose temporal arteritis, both of which are less likely based on the MRI and clinical presentation. Cerebral autosomal dominant arteriopathy with subcortical infarcts and leukoencephalopathy (CADASIL) is also less likely than MS based on the MRI appearance. (Atlas, Chapter 13)

431. The answer is A. The ultrasound beam cannot penetrate calcium, so acoustic shadowing is produced, obliterating information on structures deep to the plaque. Both the grayscale images and the Doppler signals will be lost. Calcium also produces technical limitations in CT angiography. In these cases, MRA may provide adequate information Technical improvements (mainly software) in CT are reducing this problem. With carotid duplex CTA and/or MRA, invasive catheter angiography can be avoided in most stroke and TIA patients. The MRA tends to overestimate high-grade arterial stenosis, and is most useful in moderate degrees of stenosis. Carotid duplex is less expensive than either MRA or CTA. (Johnson et al., *Neurology* 2001; Prokop et al., *JBR-BTR* 2004)

432. The answer is C. Epidural hematomas are caused by arterial hemorrhage 90% of the time, generally related to trauma. Most occur on the side of the traumatic impact, although a subdural hematoma may coexist on the opposite ("contre-coup") side. The posterior fossa is not a common site, although this is the most dangerous location if surgical decompression is not performed promptly. The CT appearance is a biconvex extra-axial hematoma. (Osborn, Chapters I, 2, 6)

433. The answer is A. This is a mixed subdural hematoma, with hemorrhagic components of different ages. There is a large subdural hematoma on the left, with both acute and chronic components. There is a smaller subacute subdural hematoma, on the right parietal. These are caused by tears in bridging veins. Trauma and atrophy are predisposing factors. Subdural hematomas are extra-axial (external to pia) collections that are most often crescent-shaped, as opposed to the biconvex shape of an epidural hematoma. Subdural hematomas are most common with age, but they occur equally in both genders. Vascular malformations or dural metastases may occasionally cause a subdural hematoma, but the most common cause is trauma. (Osborn, Chapters I, 2, 20)

434. The answer is E. The CTA captures both arteries and veins. Postprocessing procedures determine whether arteries or veins or both are seen on a particular reconstruction.. The paired veins at the midline are the internal cerebral veins. The structure between the internal cerebral veins is not an aneurysm. It is a calcified structure that is not contiguous with any vessel. It is calcified choroid plexus. This black-and-white figure is an alternate view of the same image. The veins in are now in a partial sagittal orientation. In this view, the calcification is clearly separate from the vascular structures. A review of venous structures shown: 1, confluence of sinuses; 2, straight sinus; 3, vein of Galen; 4, basal vein of Rosenthal (one of two paired veins); 5, internal cerebral vein (one of two paired veins). (Harnsberger, Section 8)

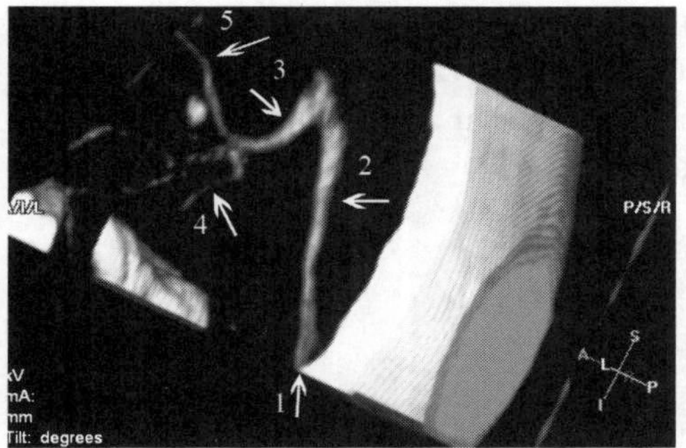

435. The answer is D. This is the typical enlarged superior temporal artery that occurs following EC-IC bypass surgery, which was performed in this patient 2 years prior to this CTA. Eighty-six percent of patients undergoing EC-IC bypass have enlargement of the superficial temporal artery. The contrast settings would need to be higher to visualize other branches of the ECA that have lower flow, such as the facial artery. The internal jugular vein is partially seen, but again, different contrast settings would be required to visualize this entire vein. The superficial temporal artery has a surgical anastomosis to the MCA. (Harnsberg, Sections 8, 9; Lee et al., *Arch Neurol* 1979)

436. The answer is D. This woman presented with multiple small infarcts in the right MCA territory. Her father died at age 28 from a myocardial infarction and was found to have diffuse atherosclerosis. She had an isolated right MCA stenosis. Recurrent TIAs were controlled for 2 years on platelet inhibition and anticoagulation, but when the stenosis progressed and became symptomatic on maximal medical therapy, an angioplasty was performed. The MCA velocities improved but, 3 years later, the stenosis had progressed and she again became symptomatic. The restenosis was longer than the initial stenosis and an EC-IC bypass was performed. The patient has been symptom-free for 4 years. Questions 435 and 415 show the intracranial and extracranial views of this patient's EC-IC bypass. Migraine headaches can result in asymmetrical flow, but not in stenotic velocities. The depth and direction of flow tell the reader that this signal is from the MCA. The ACA signal would be deeper (i.e., 68–70 mm) and would be flowing away from the probe (under the line). A left ACA stenosis with collateral flow would show a mild elevation of flow velocity in the right ACA, with the ACA velocity being slightly higher than the MCA velocity. (Hennerici, Chapter 3)

437. The answer is A. Pictured here is the same MRA with a different orientation. It is clearer from this view that the right PCA is the terminal branch of the basilar artery, with no left PCA coming off the basilar artery. The left PCA is the larger artery coming from the left ICA, otherwise known as a fetal origin of the PCA. This artery is best seen on the image provided with the question. The smaller artery, which is the final branch of the basilar artery on the left side, is the superior cerebellar artery. (Harnsberger, Section 7)

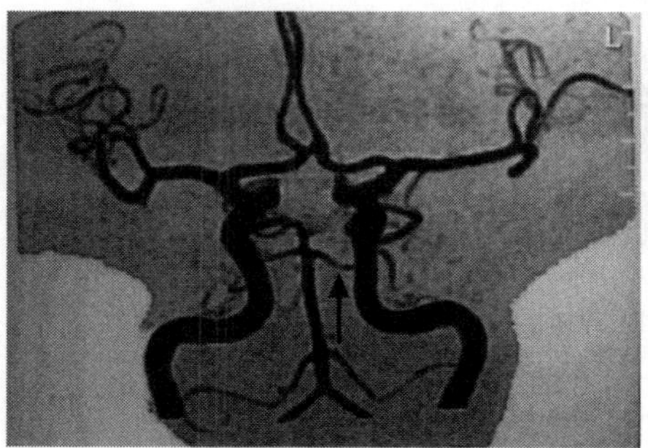

438. The answer is B. The delta sign is the appearance of the superior sagittal sinus thrombosis on contrast-enhanced CT. A triangular pattern of enhancement is apparent, surrounding a central relatively hypodense thrombus. The classic clinical complication of superior sagittal sinus thrombosis is bilateral paramedian hemorrhages. Subdural hematoma can be seen on CT scan, but is simply a distractor in this case. Transverse sinus thrombus can be seen on MRI/MRV or on cerebral angiography, but not on CT. (Ginsberg & Bogousslavsky, Chapter 107)

439. The answer is A. A developmental venous anomaly (DVA) does not bleed. In this case, there is evidence of a hemorrhage in the right cerebellum. There is also a classic "caput medusae" surrounding a large draining vein, which is the typical appearance of a DVA (venous angioma). Bleeding from a DVA is so rare that, when hemorrhage is present, an accompanying cavernoma or an AMV is usually found. Sturge-Weber syndrome includes pial angiomatosis, and these present in infancy. There is evidence of hemorrhage in the cerebellum, but this is characteristic of hemosiderin rather than acute hemorrhage. (Osborn, Chapters I, 5, 24)

440. The answer is B. This is an encapsulated cerebrospinal fluid (CSF) density, consistent with a cystic structure. It is located in the pineal gland. This lesion is too high in the neuraxis to be related to the basilar artery, and an aneurysm would have either flow void or thrombus characteristics. The central CSF density makes artifact unlikely. The pineal cyst is not related to her symptoms, but the headache was an indication for imaging. (Atlas, Chapter 14)

441. The answer is C. This patient had a malignant glioblastoma multiforme (GBM). As no vessels are seen, this should be recognized as a nonenhanced scan. Thus, the mixed density seen on T1WI (MRI on the right) represents a hemorrhagic component. The sagittal images show a globular lesion, with mass effect clear on axial images. This picture is classic for a malignant brain tumor. The shape of the lesion is more consistent with a mass than an infarct. An abscess would not contain blood. The patchiness of the hyperintensity is not consistent with lobar hemorrhage, which would be more homogeneous. Glioblastoma multiforme and oligodendrogliomas are primary brain tumors that may present with hemorrhage. (Osborn, Chapters I, 6, 20)

442. The answer is A. When the paired embryonic longitudinal arteries fail to fuse completely, a fenestrated basilar artery is formed. The vertebral arteries form the basilar; then there is a slight interruption of the fusion at the proximal portion of the basilar, leading to the "doughnut hole" appearance. A basilar dissection would appear as a narrowed basilar artery. Dolichoectasia is a large basilar artery associated with slow flow. Basilar thrombosis would cause stenosis or occlusion of the basilar artery, which is not present in this example. (Osborn, Chapter 9)

443. The answer is B. This patient had a symptomatic basilar stenosis that was successfully treated with stent placement. A vertebral stenosis would be seen at a shallower depth. Reversal of flow in a vertebral artery would again be at a shallower depth, and the waveform would be above the line, flowing toward the probe. This is a classic arterial signal, not a venous signal. (Hennerici, Chapter 2)

444. The answer is B. Nephrogenic fibrosing dermopathy/nephrogenic systemic fibrosis (NFD/NSF) has been found in patients with acute or chronic renal failure who have been exposed to gadolinium-containing contrast agents. NFD/NSF is a fibrosing cutaneous disorder that is characterized clinically by the acute onset of hardening and thickening of the skin of the extremities and trunk, often resulting in flexion contractures. Histologically, there is an increase in spindle-shaped cells, collagen, and sometimes mucin deposition in the dermis. Gadolinium has been detected in skin tissue samples of affected patients. Other organs that may be involved include lungs, myocardium, or striated muscles. (Introcaso et al., *Int J Dermatol* 2007)

445. The answer is B. This is an example of schizencephaly. With an MCA stroke, the cortical ribbon in the MCA territory would be destroyed. The borders of the infarct would be subcortical white matter. In schizencephaly, there is an open lip lined with gray matter or cortical ribbon. This is clearly seen on the MRI.

Note the deep sulcal structures on the edge of the cleft, which would not be present in an infarct. (Osborn, Chapters I, 1, 70)

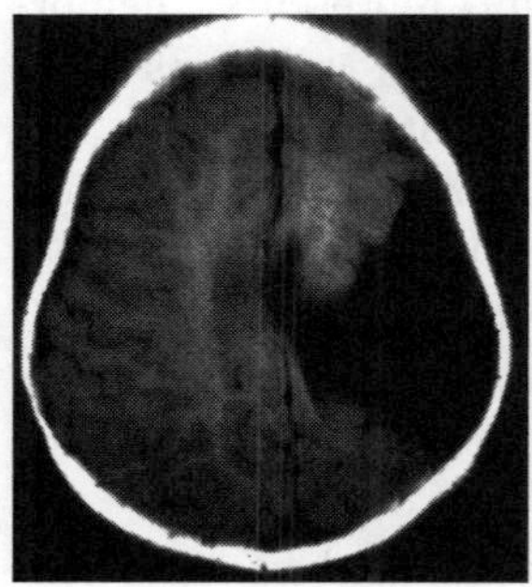

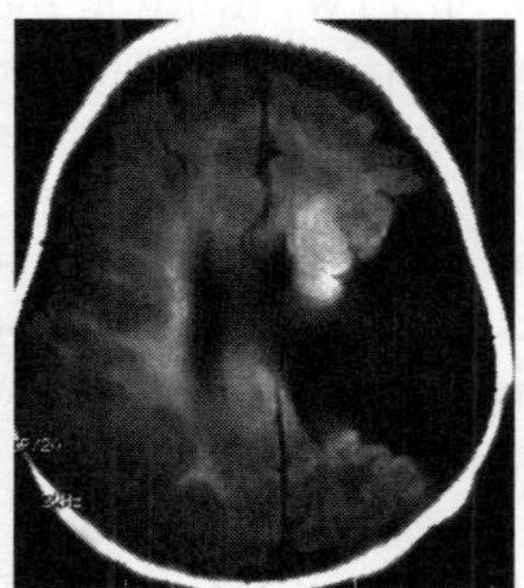

446. The answer is D. Hypodensity of more than one-third of the MCA territory was associated with increased symptomatic hemorrhage and death following thrombolysis in the European Cooperative Acute Stroke Study (ECASS). Attenuation of the lentiform nuclei is an early infarct sign with no prognostic significance. An thromboembolus in the MCA often produces a hyperdense MCA sign; this is not necessarily a bad prognostic sign and is not a contraindication to thrombolytic therapy. Calcified atherosclerosis of the MCA can also produce a hyperdense MCA. Early infarct signs are not always reliable to predict the side of an acute infarct, because old ischemia can produce hypodensity and attenuation of the lentiform nuclei. (Larrue et al., *Stroke* 1997; Manelfe et al., *Stroke* 1999)

447. The answer is C. This diagnosis is best made using MRI with contrast. The arterial phase of a MRA will generally be normal. Digital subtraction angiography is also generally normal in the arterial phase. Small DVAs can be missed on an noncontrasted MRI study. (Osborn, Chapters I, 5, 16)

448. The answer is C. The halo sign represents edema in the vessel wall. When seen in the superficial temporal artery this finding is 92% to 100% specific for temporal arteritis. Internalization of the ECA is a finding made in the proximal ECA in the neck, with a low-resistance pattern seen in this artery. (LaSar et al., *J Vasc Surg* 2002; Schimdt & Kraft, *N Engl J Med* 1997)

449. The answer is C. To the right of the diameter measurement device is the carotid bulb, so this is clearly one of the branches of the common carotid artery. This is a high-resistance waveform, typical of the ECA. The common carotid perfuses both high- and low-resistance beds. Normal waveforms of the other arteries are shown on the next page. The ICA has a low-resistance waveform, with a higher diastolic reading. The vertebral artery is smaller and of a lower velocity, with vertebral shadowing. (Hennerici, Chapter 2)

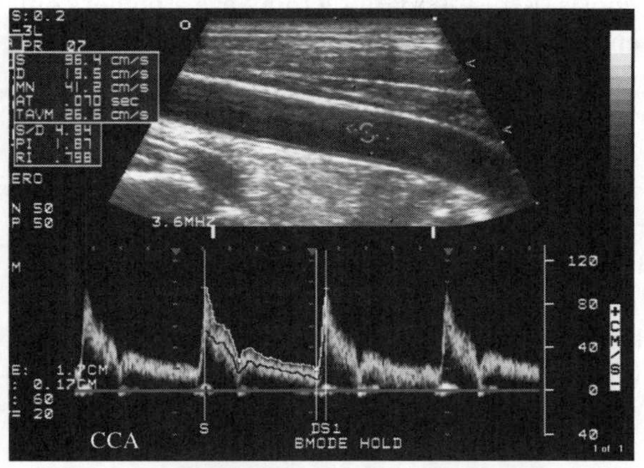

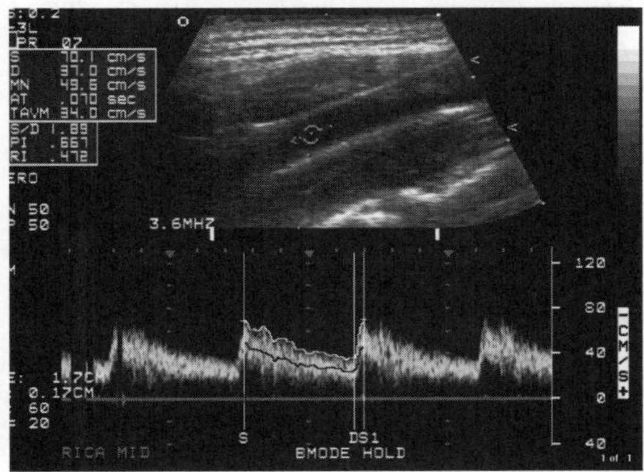

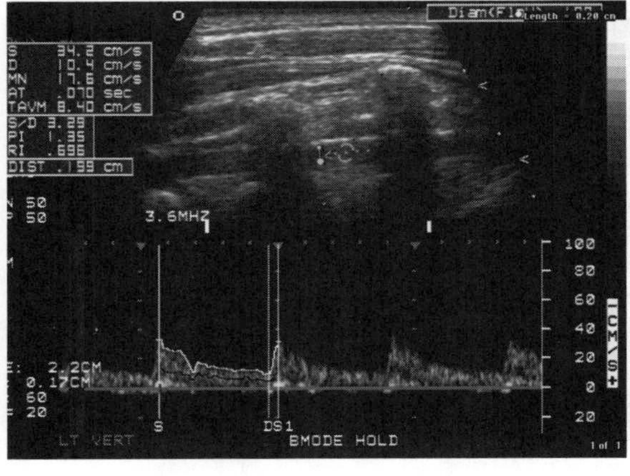

450. The answer is D. The present regimen would clearly lead to carotid occlusion, because the stenosis has progressed rapidly. Anticoagulation would do nothing to slow down the restenosis. Repeat endarterectomy has a higher complication rate than the initial endarterectomy. An EC-IC bypass has no proven role in this setting. The best option at this time would stent placement. (Yadav et al., *Stroke* 1996)

451. The answer is A. This is a normal basilar artery. The velocity is 41 cm/sec, which is at the low normal end for the basilar. It is too deep to be a vertebral artery. Bilateral fetal origin of the posterior cerebral arteries may decrease the amount of blood through the basilar artery, but this generally results in a smaller basilar artery and does not affect flow velocity. Subclavian steal would produce flow in the opposite direction in a vertebral artery, at a shallower depth. (Hennerici, Chapter 3)

452. The answer is C. This perfusion CT was performed using the CereTOM scanner. A decrease in relative cerebral flood flow is seen in the right internal carotid territory. Cerebral vasculitis would have mutifocal perfusion defects. The flow in the left hemisphere is normal. This patient indeed had a right carotid occlusion and increased oxygen extraction fraction by positron emission tomography (PET) scanning. She was symptomatic. An EC-IC bypass normalized her clinical picture and her perfusion scan. (Koenig et al., *Stroke* 2001)

453. The answer is B. This is the classic tunnel defect of a PFO. There was a left-to-right shunt, but that cannot be determined from this image, which did not use agitated saline. The other answers are distractors. In this figure, the left atrium, right atrium, left ventricle, and the long tunnel are labeled. (Fuster, Chapter 73)

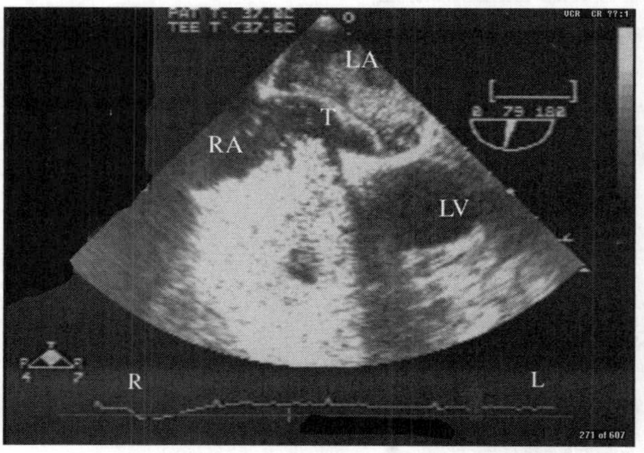

454. The answer is C. This patient is having crescendo TIAs. This situation is clinically suggestive of a tight carotid stenosis with impending occlusion. With tight stenosis, a carotid duplex can produce false-positive findings suggesting occlusion. Because residual flow would make the patient a candidate for endarterectomy, CTA or catheter angiography should be performed urgently. An MRA may not distinguish tight focal stenosis from occlusion. "Signal dropout" in high-grade stenosis is a drawback of MRA. A critical stenosis was found at angiography in this patient, and endarterectomy was performed. Had carotid occlusion been documented, Aggrenox or Plavix would have been an appropriate next therapy, in conjunction with an evaluation for other causes of stroke. (Hennerici, Chapter 2)

455. The answer is C. The CTA was obtained in clinic using the CereTom scanner. A small protrusion, seen at the bulb, represents the only evidence of the ICA. The artery seen on the CTA image is clearly the ECA, because the extracranial ICA has no branches. Internalization of the ECA is a finding on carotid duplex when the ECA is providing intracranial flow via collaterals and thus has a low-resistance waveform. This cannot be determined by angiography. The key to determining that this is a congenital occlusion is finding the narrowing or absence of the carotid canal. This can be seen on CT source images. The normal right carotid canal is designated by the arrow. Bilateral congenital absence of the ICA has also been reported, with the entire brain perfused by the "posterior circulation." (Rumboldt et al., *Eur Radiol* 2003)

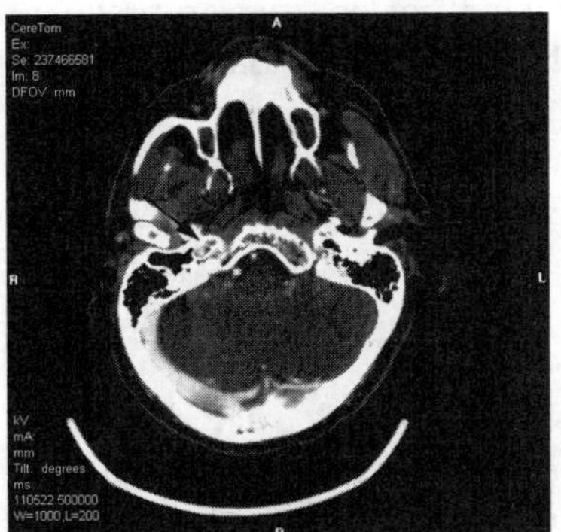

456. The answer is B. Variations in the Doppler angle can produce huge discrepancies in the reported velocity. The most commonly used angle is 60 degrees. A small sample volume is desirable, because large sample volumes will produce a wide spectrum of velocity readings. Color and power Doppler have added new dimensions to the duplex study, but these do not influence the accuracy of velocity readings. (Hennerici, Chapter 2)

457. The answer is D. This is a 95% ICA stenosis, with very high peak systolic and end diastolic velocities. The exact velocity criteria and stenosis range varies from lab to lab. A PSV of 85, EDV of 18 is normal, with stenosis of less than 40%. A PSV of 155, EDV of 35 denotes 40% to 59% stenosis. A PSV of 210, EDV of 45 denotes 60% to 90% stenosis. A PSV of 155, EDV of 35 denotes a stenosis of - above 90%. (Hennerici, Chapter 2)

458. The answer is C. This patient, who presented with transient neurologic classic crescendo TIAs, had an atretic P1 segment of the PCA on the left, consistent with fetal origin of the left PCA. In this situation, both the MCA and PCA territories are perfused by the left ICA. Multiple acute embolic strokes were noted, which probably occurred as the critical stenosis progressed toward occlusion. On MRA, this patient did have an atretic P1 segment on the left, a typical finding in a patient with a fetal origin. Because the carotid was occluded, it was not possible to document the fetal origin of the PCA, but this fits the scenario best. There are reports of "posterior circulation" infarcts from carotid emboli. Because fetal origin of the PCA is the most common vascular variant, present in at least 15% of individuals, this phenomenon is likely more frequent than is recognized. It should be remembered that the terms "posterior" and "anterior" do *not* invariably refer directly to carotid territory or basilar territory in every patient. (Chaturvedi et al., *Neurology* 1999; Pessin, *Stroke* 1989)

459. The answer is D. Intravenous contrast should not be used on pregnant women. Cardiac pacers and claustrophobia can be contraindications to MRI but not to CT. Shellfish allergy is often thought to be a contraindication to iodine contrast, but that is not always the case. A patient with "shellfish allergy" should be questioned carefully as to the nature of the reaction to shellfish. Some causes of shellfish intolerance do not necessarily represent iodine allergies. (Fergus et al., *AJR* 1997)

460. The answer is A 3, B 1, C 2, D 4. Transcranial Doppler detects flow in the anterior and posterior circulation vessels using four cranial insonation windows. The anterior, middle, and posterior cerebral arteries and the terminal internal carotid arteries are insonated through the transtemporal approach. The submandibular approach is also used to measure flow velocity in the distal ICA at the entry into the skull in patients with subarachnoid hemorrhage. The transorbital approach is used to insonate the ophthalmic artery and the ICA siphon. The transforaminal approach (also known as the nuchal or suboccipital approach) allows the insonation of the terminal vertebral arteries and the basilar artery. (Alexandrov et al., *J Neuroimaging* 2007)

461. The answer is A. Cerebral microbleeds (CMBs) are focal areas of signal loss on gradient-echo T2*-weighted MRI sequences due to focal hemosiderin deposition from previous small bleeds. They are believed to be due to previous extravasation of blood associated with bleeding-prone small-vessel disease. Increasing age and blood pressure, as well as decreased cholesterol, increase the risk for CMBs. (Fiehler, *Int J Stroke* 2006)

462. The answer is D. Diffusion-weighted imaging (DWI) has shown clinically relevant acute ischemic lesions in some patients with TIA, depending on the duration of the symptoms and the timing of the study. Perfusion-weighted imaging (PWI) is likely to be even more sensitive than DWI in detecting these changes. In a University of California, Los Angeles (UCLA) study of TIA patients, the percentage of patients with a DWI abnormality increased with a longer total duration of symptoms. As the symptom duration increased from 10 minutes to 24 hours, the percentage with a DWI lesion increased from 30% to 71%. Approximately a quarter of patients with hemispheric TIAs, with transient signs and symptoms, have cerebral infarction by imaging criteria. A small percentage of TIA patients have early DWI lesions but no later imaging evidence of infarction, with the exact numbers depending on characteristics of the TIA. (Chaturvedi & Levine, Chapter 5)

463. The answer is E. Posterior reversible encephalopathy syndrome (PRES) is a syndrome featuring loss of cerebral autoregulation and capillary leakage (vasogenic edema). It can have multiple etiologies, including hypertension and chemotherapy. It can cause multiple neurologic symptoms, both transient and fixed, including cortical blindness. Hyperintense signal on DWI may be seen in hyperacute ischemia, with both fixed and transient clinical deficits. A hyperacute ischemic lesion (early cytotoxic edema) results in increased signal intensity (restricted diffusion) on DWI and a corresponding decreased signal on apparent diffusion coefficient (ADC) mapping. The vasogenic edema in PRES may result in hypointense to mildly hyperintense signal on DWI, because these images have both T2 and diffusion contributions. However, the acute ADC map shows hyperintense signal with vasogenic edema (PRES) and hypointense signal with cytotoxic edema (acute ischemia). (Schaefer et al., *Neuroimaging Clin N Am* 2005)

464. The answer is E. Subacute and chronic infarcts may result in increased signal on DWI because of "T2 shine-through" from increased T2 signal, rather than decreased diffusion. The use of ADC mapping, with hypointense signal in acute infarction and hyperintense signal in subacute and chronic infarction, differentiates the age of the lesion. False-positive DWI can occur in multiple conditions with decreased diffusion, including those caused by increased viscosity (cerebral abscess), dense cell packing (glioblastoma multiforme), and cell necrosis (herpes encephalitis). (Schaefer et al., *Neuroimaging Clin N Am* 2005)

465. The answer is B. Susac syndrome, most often seen in young women of all races, is the clinical triad of encephalopathy, hearing loss, and branch retinal artery occlusion. The MRI picture can be confused with MS or acute disseminated encephalomyelitis with multifocal, often enhancing, lesions. All the listed areas are associated with MR lesions in Susac syndrome, but the characteristic lesions are punched out or "snowball," high-T2 signal lesions, seen best on sagittal images, in the central fibers of the corpus callosum. (Susac et al., *Neurology* 2003)

466. The answer is A. The combination of MRI and MRA is not as sensitive as angiography for dissections, but the specificity is equivalent. Thus, MR should be the first imaging modality when dissection is suspected. Duplex is also a reasonable first test if proximal ICA dissection is suspected. Intraluminal hematomas can be seen on MRI, which is the reason for combining MRI with MRA for screening. Angioplasty and stenting are controversial. Angiography should be used if screening tests are negative and dissection is still strongly suspected. (Osborn, Chapters I, 2, 9)

467. The answer is B. Although counterintuitive (at least to the authors of this book), women have thicker skulls than men. Age does increase skull thickness, and TCD insonation is easiest in young people. In teenagers and young adults, the entire circle of Willis can sometimes be traced through a single temporal window. (Grotta et al., *Stroke* 1993; Halsey, *Stroke* 1990; von Kummer, *Stroke* 2003)

8 Clinical Pathology
Questions

468. The media of arteries consists of:

A. Endothelial cells.
B. Smooth muscle cells.
C. Collagen and fibrous tissue.
D. Elastin.

469. Atherosclerotic lesions:

A. Occur most often in high-shear regions.
B. Occur most often in low-shear regions.
C. Are not related to shear effects.
D. Develop uniformly in the aorta based on shear stress.

470. Which solid tumor is generally **not** associated with intratumoral parenchymal brain hemorrhage?

A. Melanoma.
B. Germcell tumors.
C. Papillary thyroid.
D. Renal cell.
E. Leiomyosarcoma.

471. Which one of the following is the most common pathologic mechanism for the cerebrovascular manifestations of systemic lupus erythematosus (SLE)?

A. Premature atherosclerosis.
B. Arterial vasospasm.
C. Antiphospholipid antibodies.
D. Intracerebral hemorrhage.
E. Cerebral arterial dissection.

472. Where is cervicocephalic fibromuscular dysplasia most likely to occur?

A. Vertebral artery.
B. Proximal internal carotid artery.
C. Intrapetrosal internal carotid artery.
D. Middle third (C1 to C2 level) of the internal carotid artery.
E. Middle cerebral artery.

473. Cavernous malformations:

A. Are seen as collections of very small sinusoidal channels on cerebral angiography.
B. Are mainly located infratentorially.
C. Contain normal brain parenchyma between sinusoidal vascular channels.
D. Are always congenital, never arising de novo.
E. May be inherited by autosomal dominant transmission with incomplete penetrance.

474. Developmental venous anomalies (DVAs):

A. Are rare cerebral vascular malformations.
B. Commonly cause cerebral hemorrhage and should be excised when diagnosed.
C. Can be associated with cavernous malformations.
D. Are poorly imaged on contrast enhanced MRI.
E. Drain only abnormal brain.

475. The most common organism producing infective endocarditis is:

A. *Staphylococcus aureus.*
B. *Streptococcus viridans.*
C. *Streptococcus bovis/Streptococcus equines.*
D. *Enterococcus faecalis.*
E. *Pneumococcus.*

476. The following picture most likely represents:

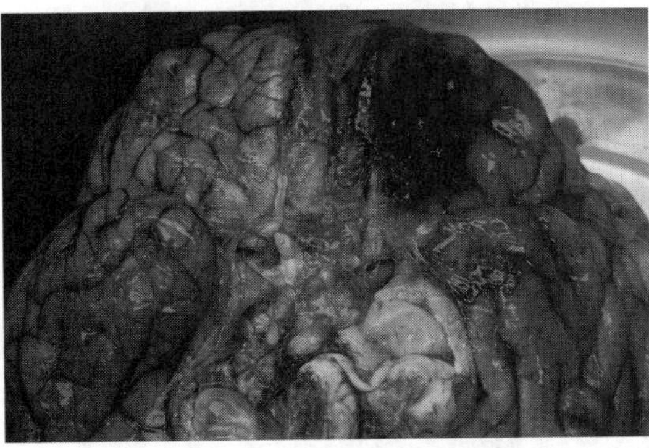

See color section following page 282.

A. Remote cerebral infarction.
B. Acute cerebral infarction.
C. Intraparenchymal hemorrhage due to disseminated intravascular coagulation.
D. Epidural hemorrhage.
E. None of the above.

477. The following picture most likely represents the following clinical scenario:

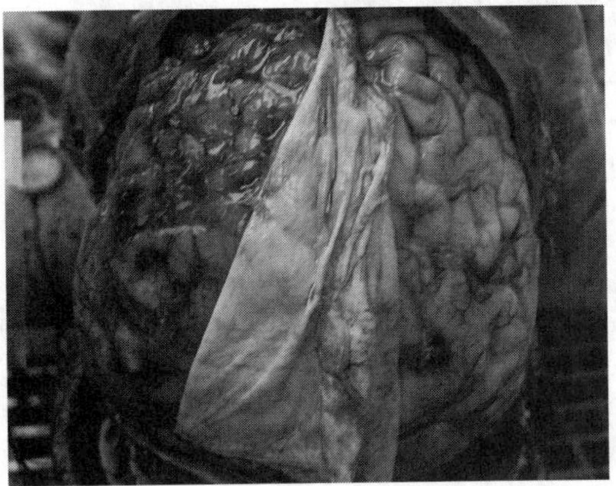

See color section following page 282.

A. Head trauma, a lucid interval followed by loss of consciousness, and evidence of rupture of the middle meningeal artery.
B. Sudden onset of right hemiplegia and aphasia, followed 2 days later by stupor and evidence of uncal herniation.
C. Minor head trauma 2 months previously and progressive right hemiparesis and headaches.
D. Sudden onset of severe headache and a stiff neck, without focal neurologic deficit.
E. Subacute onset headache, fever, stiff neck, and lethargy.

478. Fibromuscular dysplasia (FMD) is an abnormality of fibrous tissue proliferation. Which type of FMD, characterized by the dominant arterial wall involved, is the most common?

A. Intimal fibroplasia.
B. Medial dysplasia.
C. Adventitial fibroplasia.
D. Endothelial dysplasia.

479. The following picture most likely represents which of the following?

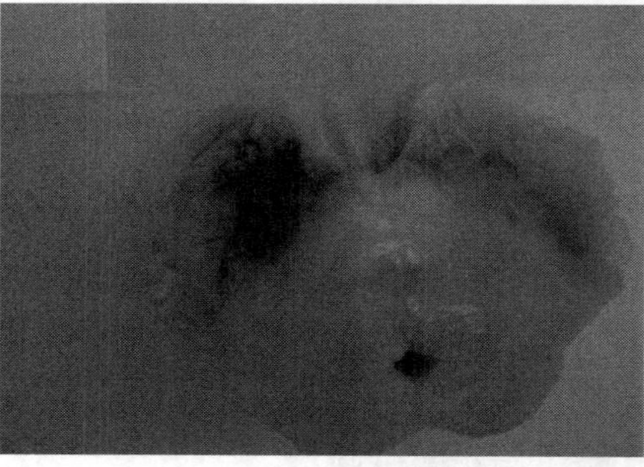

See color section following page 282.

A. Hypertrophy of the midbrain substantia nigra.
B. Metastatic carcinoma in the midbrain.
C. Normal appearance of the midbrain.
D. Midbrain damage due to global anoxia.
E. Duret hemorrhage in the midbrain due to herniation.

480. Which microbiologic agent exhibits tissue tropism to vascular endothelium resulting in vascular damage?

A. *Staphylococcus.*
B. *Loa loa.*
C. *Aspergillus.*
D. *Streptococcus.*
E. All of the above.

481. The following picture most likely represents the following clinical scenario:

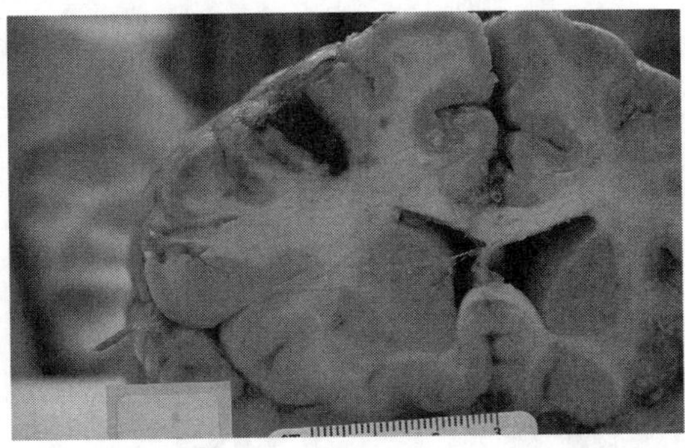

See color section following page 282.

A. A patient with a brain tumor with hemorrhage.
B. A patient with diffuse anoxic damage after cardiac arrest.
C. A patient with an acute ischemic stroke.
D. An elderly patient with ICH without chronic hypertension.
E. A younger patient with ICH with chronic hypertension.

482. The following picture is most likely associated with:

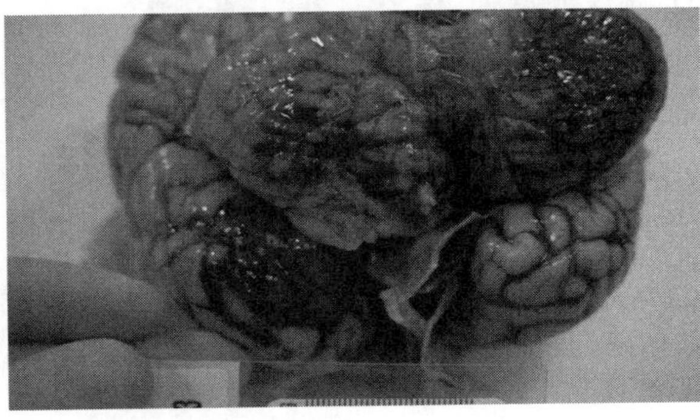

See color section following page 282.

A. Subdural hemorrhage.
B. A posterior communicating artery aneurysm.
C. Internal carotid artery stenosis.
D. Out-of-hospital cardiac arrest.
E. A vertebral artery dissection.

483. Which primary central nervous system (CNS) tumor may present with ICH?

A. Oligodendroglioma.
B. Pilocytic astrocytoma.
C. Anaplastic astrocytoma.
D. Ependymoma.
E. Ganglioglioma.

484. The following biopsy is most likely associated with:

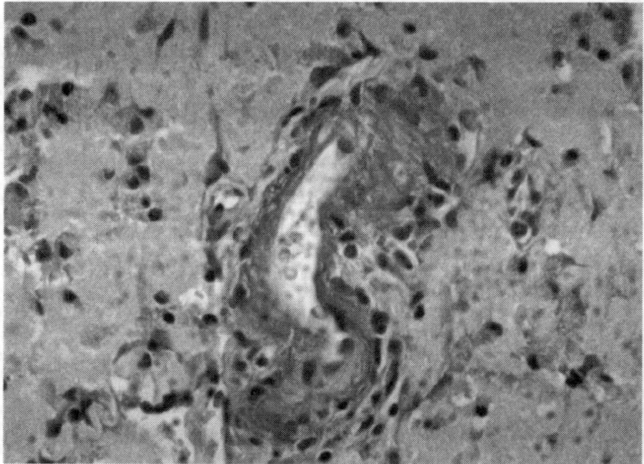

See color section following page 282.

A. A parietal lobe hemorrhage.
B. A thalamic infarct.
C. A basal ganglia hemorrhage.
D. A subdural hematoma.
E. An epidural hematoma.

485. The following picture most likely represents:

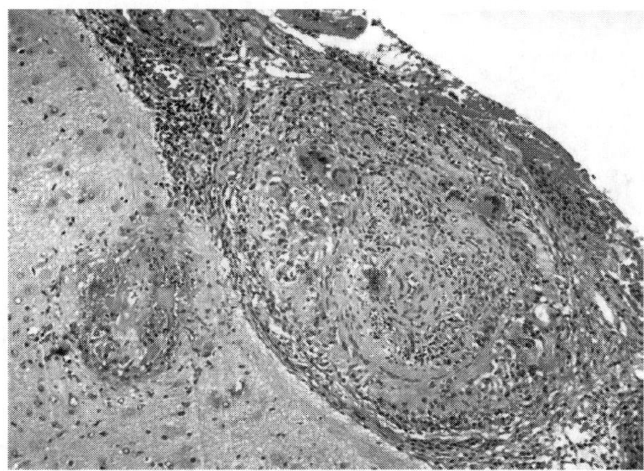

See color section following page 282.

A. Herpes encephalitis.
B. Granulomatous angiitis.
C. Acute ischemic stroke.
D. Bacterial meningitis.
E. Amyloid angiopathy.

486. What is does this brain biopsy show?

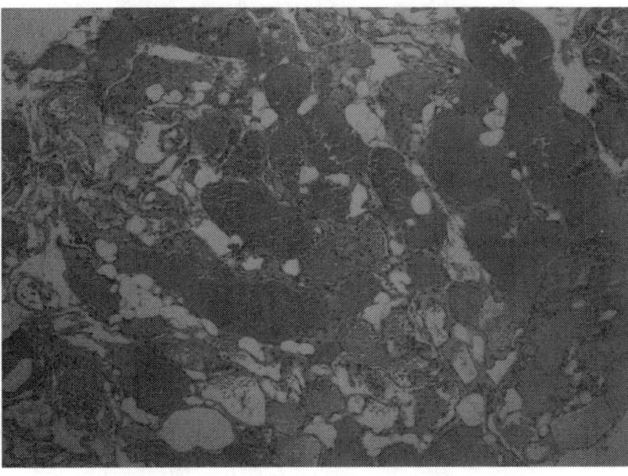

See color section following page 282.

A. Arteriovenous malformation.
B. Developmental venous anomaly.
C. Cavernous malformation.
D. Arteriovenous fistula.
E. Capillary telangiectasia.

487. Strokes due to the infectious agent shown in the image are generally caused by:

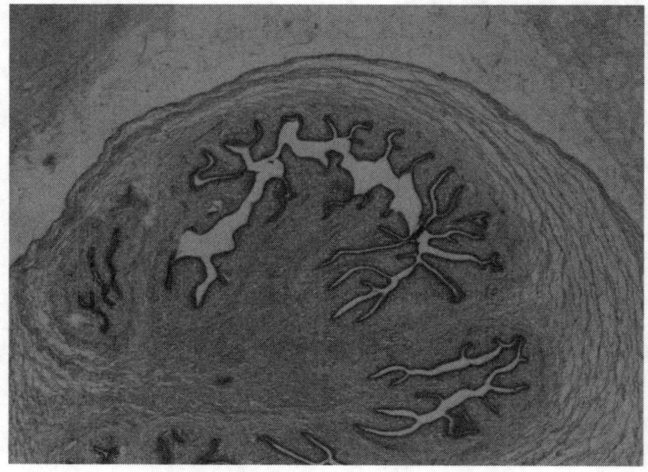

See color section following page 282.

A. Intracerebral hemorrhage.
B. Arterial dissection.
C. Cardiac embolization.
D. Cerebral arteritis.
E. Subarachnoid hemorrhage.

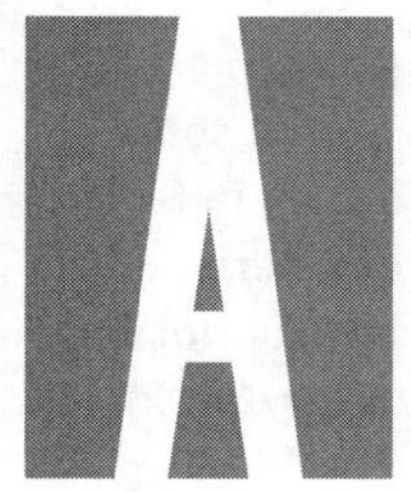

Clinical Pathology Answers

468. The answer is B. Arteries contain three distinct concentric layers. The innermost layer, the intima, consists of endothelial cells. The second layer, the media, contains smooth muscle cells. The internal elastic lamina separates the media from the third layer, the adventitia, which is composed of collagen, elastin, and fibrinous tissue. (Strandness, Chapter 9)

469. The answer is B. Atherosclerotic lesions occur most often in areas of low shear. Early intimal lesions are seen less often in areas of high shear stress. Shear stress increases prostacyclin production and endogenous tissue plasminogen activator production. The distribution and severity of atherosclerotic lesions in the aorta is not uniform, with the ascending aorta less affected by atherosclerosis than the abdominal aorta, despite low wall shear stress. (Shaaban & Duerinck, *AJR* 2000; Strandness, Chapter 9)

470. The answer is E. A variety of solid tumors are associated with metastatic intratumoral parenchymal brain hemorrhage. Melanoma, germ cell tumors, papillary thyroid cancer, renal cell cancer, hepatocellular tumors and lung cancer can all metastasize to the brain and lead to intracerebral hemorrhage. Brain metastases with hemorrhage from leiomyosarcoma have been reported but are very rare. Subdural hemorrhage can occur with dural or skull metastasis from multiple carcinomas, especially breast, prostate, and gastric carcinomas, as well as with leukemia and lymphoma. (Rogers, *Semin Neurol* 2004)

471. The answer is C. Multiple pathologic mechanisms have been suggested to explain cerebrovascular disease in systemic lupus erythematosus (SLE). Most of the known mechanisms are related to ischemic stroke in SLE patients. Although the incidence of ICH is increased in SLE, it is much less common than ischemic stroke. There is a very strong association between antiphospholipid antibodies and SLE, but antibodies to protein S are rarely seen in lupus patients. Valvular disease is common in patients with SLE, and it is a source of emboli in some patients. Cerebral vasculitis and cerebral arterial dissection occur rarely in SLE, as compared to more common mechanisms of cerebral ischemia of arterial origin involving premature cerebral atherosclerosis. Arterial vasospasm has not been associated with SLE related stroke. (Jennekens & Kater, *Rheumatology* 2002)

472. The answer is D. The majority (95%) of cases of cervicocephalic fibromuscular dysplasia involve the middle one-third of the internal carotid artery, often bilaterally. Involvement of the proximal internal carotid artery is rare. Intracranial arteries, generally the intrapetrosal internal carotid artery or carotid siphon, are involved in 7% to 20% of cases of cervicocephalic fibromuscular dysplasia. The extracranial vertebral artery may be involved in about 10% of cases. (Leary et al., *Curr Treat Opt Cardiovasc Med* 2004)

473. The answer is E. Cavernous malformations (cavernomas, cavernous malformations, cavernous hemangiomas) are composed of well-circumscribed sinusoidal vascular channels containing blood and blood products. They contain immature blood vessel wall components, lacking elastin, and an extensive smooth muscle layer. The lack of brain parenchyma intervening between the thin-walled vascular channels is characteristic of cavernous malformations. Although cavernous malformations were believed to always be congenital lesions, they can arise de novo. Previous irradiation, familial inheritance, pregnancy, viral infection, and biopsy-related seeding may be associated with development of cavernous malformations. The majority of cavernous malformations are supratentorial, most commonly in the frontal lobe, but they can occur in the infratentorial compartment or in the spinal cord. These are angiographically occult lesions that are best diagnosed on magnetic resonance imaging (MRI) with contrast, appearing as well-defined, lobulated lesions with a heterogeneous signal on T1 and T2 sequences. Their characteristic MRI picture results from thrombosis, fibrosis, calcification, and hemorrhage of varying acuity. Cavernous malformations may be found transmitted in families with localization to chromosome 7q11–22 in Hispanic Americans. De novo formation and hemorrhage may be more common in familial cavernous malformations. (Rivera et al., *Neuroimag Clin N Am* 2003)

474. The answer is C. Developmental venous anomalies (DVAs; previously known as venous angiomas) are the most common cerebral vascular malformation, occurring in approximately 4% of the population. They are sporadic anomalies that generally occur in cerebral hemispheres but rarely in the spinal cord, brainstem, or thalamus. They should not be excised as an incidental finding because they rarely hemorrhage, and they drain normal brain. Excision may compromise normal venous drainage and can result in hemorrhage. Developmental venous anomalies are commonly associated with cavernous malformations of the brain. Increased venous pressure from stenosis of the collecting vein may lead to the formation of a cavernous malformation through microhemorrhages into a capillary bed. The characteristic MRI picture of a DVA is of a group of radiating, linear flow voids (a "caput medusa") centered on a large collecting vein. (Rivera et al., *Neuroimag Clin N Am* 2003)

475. The answer is A. All the listed organisms can infect cardiac valves. In recent series *Staphylococcus aureus* surpassed *Streptococcus viridans* as the most common cause of infective endocarditis. This shift has been attributed to improved dental care and hygiene and the increase in nosocomial and healthcare-related infections. Factors associated with *S. aureus* endocarditis include chronic hemodialysis, diabetes mellitus, intravascular devices, and intravenous drug use. *Streptococcus bovis* is associated with gastrointestinal tract diseases. Pneumococcal endocarditis is rare, occurring most often in patients with splenectomy who are at risk for overwhelming pneumococcal sepsis. (Hoen, *Heart* 2006; Lindberg et al., *Scand J Infect Dis* 1998; Mylonakis et al., *N Engl J Med* 2001)

476. The answer is C. This brain was removed from a young woman who underwent chemotherapy and radiation treatment for a lymphoma. She developed a neutropenic fever with sepsis and disseminated intravascular coagulation and was intubated for respiratory distress. She was sedated and paralyzed on the ventilator, and her neurologic condition could not be assessed. When she died from the complications of her lymphoma, a left frontal hemorrhage was discovered on autopsy. (Graham & Lantos, Chapter 6)

477. The answer is B. This is an autopsy photograph of a man who occluded his left internal carotid artery, resulting in a massive left hemispheric infarct with swelling and fatal herniation. The dura on each side is resected to the center, revealing right and left hemispheres and both surfaces of the dura. Note the unilateral hemorrhage over the surface of the left hemisphere with clear parenchyma on the surface of the right hemisphere. The left hemisphere, with the dural covering peeled back, shows edema and hyperemic parenchyma consistent with a subacute infarct. There is no blood on either surface of the dura, as would be expected with a chronic subdural hematoma or an epidural hematoma. The leptomeninges are not cloudy from pus, as expected with meningitis. Subarachnoid hemorrhage would cause bleeding on the surface of both hemispheres. (Graham & Lantos, Chapter 6)

478. The answer is B. Focal or generalized intimal fibroplasia encompasses less than 10% of fibromuscular dysplasia (FMD). Angiographically, intimal fibroplasias presents as a smooth focal stenosis or a long smooth stenosis. Medial fibroplasia occurs in 75% to 80% of all FMD cases. Medial dysplasia has three subtypes: medial fibroplasia (angiographic "string of beads"), perimedial fibroplasia, and medial hyperplasia. Adventitial fibroplasia is quite rare. Endothelial dysplasia is a not a term for a type on FMD. (Leary et al., *Curr Treat Opt Cardiovasc Med* 2004)

479. The answer is E. Duret hemorrhages are found in the ventral and paramedian upper brainstem (mesencephalon and pons) after transtentorial and subfalcine herniations due to supratentorial mass lesions. During transtentorial herniation, when the uncus (the mesial hippocampus) slides under the tentorium, the midbrain is stretched; this ruptures small perforating vessels and produces hemorrhage. The precise pathophysiology of Duret hemorrhages may be both arterial (stretching and laceration of pontine perforating branches of the basilar artery) and venous (thrombosis and venous infarction). The diagnosis of Duret hemorrhages is made on computed tomography (CT) or MRI of the brain, and they presage poor outcome. The substantia nigra in the rostral midbrain is evident on this section, as a bilateral line of pigmented cells. (Parizel et al., *Intensive Care Med* 2002)

480. The answer is E. Bacteria (*Staphylococcus, Streptococcus, Salmonella*), fungi (*Aspergillus, Mucor*), and parasites (*Cysticercus, Angiostrongylus, Loa loa*) may cause direct vessel invasion and necrosis. (Mohan & Kerr, *Curr Rheum Rep* 2003)

481. The answer is D. The brain shows a hemorrhage in the cortical ribbon in a patient with cerebral amyloid angiopathy (CAA). Cerebral amyloid angiopathy is the most common cause of peripherally located ICH, particularly in elderly normotensive patients. Because of their common superficial locations, these may be associated with secondary subarachnoid hemorrhage. There is no evidence of edema or underlying mass lesion to suggest hemorrhage into a tumor. Severe diffuse anoxic damage may show laminar necrosis in the outer layer of the cortex. Less severe anoxic damage may not be evident on gross inspection. A hypertensive hemorrhage is generally found in deeper subcortical structures. (Graham & Lantos, Chapter 6)

482. The answer is E. This brain shows bilateral cerebellar and right occipital infarcts with hemorrhagic conversion. The territory of the infarction is consistent with embolization to the posterior inferior cerebellar arteries and the right posterior cerebral artery from a vertebral artery dissection. (Graham & Lantos, Chapter 6)

483. The answer is A. Oligodendrogliomas are vascular and may present as an ICH. The other primary central nervous system (CNS) tumor that is associated with hemorrhage is glioblastoma multiforme. The other tumors listed are not particularly likely to hemorrhage. (Graham & Lantos, Chapter 11)

484. The answer is A. Cerebral amyloid angiopathy (CAA) is characterized by extracellular deposition of fibrillar proteins (β-amyloid or Aβ) in the walls of blood vessels of the brain and meninges, with increased risk of lobar ICHs. This is the Congo-red stained biopsy of the brain of a patient with CAA. Thickening of the arterial wall is present, with an amorphous substance that is red with alkaline Congo stain, as seen above, and gives apple-green birefringence in polarized light. Deposition of Aβ, a cleavage product of the β-amyloid precursor protein, in the walls of cerebral blood vessels is seen in sporadic CAA, in CAA associated with Alzheimer disease, and in Down's syndrome, as well as in hereditary forms of CAA associated with ICH in young adults. (Graham & Lantos, Chapter 6)

485. The answer is B. The histopathologic picture of granulomatous angiitis is seen in Takayasu's arteritis, giant-cell arteritis, and primary angiitis of the central nervous system. This is a biopsy specimen of the leptomeninges in a case of granulomatous primary angiitis of the CNS, showing lymphocytes, histiocytes, and multinucleated giant cells. The thickened intima and adventitia are infiltrated with lymphocytes. Giant cells of Langhans' type (multinucleated giant cells) are found scattered in all layers. If the biopsy specimen were a superficial temporal artery, then this pathology would be consistent with giant cell arteritis. (Graham & Lantos, Chapter 6)

486. The answer is C. Cavernous malformations are compact vascular lesions that can be found anywhere in the brain or leptomeninges. As shown in this picture, they are composed of closely apposed, dilated, thin-walled vascular channels with little or no intervening brain parenchymal. Areas of calcification or even ossification may be present. A peripheral rim of hemosiderin deposition can be seen in the normal brain tissue, surrounding a cavernous malformation. A capillary telangiectasia is composed of dilated (ectatic) capillary-type blood vessels, separated by normal brain parenchyma. These lesions are generally found incidentally and rarely hemorrhage. The variably sized blood vessels in arteriovenous malformations are separated by normal or reactive brain parenchyma. Developmental venous anomalies are composed of dilated veins separated by normal brain tissue. (Graham & Lantos, Chapter 6)

487. The answer is D. The microscopic image is the scolex (head) of the *Taenia solium* (pork tapeworm). There are four suckers and two rows of hooks. Neurocysticercosis is the most common parasitic infection of the CNS and is endemic in tropical areas of the world. Fecal-oral contamination with eggs of *T. solium* leads to infestation of the CNS or muscles of humans, an intermediate host. Degenerated cysticerci calcify in the brain, causing multiple neurologic problems including seizures, focal signs, intracranial hypertension, or hydrocephalus. Cerebral arteritis has been reported in up to 53% of patients with neurocysticercosis. Small-vessel infarcts are the most common stroke type in neurocysticercosis. (Camargo, *Neuroimag Clin N Am* 2005)

9 Rehabilitation Questions

488. Match the stroke scale with its best measure. Use each answer only once.

A. National Institutes of Health Stroke Scale (NIHSS).
B. Barthel Index (BI).
C. Modified Rankin Scale (mRS).
D. Glasgow Outcome Scale (GOS).
E. Stroke Impact Scale (SIS).

1. Changes in emotion, communication, memory, thinking, functioning.
2. Outcome after brain injury.
3. Disability outcome after stroke.
4. Aspects of activity related to self-care and mobility.
5. Key components of a standard neurologic examination.

489. Acute inpatient stroke units:

A. Improve functional outcome from stroke but do not alter long-term survival.
B. Improve functional outcome and long-term survival and increase the number of patients who return home following a stroke.
C. Improve 6 week outcomes following a stroke but do not improve long-term independence or long-term survival.
D. Improve short-term survival but do not improve long-term survival.

490. The most important factor affecting outcome in stroke rehabilitation units is:

A. The amount and intensity of specialized therapy.
B. The provision of interdisciplinary services.
C. The provision of a multidisciplinary services.
D. Association with an acute hospital facility.

491. Which statement is correct about intermittent-pressure stockings to prevent deep venous thrombosis (DVT) following an acute ischemic stroke?

A. Stockings should be used only if a DVT develops.
B. No statistically significant effect is noted in the prevention of DVT when intermittent-pressure stockings are used.
C. Intermittent-pressure stockings should be used following acute stroke, but should be used in combination with low-dose subcutaneous heparin or low-molecular-weight heparin (LMWH).
D. Intermittent-pressure stockings should be used alone, because they are effective, and heparin is contraindicated following acute stroke.

492. Which statement is true for stroke patients who are unable to meet their own nutritional needs because of dysphagia?

A. No difference is noted in the outcome of patients fed via a percutaneous endoscopic gastrostomy (PEG) as compared to a nasogastric (NG) tube.
B. Nasogastric tube placement is preferable to PEG placement, because it is a less invasive procedure.
C. Outcomes are improved with the use of a PEG when compared to an NG tube.
D. Intravenous total parenteral nutrition is the best method of nutritional supplementation in stroke patients.

493. Which statement is true about urinary incontinence in patients hospitalized with an acute stroke?

A. Carefully managed use of Foley catheters does not increase the risk of urinary tract infections in the acute stroke.
B. Young patients have a greater incidence of urinary incontinence following an acute stroke.
C. Urodynamic studies are an essential part of the evaluation of stroke patients.
D. Fifty percent of stroke patients have urinary incontinence during the acute hospital stay, with 20% of stroke patients having incontinence 6 months following the stroke.

494. Which statement is true about speech therapy following an acute stroke in a patient with aphasia?

A. Recovery is nearly twice as good in patients with aphasia or dysarthria who receive speech therapy that begins within the first 4 weeks following a stroke.
B. Recovery is not aided by speech therapy unless it is started within the first 4 weeks following a stroke.
C. Unfortunately, speech therapy does not produce better outcomes in stroke patients with aphasia or dysarthria.
D. Inpatient speech therapy is more effective than outpatient therapy.

495. The most commonly used scale for measuring function following a stroke is also the one recommended by the American Stroke Association. It is:

A. The Barthel index (BI).
B. The Functional Independence Measure (FIM).
C. The Lawton scale.
D. The Rankin scale.
E. The Scandinavian Stroke Scale (SSS).

496. Inpatient rehabilitation services following major stroke:

A. Are only useful if continued physician and nursing care are required.
B. Are clearly more effective than outpatient rehabilitation.
C. Are not necessarily more effective than outpatient services.
D. Are not reimbursed by Medicare.

497. Constraint-induced motion therapy (constraining the normal limb to force the use of the abnormal limb) of the arm:

A. Is the most useful therapy for improving strength and fine motor skills of most patients following stroke.
B. Is extremely useful with 2 hours of training daily for 8 weeks.
C. Is useful in patients with cognitive deficits or aphasia, who will not respond well to verbal instructions.
D. Is useful only in patients with 20 degrees of wrist extension and 10 degrees of motion in each finger.

498. Functional electrical stimulation (a technique of applying electrical stimulation to a paretic muscle following stroke):

A. Improves muscle strength and motor control initially, but no evidence suggests improved function using this therapy.
B. Is most useful in patients with contractures developing several weeks after a stroke.
C. Should not be used in patients with glenohumeral subluxation.
D. All of the above.

499. Which of the following antispasticity medication is contraindicated in the acute stroke patient?

A. Tizanidine (Zanaflex).
B. Baclofen (Lioresal).
C. Dantrolene (Ditropan).
D. Diazepam (Valium).

500. Botulinum toxin:

A. Is useful in reducing spasticity and involuntary movements in several neurologic diseases, including stroke, but it is more effective in stroke patients when given with electromyographic (EMG) guidance.
B. Is more useful in controlling stroke-induced spasticity than is phenol/alcohol neurolysis.
C. Is of limited use because it produces sedation.
D. Is the treatment of choice in stroke patients with a history of myasthenia gravis.

501. Dextroamphetamine treatment in patients with severe strokes:

A. Does not improve functional recovery.
B. Improves functional recovery, but only if used in conjunction with physical therapy.
C. Improves early functional recovery if used in conjunction with physical therapy, but patients not treated with physical therapy only reach the same functional outcome with several months delay.
D. Improves functional recovery, with or without addition of physical therapy.

502. Recovery of motor function following stroke with severe hemiparesis:

A. May improve significantly between 6 and 24 months.
B. Cannot be predicted at 1 month.
C. Is essentially complete at 6 months.
D. Is independent of patient age.

503. The Extremity Constraint-Induced Therapy Evaluation (EXCITE) trial:

A. Used constraint-induced movement therapy (CIMT) on patients in the first 3 months after ischemic stroke.
B. Constrained the nonparetic leg to maximize function in the paretic leg.
C. Found benefit with CIMT that persisted for at least a year.
D. Used CIMT for 6 months to show any benefit.
E. Found no statistically significant difference between the two therapies that were compared.

504. The Barthel scale:

A. Measures acute neurologic dysfunction.
B. Measures activities of daily living.
C. Is a predictor of functional independence when the score is below 20.
D. Must be administered by a physician.
E. Requires face-to-face contact with the patient to administer.

505. Which of the following may be an effective adjunct to speech and language therapy in post-stroke aphasia?

A. Transcranial magnetic stimulation.
B. Piracetam (Nootropil, Myocalm).
C. Donepezil (Aricept).
D. Bromocriptine (Parlodel).
E. All of the above.

506. Match the disorder of speech and language with its best definition. Use each answer only once.

A. Aphasia	1. Impairment of speech intelligibility.
B. Dysarthria	2. Disturbance of semantics, phonology or syntax.
C. Apraxia	3. Impaired speech planning and programming.
D. Aphonia	4. Inability to speak.
E. Abulia	5. Decreased speech and movement.

507. Which statement best describes recovery after rehabilitation following cerebellar infarction?

A. Patients with cerebellar infarcts in general have poor functional recovery.
B. Patients with cerebellar hemorrhage have better functional outcome than do patients with ischemic cerebellar infarcts.
C. Patients with infarcts in the territory of the posterior inferior cerebellar artery (PICA) have better outcomes than do patients with infarcts of the superior cerebellar artery (SCA).
D. Functional Independence Measure (FIM) scores generally do not reach a level compatible with independence by the time of discharge from rehabilitation.

508. Which statement best describes post-stroke depression?

A. The definition of post-stroke depression is a worsening of the Hamilton depression scale by 10% of the estimated pre-stroke score.
B. Approximately 25% of potential patients are excluded from trials of post-stroke depression treatment because of communication problems/aphasia.
C. Antidepressants should be used with caution following stroke, because many of these agents hamper recovery.
D. According to the American College of Physicians, a new antidepressant should be changed after 6 weeks if no improvement is noted. Antidepressants should be continued for at least 4 months following recovery of symptoms.

509. Which statement about brain plasticity is true?

A. Stimulation of *N*-methyl-D-aspartate (NMDA) receptors may be detrimental.
B. γ-Aminobutyric acid ($GABA_A$) receptor antagonists may increase plasticity by enhancing long-term potentiation (LTP).
C. Serotonin has no impact on plasticity.
D. Mechanisms involved in plasticity are consistent throughout brain cortical regions.

510. Which statement best describes brain plasticity?

A. Animal studies have demonstrated improved performance in animals exposed to an enriched environment (one with general activities and game playing) following stroke, but only if this exposure occurs during the first weeks following the ischemic insult.
B. Animal studies suggest motor activity (e.g., wheel running, etc.) is more important to recovery following stroke than social interaction.
C. Learning and repetition will increase the number of dendritic spines in cortical areas representing the specific activities, but the volume of cortex related to these activities is unchanged.
D. Transient alterations of cortical representation areas may be common in everyday life.

511. Stem cells:

A. Are found in the brains of adult rodents but not adult humans.
B. Are found in adult human brains but are not capable of differentiating.
C. Are found in adult human brains and can differentiate into glial cells but not neurons.
D. Are found in adult human brains and can differentiate into neurons.

512. Pilot studies with hyperbaric oxygen following acute stroke suggest:

A. A trend toward improved outcome that does not reach statistical significance in treated versus sham patients.
B. A trend toward worsened outcome that does not reach statistical significance in treated versus sham patients.
C. Increased incidence of claustrophobia in treated versus sham patients.
D. The occurance of significant barotrauma in approximately half of treated patients.

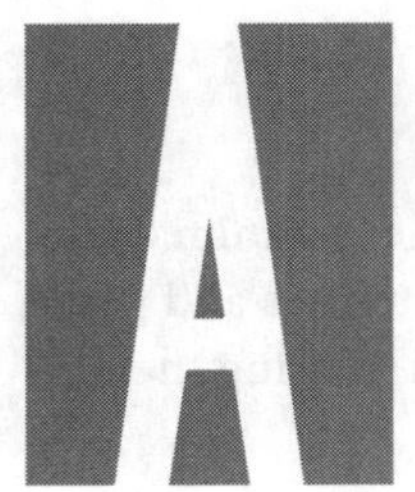

Rehabilitation Answers

488. The answer is A 5, B 4, C 3, D 2, E 1. The National Institutes of Health Stroke Scale (NIHSS) is a 15-item impairment scale that provides a quantitative measure of the key components of a standard neurologic examination. The best score is 0, with higher scores indicating increased neurologic impairment. The "maximum" score is not a useful concept because of the nature of the scale. For example, if hemiplegia is present, with the maximum score for motor dysfunction, the score for ataxia on the plegic side must be zero. Items involving aphasia will be scored generally with dominant hemispheric strokes, but neglect will be scored with nondominant hemispheric strokes. Some neurologic deficits found in patients with an ischemic stroke are not scored on the NIHSS. A flaw of this scale is that dominant strokes in general get higher scores than nondominant strokes with similar infarcted tissue volume. The Barthel Index (BI) is a scale that measures ten basic aspects of activity related to self-care and mobility, with a normal score of 100. The modified Rankin Scale (mRS) is a 0 (no symptoms) to 6 (death) score used to assess disability after a stroke. The Glasgow Outcome Scale (GOS) ranges from 1 (good recovery) to 5 (death) in the assessment of outcomes after acute brain injury. The Stroke Impact Scale (SIS) was developed from the prospective of patient and caregivers and asks multiple questions about emotional, cognitive, and functional aspects of the patients' stroke. (Kasner, *Lancet Neuro* 2006)

489. The answer is B. Stroke units provide both short- and long-term benefits, when compared to the outcomes of patients who are treated in standard hospital wards. All aspects of patient outcomes are improved, including functional scores, returning to home, quality-of-life scales, and long-term survival. Although the differences in treatment occur only during the first 6 weeks following the stroke, the differences in outcomes hold over the long-term. (Indredavik et al., *Stroke* 1999)

490. The answer is B. Interdisciplinary services are provided by a team that includes various types of rehabilitation professionals who communicate and plan carefully toward a common goal. The multidisciplinary team includes a similar spectrum of rehabilitation services, without the communication and common goals. The outcome of these services, independently delivered, is not as good as the results from teams that work closely together. Only a weak correlation with improved outcomes was related to the intensity of rehabilitation services. (Cifu & Stewart, *Arch Phys Med Rehab* 1999)

491. The answer is C. The use of pressure stockings alone is associated with a slight decrease in the incidence of DVT in patients with acute stroke, but this is not statistically significant. Only when used in combination with low-dose subcutaneous heparin or low-molecular-weight heparin (LMWH) is the difference significant. The combination is clearly more effective than either heparin/LMWH or pressure stockings alone. Low-dose heparin/LMWH is not contraindicated following an ischemic stroke. Intermittent-pressure stockings should *not* be used following development of a DVT, because this could dislodge a clot and produce a pulmonary embolus. (Kamran et al., *Neurology* 1998)

492. The answer is C. Percutaneous endoscopic gastrostomy (PEG) improves nutritional status (measured by weight, mid-arm circumference, and serum albumin) when compared to a nasogastric (NG) tube. This review suggests that the optimal time for post-stroke feeding and both drug and rehabilitation therapy for dysphagia has not been adequately studied. (Bath et al., *Cochrane Database Syst Rev* 2000)

493. The answer is D. Foley catheters can be useful in preventing skin breakdown, but removal should be considered after 48 hours to avoid risk of urinary tract infections. Patients with more severe strokes, diabetes, increased age, and the presence of other disabling conditions have an increased risk of urinary incontinence following stroke. There is no evidence for or against the routine usage of urodynamic studies in the stroke patient. (Duncan et al., *Stroke* 2005)

494. The answer is A. Individual studies and meta-analyses document improved outcomes in patients who receive speech therapy compared with those who do not. Although speech therapy starting more than 4 weeks following a stroke is still useful, earlier intervention is most successful. Centers that were previously inpatient facilities are now providing outpatient care instead, with decreased cost and comparable results. (Duncan et al., *Stroke* 2005)

495. The answer is B. The BI is a measurement of activities of daily living, including walking and grooming, but it does not measure other important functions such as balance, cognition, and muscle performance. The Functional Independence Measure (FIM) includes measures of social interactions and cognitive function, along with activities of daily living. The Lawton scale, developed in 1969, was the first activities-of-daily-living scale, but it is used infrequently now. The Rankin scale is a disability scale, not a measure of function. The SSS is a scale based on portions of the neurologic exam, similar to the NIHSS. (Duncan et al., *Stroke* 2005)

496. The answer is C. No study has demonstrated the superiority of one type of rehabilitation setting compared to others. Clearly, when continued physician and nursing services are required, inpatient rehabilitation is preferable, because these services are rarely available in the outpatient setting. Inpatient services do improve short-term outcomes, most likely because of the availability of physician and nursing staff, but long-term outcomes are not different. The multidisciplinary approach of the rehabilitation team is more important than the setting. The decision for inpatient rehabilitation depends in large part on patient safety issues and on the amount of social and family support available at home. Factors that often require inpatient services include incontinence, risks for skin breakdown, immobility, inability to perform activities of daily living, nutritional problems, and inability to manage medications. (Duncan et al., *Stroke* 2005)

497. The answer is D. Constraint-induced motion therapy is not recommended in all patients. The published trial included a relatively small number of patients. There are significant limitations to the therapy, including the need for 6 to 8 hours of training daily for 6 weeks. Patients with aphasia or cognitive deficits do not do well with this therapeutic approach. The therapy is not useful in patients who are plegic or who have movement restricted by contractures. The treatment is probably useful for a subgroup of patients, but this is not a standard recommendation for all stroke patients. More trials of this therapy are under way. (Duncan et al., *Stroke* 2005)

498. The answer is A. This technique has been used for years but is not considered the routine standard care. This technique is only useful in the first few weeks following an acute stroke. The populations in which it has shown utility include patients with shoulder subluxation and in gait training. (Duncan et al., *Stroke* 2005)

499. The answer is D. All the listed medications are approved by the U.S. Food and Drug Administration (FDA) for treatment of spasticity. They improve spasticity, but little evidence suggests an improvement of long-term function. Valium is contraindicated in the acute period because of evidence of the drug's interference with functional recovery following acute stroke. (Duncan et al., *Stroke* 2005)

500. The answer is B. Botulinum toxin is very useful in stroke-related spasticity, but there is no evidence of increased effectiveness when given with electromyographic (EMG) guidance. Phenol/alcohol is useful in reversing spasticity in stroke patients, but it is irreversible and has side effects that make it a less desirable choice. Botulinum toxin does not produce sedation, but it is absolutely contraindicated in patients with myasthenia gravis because it can increase the neuromuscular blockage that is already present in patients with this disorder. (Duncan et al., *Stroke* 2005)

501. The answer is A. Animal studies have suggested the utility of dextroamphetamine in recovery from stroke, but as yet no good clinical data support its use in stroke patients in general. One setting in which positive data is available is in the improvement of aphasia when used in conjunction with speech and language therapy. In patients with severe strokes, no motor improvement was noted with the addition of dextroamphetamine. (Gladstone et al., *Stroke* 2006)

502. The answer is C. Although improvement over years is recognized, functional recovery generally remains constant after 6 months. The level of 6-month recovery can be reliably predicted at 1 month to within 86%. Recovery is better in younger patients. (Umphred, 2001)

503. The answer is C. The Extremity Constraint-Induced Therapy Evaluation (EXCITE) trial was a randomized multicenter trial comparing usual rehabilitation therapy with constraint-induced movement therapy (CIMT). The patients wore a restraining mitt on the nonparetic hand for 3 to 9 months after an ischemic stroke. Therapy was continued for 2 weeks and showed persistent, statistically significant benefits. (Wolf et al., *JAMA* 2006)

504. The answer is B. The Barthel score measures walking, dressing, feeding, grooming, and bowel and bladder control. The maximum score is 100. A score of above 60 represents relative independence, with a score of 100 being the best level of function. It does not measure acute neurologic dysfunction. It is relatively simple to administer, not requiring specialized medical training, and can be determined by telephone with a reliable patient or a caretaker. It is frequently used in clinical trials as an outcome measure. (Ginsberg & Bogousslavsky, Chapter 90)

505. The answer is E. The supplementation of those neurotransmitters required for synaptic plasticity is an attractive idea for the pharmacotherapy of aphasia, and there have been some reports of utility for all of the agents listed However, clinical trial results are not particularly encouraging. Although some studies using transcranial magnetic stimulation have shown benefit, difficulties with treatment blinding hamper interpretation of the data. Piracetam, a γ-aminobutyric acid (GABA) derivative, has shown some weak benefit but the drug is not readily available in the United States. Donepezil, a centrally acting reversible acetyl cholinesterase inhibitor, may be of benefit but there have been no randomized trials in aphasic stroke patients. The dopamine D_2 receptor agonist, bromocriptine, has been evaluated with conflicting results. (Jordan & Hillis, *Curr Opin Neurol* 2006)

506. The answer is A 2, B 1, C 3, D 4, E 5. Cerebrovascular disease can cause multiple speech disorders. Aphasia and apraxia of speech are caused by dominant hemispheric lesions. Dysarthria can be due to multiple different upper or lower motor neuron lesions. Bilateral subcortical infarcts can cause aphonia. Abulia, a decrease in spontaneous speech and movement, is associated with lesions of the cingulate gyrus or the supplementary motor area. (Jordan & Hillis, *Curr Opin Neurol* 2006; Mohr et al., Chapters 6, 7, 11)

507. The answer is C. Patients with posterior inferior cerebellar artery (PICA) infarcts (Wallenberg syndrome) generally have better recovery than patients with superior cerebellar artery (SCA) infarcts. Patients with cerebellar infarcts in general have good recovery, with FIM scores compatible with independence at the time of discharge and continued improvement after discharge. Patients with ischemic cerebellar infarcts have shorter inpatient stays and better outcome following rehabilitation than do patients with cerebellar hemorrhages. Cerebellar edema from either hemorrhage or infarction, with herniation and hydrocephalus that is not surgically treated, can significantly worsen outcome. (Kelly et al., *Stroke* 2001)

508. The answer is D. Trials of depression after stroke have failed to yield clear treatment recommendations for several reasons. The use of appropriate diagnostic criteria, including depression scales, has not been systematically applied to post-stroke depression patients. A full 50% of stroke patients have been excluded from trials because of communication problems. The duration of treatment has been inadequate, with the average total duration of treatment being only 6 weeks. There has also been inadequate duration of follow-up to determine relative outcomes following treatment. The American College of Physicians suggests that antidepressants should be continued for 4 months or more beyond improvement and that treatment should be switched if no clinical improvement is seen by 6 weeks. Several antidepressive agents may have neuroprotective effects, but clinical efficacy for the prevention of depression after stroke or for improved stroke recovery has not been proven. (Hackett et al., *Stroke* 2005)

509. The answer is B. γ-Aminobutyric acid ($GABA_A$) antagonism stimulates long-term potentiation (LTP). Glutamate is an important excitatory neurotransmitter that has multiple mechanisms related to acute brain injury and recovery. Animal studies have shown *N*-methyl-D-aspartate (NMDA) receptor antagonists to be neuroprotective in acute cerebral ischemia, but translational studies to humans have been disappointing. Glutamate is an excitatory neurochemical that excites NMDA receptors and *enhances* brain plasticity. The inhibition of glutamate following stroke is a complex topic, because glutamate may enhance acute neuronal damage but may be necessary for recovery and plasticity. Serotonin may enhance plasticity, and trials of this category of antidepressant are underway as a treatment to ameliorate post-stroke depression while enhancing recovery. The mechanisms for brain plasticity are highly variable among different cortical regions of the brain. (Johansson, *Stroke* 2003)

510. The answer is D. Transient alterations of cortical representation areas have been demonstrated with learning tasks in human volunteers. Animal studies have demonstrated that an enriched environment is useful to stroke recovery, even when introduced as late as 15 days following stroke. Social interaction appears more important than motor activities. Repetitive activities do result in an enlarged area of cortical representation for that activity. (Johansson, *Stroke* 2003)

511. The answer is D. Stem cells in adult brains were first identified in rodents but have now been found in human brains. Differentiation into neurons has been observed in the dentate gyrus. The clinical implications of manipulation of endogenous stem cells is a subject of speculation at present. (Johansson, *Stroke* 2003)

512. The answer is B. Although statistical significance was not reached, the trend suggests that hyperbaric oxygen treatment does not help patients with acute stroke and may result in clinical worsening. Claustrophobia was the same in treated and sham patients as all entered the hyperbaric chamber. Only a single treated patient had symptoms of barotrauma. Trials of hyperbaric oxygen to improve chronic, established neurologic deficits due to ischemia are underway. (Rusyniak & Kirk, *Stroke* 2003)

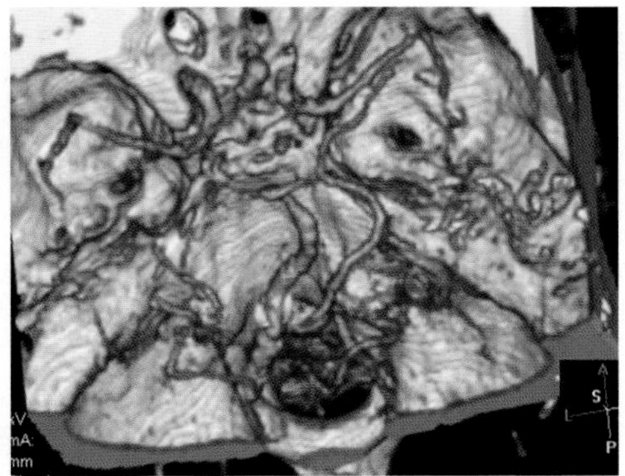

Answer 404

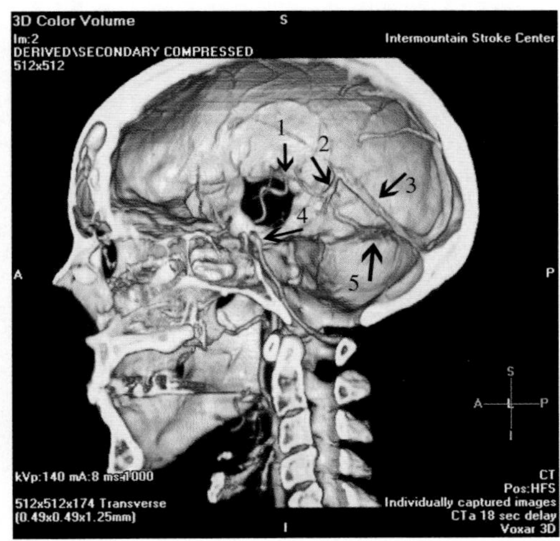

Question 415

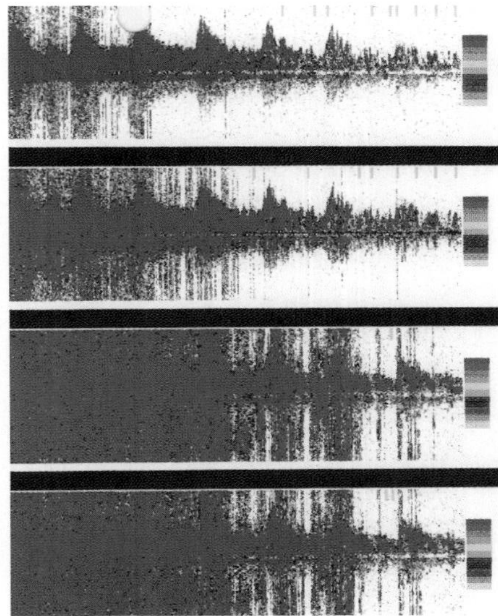

Question 422

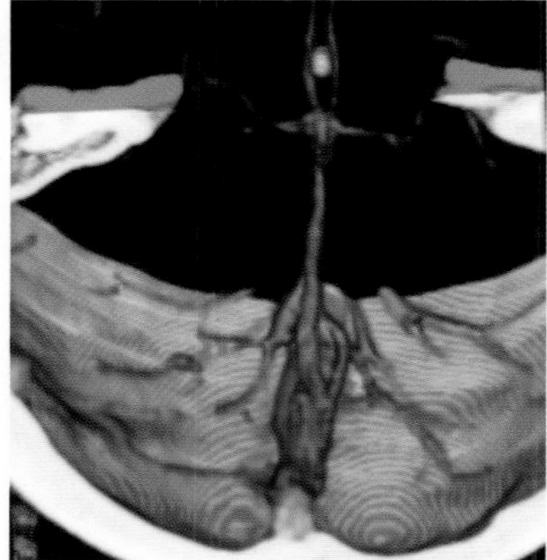

Question 434

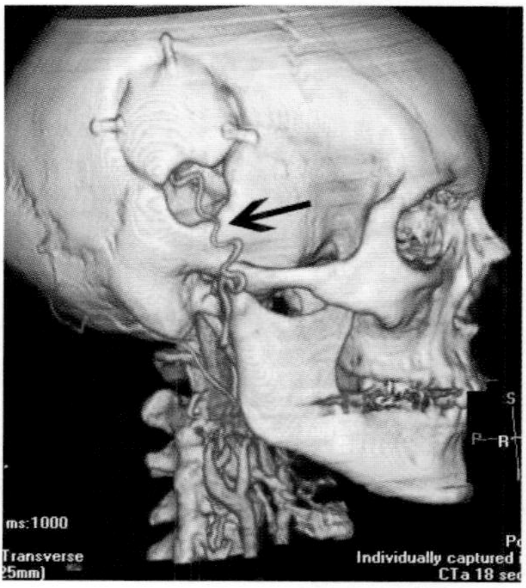

Question 435

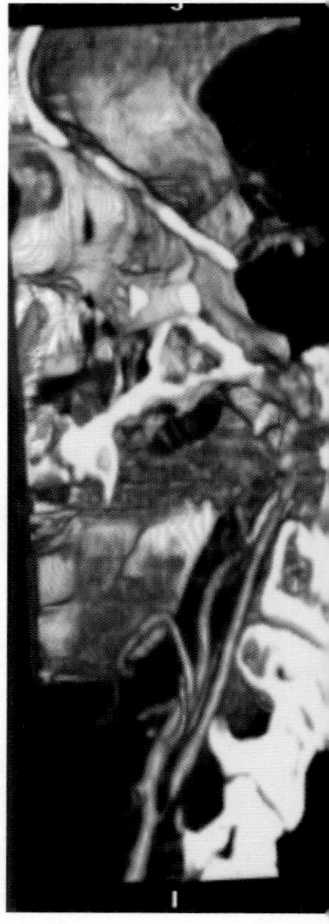

Question 450

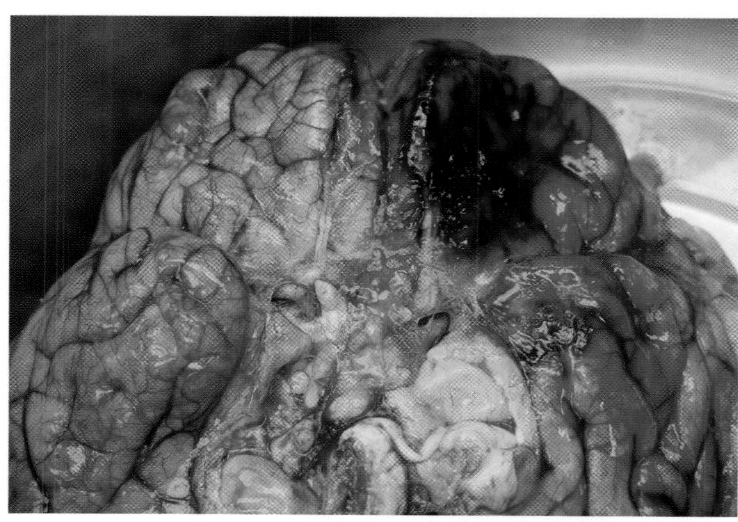

Question 476

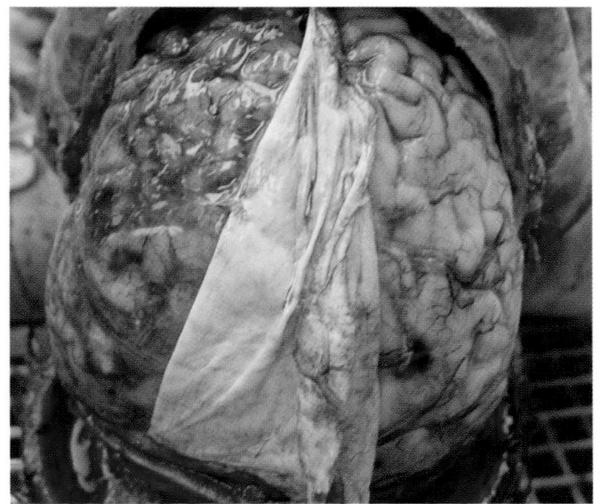
Question 477

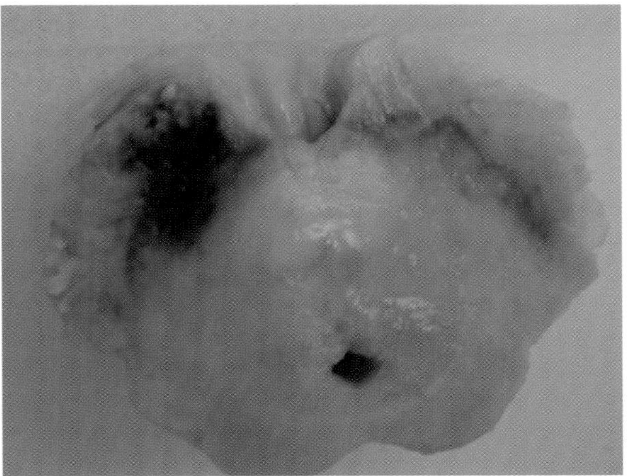
Question 479

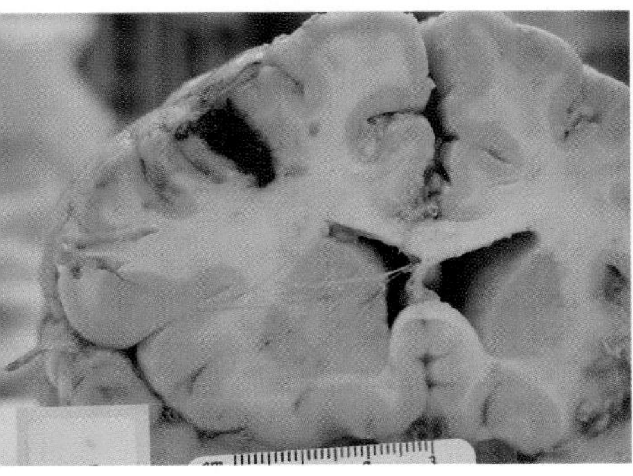
Question 481

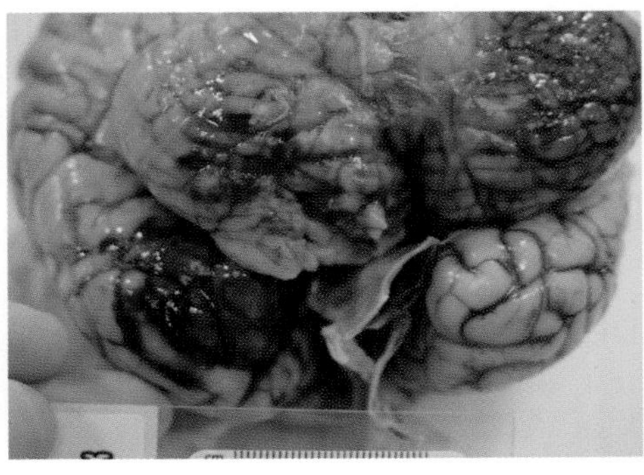
Question 482

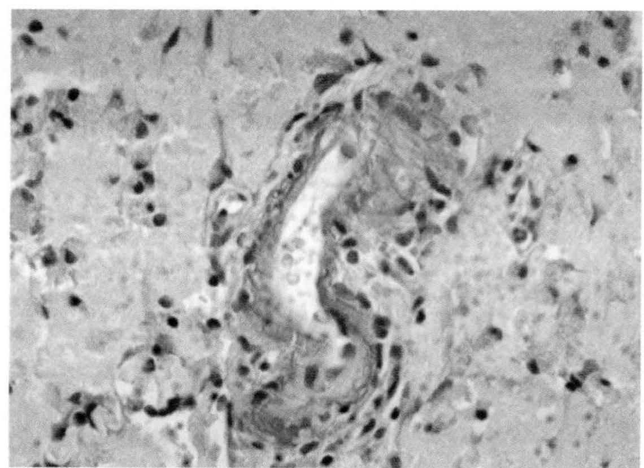

Question 484

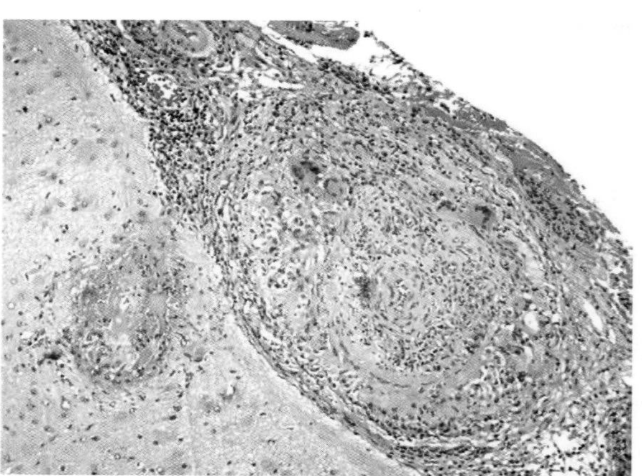

Question 485

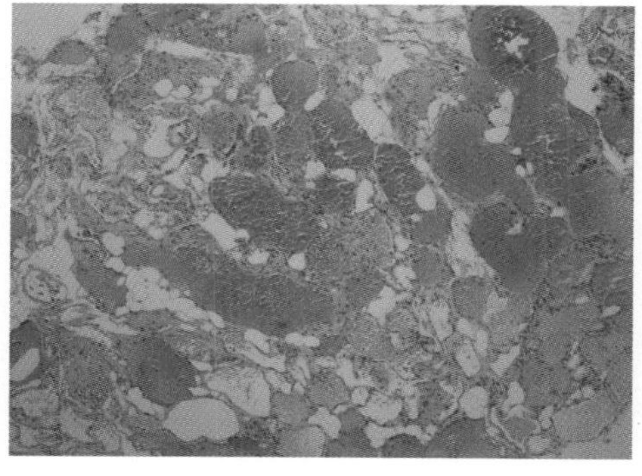

Question 486

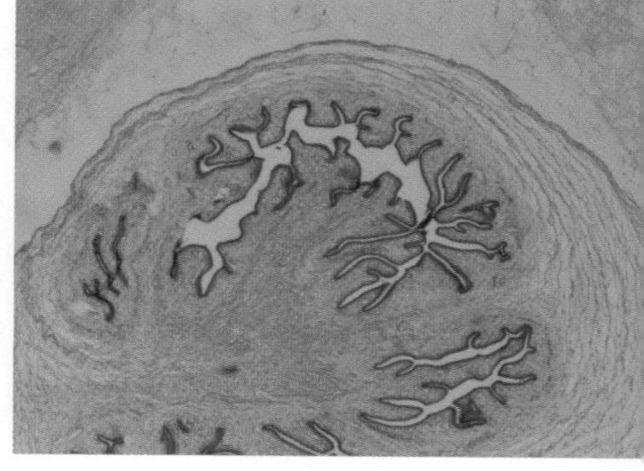

Question 487

REFERENCES

Adams HL, Jr., del Zoppo G, Alberts MJ, et al. Guidelines for the early management of adults with ischemic stroke. *Stroke* 2007;38:1655.

Adams HP, Powers WJ, Grubb RL, et al. Preview of a new trial of extracranial-to-intracranial arterial anastomosis: The carotid occlusion surgery study. *Neurosurg Clin N Am* 2001;12(3):613–661.

Adams RD, Victor M, Mancall EL. Central pontine myelinolysis: A hitherto undescribed disease occurring in alcoholic and malnourished patients. *Arch Neurol Psychiatry* 1959; 81(2):154–172.

Aguilar M, Hart RG, Kase CS, et al. Treatment of warfarin-associated intracerebral hemorrhage: Literature review and expert opinion. *Mayo Clin Proc* 2007;82(1):82–92.

Albers GW, Amarenco P, Easton JD, Sacco RL, Teal P. Antithrombotic and thrombolytic therapy for ischemic stroke. The Seventh ACCP conference on antithrombotic and thrombolytic therapy. *Chest* 2004;126;483S–521S.

Albers GW, Caplan LR, Easton JD, et al. Transient ischemic attack—proposal for a new definition. *N Engl J Med* 2002;347:1713–1716.

Alexandrov AV, Sloan MA, Wong LK, et al. Practice standards for transcranial Doppler ultrasound: Part 1 – Test performance. *J Neuroimaging* 2007;17:11–18.

Almawi WY, Tamim H, Kreidy R, et al. A case control study on the contribution of factor V-Leiden, prothrombin G20210A, and MTHFR C677T mutations to the genetic susceptibility of deep venous thrombosis. *J Thromb Thrombolysis* 2005;19(3):189–196.

Amarenco P, Bogousslavsky J, Callahan A, et al. for SPARCL Investigators. High-dose atorvastatin after stroke or transient ischemic attack. *N Engl J Med* 2006;355:549–559.

American Heart Association Statistics Committee and Stroke Statistics Subcommittee. Heart Disease and Stroke Statistics—2006 Update: A Report from the American Heart Association Statistics Committee and Stroke Statistics Subcommittee. *Circulation* 2006;113:85–151.

Anile C, Zahngi F, Bracali A, et al. Sodium nitroprusside and intracranial pressure. *Acta Neurochir* 1981;58:203–211.

Ansell J, Hirsch J, Dalen J, et al. Managing oral anticoagulant therapy. *Chest* 2001;119–122.

Arepally GM, Ortel TL. Heparin-induced thrombocytopenia. *N Engl J Med* 2006;355:809–817.

Ariyo A, Thach C, Tracy R, for the Cardiovascular Health Study Investigators. Lp(a) lipoprotein, vascular disease, and mortality in the elderly. *N Engl J Med* 2003;349:2108–2115.

Atlas SW, ed. *Magnetic Resonance Imaging of the Brain and Spine*, 3rd ed. Philadelphia: Lippincott, Williams, Wilkins, 2002.

Atmaca LS, Batioglu F, Atmaca Sonmez P. A long-term follow-up of Eales' disease. *Ocular Immunol Inflamm* 2002;10:213–221.

Attems J. Sporadic cerebral amyloid angiopathy: Pathology, clinical implications, and potential pathomechanisms. *Acta Neuropathol* 2005;110:345–359.

Bang OY, Saver JL, Liebeskind DS, et al. Cholesterol level and symptomatic hemorrhagic transformation after ischemic stroke thrombolysis. *Neurology* 2007;68:737–742.

Barnett H, Taylor DW, Eliasziw M, et al. Benefit of carotid endarterectomy in patients with symptomatic moderate or severe stenosis. *N Engl J Med* 1998;339:1415–1425.

Bartsch T, Alfke K, Stingele R, et al. Selective affection of hippocampal CA-1 neurons in patients with transient global amnesia without long-term sequelae. *Brain* 2006;129:2874–2884.

Bateman BT, Schumacher HC, Bushnell CD, et al. Intracerebral hemorrhage in pregnancy: Frequency, risk factors, and outcome. *Neurology* 2006;67:424–429.

Bath PM, Bath FJ, Smithard DG. Interventions for dysphagia in acute stroke. *Cochrane Database Syst Rev* 2000;CD000323.

Behrman RE. *Nelson's Textbook of Pediatrics*, 17th ed. Philadelphia: Saunders, 2004.

Belvis R, Leta RG, Marti-Fabregas J. Almost perfect concordance between simultaneous transcranial Doppler and transesophageal echocardiography in the quantification of right-to-left shunts. *J Neuroimaging* 2006;16(2):133–138.

Benseler SM. Central nervous system vasculitis in children. *Curr Rheumatol Rep* 2006;8:442–449.

Berge E, Haug KB, Sandset EC, et al The factor V Leiden, prothrombin gene 20210GA, methylenetetrahydrofolate reductase 677CT and platelet glycoprotein IIIa 1565TC mutations in patients with acute ischemic stroke and atrial fibrillation. *Stroke* 2007;38:1069–1071.

Berger C. Neurochemical monitoring of glycerol therapy in patients with ischemic brain edema. *Stroke* 2005;34;e4.

Berger JS, Roncaglioni MC, Avanzini F, et al. Aspirin for the primary prevention of cardiovascular events in women and men. *JAMA* 2006;295:306–313.

Bernstein RA. Reversible cerebral vasoconstriction syndromes. *Curr Treat Opt Cardiovasc Med* 2006;8:229–234.

Bertolaccini ML, Hughes GR. Antiphospholipid antibody testing: Which are most useful for diagnosis? *Rheum Dis Clin North Am* 2006;32(3):455–463.

Black DF, Bartleson JD, Bell ML, Lachance DH. SMART: Stroke-like migraine attacks after radiation therapy. *Cephalalgia* 2006;26:1137–1142.

Black DF. Sporadic and familial hemiplegic migraine: Diagnosis and treatment. *Semin Neurol* 2006;26:208–216.

Bodensteiner JB, Johnsen SD. Magnetic resonance imaging findings in children surviving extremely premature delivery and extremely low birthweight with cerebral palsy. *J Child Neurol* 2006;21:743.

Bogousslavsky J, Boller F. *Neurologic Disorders in Famous Artists.* Basel, Switzerland: Krager, 2005.

Bonaa KH, Njolstad I, Ueland PM, et al. Homocysteine lowering and cardiovascular events after acute myocardial infarction. *N Engl J Med* 2006;345:1578–1588.

Bousser M-G, JM Ferro. Cerebral venous thrombosis: An update. *Lancet Neuro* 2007:6;162–170.

Breen RA, Swaden L, Ballinger J, Lipman MC. Tuberculosis and HIV co-infection: a practical therapeutic approach. *Drugs* 2006;66(18):2299–2308.

Broderick JP, Adams HP, Barsan W, et al. AHA scientific statement: Guidelines for the management of spontaneous intracerebral hemorrhage. *Stroke* 1999;30:905–915.

Brott T, Broderick J, Kothari R, et al. Early hemorrhage growth in patients with intracerebral hemorrhage. *Stroke* 1997;281:1–5.

Brown DL. Sleep disorders and stroke. *Sem Neurol* 2006;26:117–122.

Brown DW, Dueker N, Jamieson DJ, et al. Preeclampsia and the risk of ischemic stroke among young women: Results from the Stroke Prevention in Young Women Study. *Stroke* 2006;37:1055–1059.

Brown RD, Flemming KD, Meyer FB, et al. Natural history, evaluation, and management of intracranial vascular malformations. *Mayo Clin Proc* 2005;80:269–281.

Brunton, LL, ed. *Goodman and Gilman's, The Pharmacological Basis of Therapeutics,* 11th ed. New York: McGraw-Hill, 2006.

Brust JC. The diagnosis and treatment of cerebral mycotic aneurysms. *Ann Neurol* 1990;28:590.

Buis, D.R., et al. Intracranial aneurysms in children less than 1 year of age; a systematic review of the literature. *Childs Nervous System 22;*2006:1395.

Burling JE. Aspirin prevents stroke but not MI in women; vitamin E has no effect on CV disease or cancer. *Clev Clin J Med* 2006;73:863–870.

Bushnell CD, Goldstein LB. Risk of ischemic stroke with tamoxifen treatment for breast cancer. *Neurology* 2004;63:1230–1233.

Bushnell CD. Hormone replacement therapy and stroke: The current state of knowledge and directions for future research. *Sem Neurol* 2006;26:123–130.

Cacoub P, Saadoun D, Limal N, et al. Hepatitis C virus infection and mixed cryoglobinaemia vasculitis: A review of neurologic complications. *AIDS* 2005;19: S128–S134.

Calabrese AT, Coley KC, DaPos SV, et al. Evaluation of prescribing practices: Risk of lactic acidosis with metformin therapy. *Arch Intern Med* 2002;162:434–437.

Call GK, Fleming MC, Sealfon S, et al. Reversible cerebral segmental vasoconstriction. *Stroke* 1988;19:1159–1170.

Camargo EC, Bacheschi LA, Massaro AR. Stroke in Latin America. *Neuroimag Clin N Am* 2005;15:283–296.

Caress JB, Cartwright MS, Donofrio PD, Peacock JE. The clinical features of 16 case of stroke associated with administration of IVIG. *Neurology* 2003;60:1822–1824.

Carrera E, Bogousslavsky J. The thalamus and behavior: Effects of anatomically distinct strokes. *Neurology* 2006;66:1817–1823.

Chagan L, Ioselovich A, Asherova L, Cheng JW. Use of alternative pharmacotherapy in management of cardiovascular disease. *Am J Manag Care* 2002;8:270–285.

Chan KC. Morphological variations of fossa ovalis atrial septal defects (secundum): feasibility for transcutaneous closure with the clam-shell device. *Br Heart J* 1993;69(1):52–55.

Chaturvedi S, Levine S (eds.). *Transient ischemic attacks.* Malden MA: Blackwell Futura, 2004.

Chaturvedi S, Lukovits TG, Chen W, Gorelick PB. Ischemic in the territory of a hypoplastic vertebrobasilar system. Neurology 1999;52:980–983.

Chavez-Vischer, V., et al. Benign nocturnal alternating hemiplegia of childhood: Six patients and long-term follow-up. *Neurology* 2001;57:1491.

Cheung AT, Pochettino A, McGarvey ML, et al. Strategies to manage paraplegia risk after endovascular stent repair of descending thoracic aortic aneurysms. *Ann Thorac Surg* 2005;80:1288–1289.

Chimowitz MI, Lynn MJ, Howlett-Smith H, et al. Comparison of warfarin and aspirin for symptomatic intracranial arterial stenosis. *N Engl J Med* 2005;352:1305–1316.

Chobanian A, Bakris GL, Black HR, et al. The seventh report of the Joint National Committee on Prevention Detection, Evaluation, and Treatment of High Blood Pressure. *JAMA* 2003;289:2560–2572.

Cifu DX, Stewart DG. Factors affecting functional outcome after stroke: A critical review of rehabilitation interventions. *Arch Phys Med Rehabil* 1999;80 (5 Suppl 1): S35–S39.

Coates DK, Paysse EA, Levy ML. PHACE: A neurocutaneous syndrome with important ophthalmologic implications. *Ophthalmology* 1999;106:1739–1741.

Comu S, Verstraeten T, Rinkoff JS, Busis NA. Neurologic manifestations of acute posterior multifocal placoid pigment epitheliopathy. *Stroke* 1996;27:996–1001.

Currier RD. Some aspects on Wallenberg's lateral medullary syndrome. *Neurology* 1961;11:778.

Cywinski JB, Parker BM, Lozada LJ, et al. Spontaneous spinal epidural hematoma in a pregnant patient. *J Clin Anesth* 2004;16:371–375.

D'Cruz DP, Khamaschta MA, Hughes GRl. Systemic lupus erythematosus. *Lancet* 2007;369:587–596.

Danik JS, Rifai N, Buring JE, Ridker PM. Lipoprotein(a), measured with an assay independent of apolipoprotein(a) isoform size, and risk of future cardiovascular events among initially healthy women. *JAMA* 2006;296:1363–1370.

Derdeyn CP. Positron emission tomography imaging of cerebral ischemia. *Neuroimag Clin N Am* 2005;15:341–350.

Di Nisio M, Middledorp S, Buller HR. Direct thrombin inhibitors. *N Engl J Med* 2005;353:1028–1040.

Dichgans M. Genetics of ischaemic stroke. *Lancet Neurol* 2007;6:149–161.

Diener HC, et al. European Stroke Prevention Study 2. Dipyridamole and acetylsalicylic acid in the secondary prevention of stroke. *J Neuro Sci* 1996:143;1–13.

Do TH, Fisch C, Evoy F. Susac syndrome: Report of four cases and review of the literature. *Am J Neuroradiol* 2004:25:382–388.

Drolet BA, Dohil M, Golomb MR, et al. Early stroke and cerebral vasculopathy in children with facial hemangiomas and PHACE association. Pediatrics 2006;117:959–964.

Droste DW, Kriete JU, Stypmann J, et al. Contrast transcranial Doppler ultrasound in the detection of right-to-left shunts. *Stroke* 1999;30:1827–1832.

Duncan PW, Zorowitz R, Bates B, et al. Management of adult stroke rehabilitation care: A clinical practice guideline. Stroke. 2005;36:e100.

Dussailant GR, Mintz GS, Pichard AD, et al. Small stent size and intimal hyperplasia lead to restenosis. *J Am Coll Cardiol* 1995;26:720–724.

Ehtisham A, Stern B. Cerebral venous thrombosis: A review. *Neurologist* 2006;12:32–38.

Elkind MSV, Cole JW. Do common infections cause strokes? *Sem Neurol* 2006;26:88–99.

Engelter ST, Fluri F, Buitrago-Tellez C, et al. Life-threatening orolingual angioedema during thrombolysis in acute ischemic stroke. *J Neurol* 2005;252:1167–1170.

ESPRIT Study Group Medium intensity oral anticoagulants versus aspirin after cerebral ischemia of arterial origin (ESPRIT): A randomized controlled trial. *Lancet Neurol* 2007;6:115–124.

Coakley FV, Panicek DM. Iodine allergy: An oyster without a pearl? *AJR* 1997;169:951–952.

Fiehler J. Cerebral microbleeds: Old leaks and new hemorrhages. *Int J Stroke* 2006:1:122–130.

Fields W, Lemak N. *A History of Stroke.* New York: Oxford University Press, 1989.

Fink JN, Selim MH, Kumar S, et al. Is the association of National Institutes of Health Stroke Scale Scores and Acute magnetic resonance imaging stroke volume equal for patients with right- and left-hemisphere ischemic stroke? *Stroke* 2002;33:954–958.

Flossman E. Genetics of ischaemic stroke: Single gene disorders. *Int J Stroke* 2006;1:131–139.

Franchini M. Advances in the diagnosis and management of von Willebrand disease. *Hematology* 2006;11:219–225.

Frangos SG, Chen AH, Sumpio B. Vascular drugs in the new millennium. *J Am Coll Surg* 2000;191:76.

Friedrich CA. Von Hippel-Lindau syndrome. A pleomorphic condition. *Cancer* 1999;86(11 Suppl):2478–2482.

Fukui M, Kono S, Sueishi K, Ikeazaki K. Moyamoya disease. *Neuropathology* 2000;20:S61–S64.

Fullerton HJ, Johnston SC, Smith WS. Arterial dissection and stroke in children. *Neurology* 2001;57:1155–1160.

Fullerton HJ, Chetkovich DM, Wu YW, et al. Deaths from stroke in US children, 1979–1998. *Neurology* 2002;59:34–39.

Furlan AJ. Unilateral visual loss in bright light. An unusual symptom of carotid occlusive disease. *Arch Neurol* 1979;36:675.

Fuster V, Ryden LE, Cannom DS, et al. ACC/AHA/ ESC Guidelines for the Management of Patients with Atrial Fibrillation. *Circulation* 2006;113:700–752.

Fuster V, ed. *Hurst's The Heart,* 11th ed. New York: McGraw-Hill, 2004.

Futrell N, Schultz LR, Millikan C. Central nervous system disease in patients with systemic lupus erythematosus. *Neurology* 1992;42:1649–1657.

Futrell N, Millikan C. Frequency, etiology, and prevention of stroke in patients with systemic lupus erythematosus. *Stroke* 1989;20(5):583–591.

Garcia-Monaco R, De Victor D, Mann C, et al. Congestive cardiac manifestations from cerebrocranial arteriovenous shunts. *Childs Nerv Syst* 1991;7:48–52.

Gardiner C, Williams M, Longair I, et al,. A randomised control trial of patient self-management of oral anticoagulation compared with patient self-testing. *Br J Haematol* 2006;132:598–603.

Garza CA, Montori VM, McConnell JP, et al. Association between lipoprotein-associated phospholipase A2 and cardiovascular disease: A systemic review. *Mayo Clin Proc* 2007;82(2):159–165.

Geisterfer AA, Peach MJ, Owens GK. Angiotensin II induces hypertrophy, not hyperplasia, of cultured rat smooth muscle cell *Circulation Res* 1988;62:749.

Gilman S, Newman SW. *Essentials of Clinical Neuroanatomy and Neurophysiology,* 10th ed. Philadelphia: F.A. Davis, 2003.

Ginsberg MD, Bogousslavsky J, eds. *Cerebrovascular Disease: Pathophysiology, Diagnosis, and Management.* Malden MA: Blackwell Science, 1998.

Gladstone DJ, Danells CJ, Armesto A, et al. Physiotherapy coupled with dextroamphetamine for rehabilitation after hemiparetic stroke : A randomized, double-blind, placebo-controlled trial. *Stroke* 2006;37:179.

Goldenberg-Cohen N, Curry C, Miller NR, et al. Long term visual and neurologic prognosis in patients with treated and untreated cavernous sinus aneurysms. *J Neurol Neurosurg Psychiatry* 2004;75:863–867.

Gonzales D, Rennard SI, Nides M, et al. Varenicline, an alpha4beta2 nicotinic acetylcholine receptor partial agonist, vs sustained-release bupropion and placebo for smoking cessation: A randomized controlled trial. *JAMA* 2006;296:47–55.

Gottesman RF, Sherman PM, Grega MA, et al. Watershed strokes after cardiac surgery: Diagnosis, etiology, and outcome. *Stroke* 2006;37(9):2306–2311.

Graham D, Lantos PL. *Greenfield's Neuropathology*. London: Arnold, 2002.

Grasland A, Pouchot J, Hachulla E, et al. Typical and atypical Cogan's syndrome: 32 cases and review of the literature. *Rheumatology* 2004:43;1007–1015.

Greenberg DA, Jin K. From angiogenesis to neuropathy. *Nature* 2005:438;954–959.

Greer IA. Anticoagulants in pregnancy. *J Thromb Thrombolysis* 2006;21:57.

Greer JP, Foerster J, Lukens JN, et al., eds. *Wintrobe's Hematology*, 11th ed. Philadelphia: Lippincott, Williams, Wilkins, 2004.

Gregoratos G, et al Cheitlin MD, Conill A, et al. ACC/AHA guidelines for implantation of cardiac pacemakers and antiarrhythmia devices. *J Am Coll Cardiol* 1998;31:1175–1209.

Grotta JC, Chiu D, Lu M, et al. Agreement and variability in the interpretation of early CT changes in stroke patients qualifying for intravenous rtPA therapy. *Stroke* 1999;30:1528–1533.

Gruhn N, Larsen FS, Boesgaard S, et al. Cerebral blood flow in patients with chronic heart failure before and after heart transplantation. *Stroke* 2001;32:2350–2353.

Guallar E, Hanley D, Miller ER. An editorial update: Annus horribilis for Vitamin E. *Ann Int Med* 2005;143:143–145.

Guttmacher AE, Callahan JR. Did Robert Louis Stevenson have hereditary hemorrhagic telangiectasia? *Am J Med Genet* 2000;91:62–65.

Hackett ML, Anderson CS, House AO. Management of depression after a stroke: A systematic review of pharmacological therapies. *Stroke* 2005;36:1092–1103.

Haines DE. *Neuroanatomy: An Atlas of Structures, Sections, and Systems*, 6th ed. Philadelphia: Lippincott Williams & Wilkins, 2004.

Halsey JH. Effect of emitted power on waveform intensity on transcranial Doppler. *Stroke* 1990;21:1573.

Hankey G, Eikelboom J. Aspirin resistance. *Lancet* 2006;367:606–617.

Harnsberger HR, Hudgins PA, MD, Wiggins RH, III, Davidson HC, eds. *Diagnostic Imaging: Head and Neck*. Philadelphia: Amirysys-Elsevier Saunders, 2005.

Hayward CP, Rao AK, Cattaneo M. Congenital platelet disorders: Overview of their mechanisms, diagnostic evaluation and treatment. *Haemophilia* 2006;12 Suppl 3:128–136.

Heart Protection Collaborative Study Group. Effects of cholesterol-lowering with simvastatin on stroke and other major vascular events in 20,536 people with cerebrovascular disease or other high-risk conditions. *Lancet* 2004;363:757–767.

Helgason CM, Bolin KM, Hoff JA, et al. Development of aspirin resistance in persons with pervious acute ischemia stroke. *Stroke* 1994;25:2331–2336.

Hennerici M, et al. *Vascular Diagnosis with Ultrasound.* Stuttgart: Thieme, 1998.

Heyer GL, Millar WS, Ghatan S, Garzon MC. The neurologic aspects of PHACE: Case report and review of the literature. *Pediatric Neurol* 2006;35:419–424.

Hirsh J, Warkentin TE, Shaughnessy SG, et al. Heparin and low-molecular-weight heparin mechanisms of action, pharmacokinetics, dosing, monitoring, efficacy, and safety. *Chest* 2001;119:64S–94S.

Hirsh J, Fuster v, Ansell J, et al. American Heart Association/American College of Cardiology Foundation Guide to Warfarin Therapy. AHA/ACC Scientific Statement. *J Am Coll Cardiol* 2003;41:1633–1652.

Hoen B. Epidemiology and antibiotic treatment of infective endocarditis: An update. Heart 2006;92:1694–1700.

Holmes KW, Kwiterovich PO Jr. Treatment of dyslipidemia in children and adolescents. *Curr Cardiol Rep* 2005;6:445.

Howington JU, Kutz SC, Wilding GE, Awasthi D. Cocaine use as a predictor of outcome in aneurysmal subarachnoid hemorrhage. *J Neurosurg* 2003;99(2): 271–275.

Hudson SJ, Brett SJ. Heterotopic ossification—a long-term consequence of prolonged immobility. *Crit Care* 2006;10(6):174.

Hugl B, Oldenburg WA, Neuhauser B, Hakaim AG. Effect of age and gender on restenosis after carotid endarterectomy. *Ann Vasc Surg* 2006;20:602.

Hunt WE, Hess RM. Surgical risk as related to the time of intervention in the repair of intracranial aneurysms. *J Neurosurg* 1968;28:14–20.

Indredavik B, Bakke F, Slordahl SA, et al. Treatment in a combined acute and rehabilitation stroke unit: Which aspects are most important? *Stroke* 1999;30: 917–923.

Intersocietal Accrediation Commission. www.intersocietal.org

Introcaso CE, Hivnor C, Cowper S, et al. Nephrogenic fibrosing dermopathy/nephrogenic systemic fibrosis: a case series of nine patients and review of the literature. *Int J Dermatol* 2007;46:447-452.

Jamieson DG, Fu L, Usher DC, et al. Detection of lipoprotein(a) in intraparenchymal cerebral vessels: Correlation with vascular pathology and clinical history. *Exp Mol Pathol* 2001;71(2):99–105.

Jamieson DG, Parekh A, Ezekowitz MD. Review of antiplatelet therapy in secondary prevention of cerebrovascular events: A need for direct comparisons between antiplatelet agents. *J Cardiovasc Pharmacol Ther* 2005;10;153.

Jennekens FGI, Kater L. The central nervous system in systemic lupus erythematosus. Part 1. Clinical syndromes: A literature investigation. *Rheumatology* 2002a;41:605–618.

Jennekens FGI, Kater L. The central nervous system in systemic lupus erythematosus. Part 2. Pathogenic mechanisms of clinical syndromes: A literature investigation. *Rheumatology* 2002b;41:619–630.

Jensen MB, St Louis EK. Management of acute cerebellar stroke. *Arch Neurol* 2005;62:537–544.

Johansson BB. Brain Plasticity and stroke rehabilitation. *Stroke* 2000;31:223.

Johnson DM, Kramer DC, Cohen E, et al. Thrombolytic therapy for acute stroke in late pregnancy with intra-arterial recombinant tissue plasminogen activator. *Stroke* 2005;36:e53–e55.

Johnston DC, Goldstein LB. Clinical carotid endarterectomy decision making: Noninvasive vascular imaging versus angiography. *Neurology* 2001;56(8): 1009–1015.

Johnston SC, Nguyen-Huynh MN, Schwarz ME, et al. National Stroke Association Guidelines for the Management of Transient Ischemic Attacks. *Ann Neurol* 2006;60:301–313.

Johnston SC, Rothwell PM, Nguyen-Huynh MN, et al. Validation and refinement of scores to predict very early stroke risk after transient ischemic attack. *Lancet* 2007;369:283–292.

Joo SP, Kim TS, Kim YS, et al. Clinical utility of multislice computed tomographic angiography for detection of cerebral vasospasm in acute subarachnoid hemorrhage. *Minim Invasive Neurosurg* 2006;49(5):286–290.

Jordan L, Hillis A. Hemorrhagic stroke in children. *Pediatr Neurology* 2007;36;73–80.

Jordan LC, Hillis AE. Disorders of speech and language: Aphasia, apraxia and dysarthria. *Curr Opin Neurol* 2006:19:580–585.

Jordan LC. Stroke in childhood. *Neurologist* 2006;12:94–102.

Juvela S, Kase C. Advances in intracerebral hemorrhage management. *Stroke* 2006;37:301–304.

Kallenberg CG, Heeringa P, Stegeman CA. Mechanisms of disease: Pathogenesis and treatment of ANCA-associated vasculitides. *Nat Clin Pract Rheumatol* 2006;2(12):661–670.

Kamran SI, Downey D, Ruff RL. Pneumatic sequential compression reduces the risk of deep vein thrombosis in stroke patients. *Neurology*. 1998;50: 1683–1688.

Kasner S. Clinical use and interpretation of stroke scales. *Lancet Neuro* 2006:5;603–12

Kasner SE, Gorelick PB, eds. *Prevention and Treatment of Ischemic Stroke*. Philadelphia: Butterworth Heinemann, 2004.

Katz U, Achiron A, Sherer Y, Shoenfeld Y. Safety of intravenous immunoglobulin (IVIG) therapy. *Autoimmun Rev*. 2007, 6:257–259.

Keane JR. Bilateral ocular paresis. *Arch Neurol* 2007;64:178.

Kelly PJ, Stein J, Shafgat S, et al. Functional recovery following rehabilitation for cerebellar stroke. *Stroke* 2001;32:530–534.

Kent DM. Stroke—An equal opportunity for the initiation of statin therapy. *N Engl J Med* 2006;355:613–615.

Khan IA, Nair CK. Clinical, diagnostic, and management perspectives of aortic dissection. *Chest* 2002;122(1):311–328.

Khuseyinova N, Keonig W. Apolipoprotein A-1 and risk for cardiovascular diseases. *Curr Athero Rep* 2006;8:365–373.

Kim JS. Internuclear ophthalmoplegia as an isolated or predominant symptom of brainstem infarction. *Neurology* 2004;62:1491–1496.

Kittner S, et al. Pregnancy and the risk of stroke. *N Engl J Med* 1996;335(11):768–774.

Koch C. Spinal dural arteriovenous fistula. *Curr Opin Neurol* 2006;19:69–75.

Koenig M, Kraus M, Theek C, et al. Quantitative assessment of the ischemic brain by means of perfusion-related parameters derived from perfusion CT. *Stroke* 2001:32:431–437.

Koenneck H-C. Cerebral microbleeds on MRI: Prevalence, associations, and potential clinical implications. *Neurology* 2006;66:165–171.

Kupersmith M. *Neurovascular Neuroophthalmology.* Berlin: Springer Verlag, 1993.

Kurnik K, Kosch A, Sträter R, et al. Recurrent thromboembolism in infants and children suffering from symptomatic neonatal arterial stroke. *Stroke*;2003:23;2887–2892.

Kurth T, Moore S, Gaziano JM, et al. Healthy lifestyle and risk of stroke in women. *Arch Intern Med* 2006;166:1403–1409.

Kurth T, Gaziano JM, Cook NR, et al. Migraine and risk of cardiovascular disease in women. *JAMA* 2006;296:283–291.

Kushner MJ. The clinical manifestations of pontine hemorrhage. *Neurology* 1985;35:687.

Laigle-Donadey F, Taillibert S, Mokhtari K, et al. Dural metastases. *J Neurooncol* 2005;75(1):57–61.

Lanthier S, Armstrong D, Domi T, deVeber G. Post-varicella arteriopathy of childhood. *Neurology* 2005;64:660–663.

Larrue V, von Kummer R, del Zoppo G, Bluhmki E. Hemorrhagic transformation in acute ischemic stroke. Potential contributing factors in the European Cooperative Acute Stroke Study. *Stroke* 1997; 28(5):957–960.

LaSar, CJ, Meier, GH, DeMasi RJ, et al. The utility of color duplex ultrasonography in the diagnosis of temporal arteritis. *J Vasc Surg* 2002;36:1154–1160.

Lavi E, Jamieson DG, Granat M. Epidural haemangiomas during pregnancy. *J Neurol Neurosurg Psychiatry* 1986; 49(6):709-712.

Leary MC, Finley A, Caplan LR, et al. Cerebrovascular complications of fibromuscular dysplasia. *Curr Treat Opt Cardiovasc Med* 2004;6: 237–248.

Lee MS. Movement disorders after lesions of the thalamus or subthalamic region. *Mov Disord* 1995;9:493.

Lee MC, Ausman JI, Geiger JD, et al. Superficial temporal to middle cerebral artery anastomosis. Clinical outcome in patients with ischemia of infarction in internal carotid artery distribution. *Arch Neurol* 1979;36(1):1-4.

Leikin JB, Clifton JC, Hanashiro PK, et al. Carbon monoxide poisoning. *N Engl J Med* 1999;340:1290.

Leonhardt G, Gaul C, Nietsch HH, et al. Thrombolytic therapy in pregnancy. *J Thromb Thrombolysis* 2006;21(3):271–276.

Levy A. Pituitary disease: Presentation, diagnosis and management. *J Neurol Neurosurg Psychiatry* 2004:75:iii47.

Lindberg J, Prag J, Schønheyder HC. Pneumococcal endocarditis is not just a disease of the past. *Scand J Infect Dis* 1998;5:469–472.

Long-Term Intervention with Pravastatin in Ischemic Disease (LIPID) Study Group, The. Prevention of cardiovascular events and death with pravastatin in patients with coronary heart disease and a broad range of initial cholesterol levels. *N Engl J Med* 1998:339;1349–1357.

Lonn E, Yusuf S, Arnold MJ, for HOPE 2 Investigators. Homocysteine lowering with folic acid and B vitamins in vascular disease. *N Engl J Med* 2006; 345:1567–1577.

Lopaciuk S, Bykowska K, Kwiecinski H, et al. Factor V Leiden, prothrombin gene G20210A variant, and methylenetetrahydrofolate reductase C677T genotype in young adults with ischemic stroke. *Clin Appl Thromb Hemost* 2001;7(4):346–350.

Loscalzo J. Homocysteine trials—unclear outcomes for complex reasons. *N Engl J Med* 2006;354:1629.

Love S. Apoptosis and brain ischemia. *Prog Neuro-Psychopharmacol Biol Psychiatry* 2003;27:267–282.

MacDonald MG, Mullet MD, Seshia MMK. *Avery's Neonatology*, 6th ed. Philadelphia: Lippincott, Williams, Wilkins, 2005.

Manco-Johnson MJ, Grabowski EF, Hellgren M. Recommendations for t-PA thrombolysis in chirldren. *Thromb Haemost* 2002;88:157–158.

Manelfe C, Larrue V, von Kummer R, et al, Association of hyperdense MCA sign with clinical outcome in patients treated with tissue plasminogen activator. *Stroke* 1999;4:769–772.

Maron DJ, Fazio S, Linton MF. Current perspectives on statins. *Circulation* 2001;101:207.

Marquez J, Flores D, Candia L, Espinoza LR. Granulomatous vasculitis. *Curr Rheum Rep* 2003;5:128–135.

Masdeu JC, Irimia P, Asenbaum S, et al. EFNS guideline on neuroimaging in acute stroke. Report of an EFNS task force. *Eur J Neurol* 2006;13(12):1271–1283.

Matsumoto M. Cilostazol in secondary prevention of stroke: Impact of the Cilostazol Stroke Prevention Study. *Atheroscler Suppl* 2005;6:33.

Matsumura A, Namikawa T, Hashimoto R, et al. Clinical management for spontaneous spinal epidural hematoma: Diagnosis and treatment. *Spine J* 2007;epublished.

Maxfield FR, Tabas I. Role of cholesterol and lipid organization in disease. *Nature* 2005;438: 612–621.

Mayer S, Brun NC, Begtrup K, et al. Recombinant activated factor VII for acute intracerebral hemorrhage. *N Engl J Med* 2005;352:777–785.

Mayer SA, Rincon F. Treatment of intracerebral haemorrhage. *Lancet Neurol* 2005;4:662–672.

Mehta SH, Adams RJ. Treatment and prevention of stroke in children with sickle cell disease. *Curr Treat Opt Neurol* 2006;8:503–512.

Messe SR, Silverman IE, Kizer JR, et al. Practice parameter: recurrent stroke with patent foramen ovale and atrial septal aneurysm: report of the Quality Standards Subcommittee of the American Academy of Neurology. *Neurology* 2004;62(7):1042–1050.

Mettinger KL, Ericson K. Fibromuscular dysplasia and the brain. *Stroke* 1982;13: 46–52.

Miyakis S, Lockshin MD, Atsumi T, et al. International consensus statement on an update of the classification criteria for definite antiphospholipid syndrome (APS). *J Thromb Haemost* 2006;4:295–306.

Mohan N, Kerr G. Infectious etiology of vasculitis: Diagnosis and management. *Curr Rheum Rep* 2003;5:136–141.

Mohr JP, Choi DW, Grotta JC, et al., eds. *Stroke: Pathophysiology, Diagnosis, and Management*, 4th ed. Philadelphia: Churchill Livingstone, 2004.

Molyneux AJ. Ruptured intracranial aneurysms—clinical aspects of subarachnoid hemorrhage. and the International Subarachnoid Aneurysm Trial. *Neuroimag Clin N Am* 2006;16:391–396.

Moore PM. Diagnosis and management of isolated angiitis of the central nervous system. *Neurology* 1989;39;167–173.

Morgenstern LB, Viscoli CM, Kernan WN, et al. Use of ephedra-containing products and risk for hemorrhagic stroke. *Neurology* 2003;60:132–135.

The Multi-Society Task Force on PVS. Medical aspects of the persistent vegetative state: First of two parts. *N Engl J Med* 1994;330:1499–1508.

Murugappan A, Coplin WM, Al-Sadat AN, et al. Thrombolytic therapy of acute ischemic stroke during pregnancy. *Neurology* 2006;66:768–770.

Mylonakis E, Calderwood SB. Infective endocarditis in adults. *N Engl J Med* 2001;345:1318–1330.

National Institutes of Neurologic Disorders and Stroke rt-PA Stroke Study Group. Tissue plasminogen activator for acute ischemic stroke. *N Engl J Med* 1995;333:1581–1587.

Nelson KB, Lynch JK. Stroke in newborn infants. *Lancet Neurol* 2004;3:150–158.

Newman MT, Matthew JP, Grocott HP, et al. Central nervous system injury associated with cardiac surgery. *Lancet* 2006;368:694–703.

North KN, Whiteman DA, Pepin MG, et al. Cerebrovascular complications in Ehlers-Danlos syndrome type IV. *Ann Neurol* 1995;38:960–964.

Ohira T, Schreiner PJ, Morrisett LE, et al. Lipoprotein(a) and incident ischemic stroke: The Atherosclerosis Risk in Communities (ARIC) Study. *Stroke* 2006;37:1407–1412.

Olesen J, Goadsby PJ, Ramadan NM, Tfelt-Hansen P, Welch KMA, eds. *The Headaches,* 3rd ed. Philadelphia: Lippincott Williams & Wilkens, 2006.

Ortiz G, Koch S, Romano JG, et al. Mechanisms of ischemic stroke in HIV-infected patients. *Neurology* 2007:68:1257–1261.

Osborn AG. *Diagnostic Cerebral Angiography*. Philadelphia: Lippincott Williams & Wilkins, 1999.

Osborn AG, Blaser SI, Salzman KL, eds. *Diagnostic Imaging: Brain*. Philadelphia: Amirsys-Elsevier Saunders, 2004.

Palumbo V, Boulanger JM, Hill MD, et al. Leukoaraiosis and intracerebral hemorrhage after thrombolysis in acute stroke. *Neurology* 2007;68:1020–1024.

Parizel PM, Makkat S, Jorens PG, et al. Brainstem hemorrhage in descending transtentorial herniation (Duret hemorrhage). *Intensive Care Med* 2002;28(1):85–88.

Pasqualin, A, et al. Intracranial aneurysms and subarachnoid hemorrhage in children and adolescents. *Childs Nervous System* 1986;2:185.

Pasternak RC, Smith CS, Bairey-Merz CN, et al. ACC/AHA/NHBI clinical advisory on the use and safety of statins. *J Am Coll Cardiol* 2002;40:567–572.

Patrono C, Coller B, Fitzgerald GA, et al. Platelet-active drugs: The relationships among dose, effectiveness, and side effects: The Seventh ACCP Conference on Antithrombotic and Thrombolytic Therapy. *Chest* 2004;126:234S–264S.

Patsalos PM, Fröscher W, Pisani F, van Rijn CM. The importance of drug interactions in epilepsy therapy. *Epilepsia* 2002;43:365–385.

Pessin MS, Kwan ES, Scott RM, Hedges TR III. Occipital infarction with hemianopsia from carotid occlusive disease. *Stroke* 1989;20:409–411.

Peter DA, Saxman C. Preventing air embolism when removing CVCs: An evidence-based approach to changing practice. *Medsurg Nurs* 2003;12(4):223–228.

Peyvandi F, Jayandharan G, Chandy M, et al. Genetic diagnosis of haemophilia and other inherited bleeding disorders. *Haemophilia* 2006;12 Suppl 3:82–89.

Physician's Desk Reference. Montvale NJ: Thompson, 2007.

Plehn JF, Davis BR, Sacks FM, et al. Reduction of stroke incidence after myocardial infarction with pravastatin: The Cholesterol and Recurrent Events (CARE) Study. *Circulation* 1999;99:216–223.

Pohl C, Kredteck A, Bastians B, et al. Heparin-induced thrombocytopenia in neurologic patients treated with low-molecular-weight heparin. *Neurology* 2005;64:1285–1287.

Pollick C, Taylor D. Assessment of left atrial appendage function by transesophageal echocardiography: Implications for the development of thrombus. *Circulation* 1991; 84: 223–231.

PROGRESS Collaborative Group. Randomised trial of a perindopril-based blood-pressure lowering regimen among 6105 individuals with previous stroke or transient ischaemic attack. *Lancet* 2001;358: 1033–1041.

Prokop M, Waaijer A, Kreuzer S. CT angiography of the carotid arteries. *JBR-BTR* 2004;87(1):23–29.

Qureshi A, Alexandrov AV, Tegeler CH, et al. Guidelines for screening of extracranial carotid artery disease: A statement for healthcare professionals from the multidisciplinary practice guidelines committee of the American Society of Neuroimaging. *J Neuroimaging* 2007;17:19–47.

Qureshi AI, Tuhrim S, Broderick JP, et al. Spontaneous intracerebral hemorrhage. *N Engl J Med* 2001;344:1450–1460.

Raphaeli G, Liberman A, Gomori JM, Steiner I. Acute bilateral paramedian thalamic infarcts after occlusion of the artery of Percheron. *Neurology* 2006;66:E7.

Rich RR, et al. *Clinical Immunology,* 2nd ed. New York: Elsevier, Mosby, 2001.

Ridker PM, Cook NR, Lee IM, et al. A randomized trial of low-does aspirin in the primary prevention of cardiovascular disease in women. *N Engl J Med* 2005;352:1293–1304.

Ringelstein EB, Knecht S. Cerebral small vessel diseases: Manifestations in young women. *Curr Opin Neurol* 2006;19:55–62.

Rivera PP, Willinsky RA, Porter PJ. Intracranial cavernous malformations. *Neuroimag Clin N Am* 2003;13:27–40.

Roach ES. Transient global amnesia: Look at mechanisms not causes. *Arch Neurol* 2006;63:1338–1339.

Rogers LR. Cerebrovascular complications in patients with cancer. *Semin Neurol* 2004;24:453–460.

Rolfs A, Bottcher T, Zschiesche M, et al. Prevalence of Fabry disease in patients with cryptogenic stroke: Prospective study. *Lancet* 2005;366:1794–1796.

Roman GC. Vascular dementia revisited: Diagnosis, pathogenesis, treatment, prevention. *Med Clin North Am* 2002;86:477.

Ronkainen A, Hernesniemi J, Puranen M, et al. Familial intracranial aneurysms. *Lancet* 1997;349:380–384.

Ropper AH, Brown RJ, eds. *Adams and Victor, Principles of Neurology,* 8th ed. New York: McGraw-Hill, 2005.

Ropper AH, ed. *Neurologic and Neurosurgical Intensive Care,* 4th ed. Philadelphia: Lippincott Williams & Wilkins, 2004.

Rose J, Mayer S. Optimizing blood pressure in neurologic emergencies. *Neuro Crit Care* 2004;3:287–300.

Rosen CL, DePalma L, Morita A. Primary angiitis of the central nervous system as a first presentation in Hodgkin's disease: A case report and review of the literature. *Neurosurgery* 2000;46(6):1504–1508.

Rosenschein U, Roth A, Rassin T, et al. Analysis of coronary ultrasound thrombolysis endpoints in acute myocardial infarction. *Circulation* 1997;95:1411–1416.

Rosenthal AD. Coronary hemodynamic effects of atrial natriuretic peptide in humans. *J Am Coll Cardiol* 1990;16:1107.

Rothwell P. Medical and surgical management of symptomatic carotid stenosis. *Int J Stroke* 2006;1:140–149.

Ruigrok YM, Rinkel GJ, Algra A, et al Characteristics of intracranial aneurysms in patients with familial subarachnoid hemorrhage. *Neurology* 2004;62:891–894.

Rumboldt Z, Castillo M, Solander S. Bilateral congenital absence of the internal carotid artery. *Eur Radiol* 2003;12:130–132.

Rusyniak DE, Kirk MK. Hyperbaric oxygen therapy in acute ischemic stroke. *Stroke* 2003;34;571.

Ryvlin P, Montavont A, Nighoghossian N. Optimizing therapy of seizures in stroke patients. *Neurology* 2006;67(Suppl 4):S3–S9.

Sacco RL, Adams R, Albers G, et al. Guidelines for prevention of stroke in patients with ischemic stroke or transient ischemic attack: A statement for healthcare professionals from the American Heart Association/American Stroke Association Council on Stroke: Co-sponsored by the Council on Cardiovascular Radiology and Intervention. *Stroke* 2006;37:577–617.

Sachdev GP, Ohlrogge KD, Johnson CL. Review of the Fifth American College of Chest Physicians Consensus Conference on Antithrombotic Therapy: Outpatient management for adults. *Am J Health Syst Pharm* 1999;56(15):1505–1514.

Salarani C. Polymyalgia rheumatica and giant cell arteritis. *N Engl J Med* 2002;347:261.

Sanna G, Bertolaccini ML, Cuadrado MJ, Khamashta MA, et al. Central nervous system involvement in the antiphospholipid (Hughes) syndrome. *Rheumatology* 2003:42:200–213.

Savitz SI, Caplan LR. Vertebrobasilar disease. *N Engl J Med* 2005;352:2618–2626.

Scandinavian Simvastatin Survival Study (4S), The. Randomised trial of cholesterol-lowering in 4444 patients with coronary heart disease. *Lancet* 1994;344:1383–1389.

Schaefer PW, Copen WA, Lev MH, Gonzalez RG. Diffusion-weighted imaging in acute stroke. *Neuroimag Clin N Am* 2005;15:503–530.

Schmahmann JD. Vascular syndromes of the thalamus. *Stroke* 2003;34:2264–2278.

Schrader J, Lüders S, Kulschewski A, et al. Morbidity and Mortality After Stroke, Eprosartan Compared with Nitrendipine for Secondary Prevention (MOSES). *Stroke* 2005;36:1218–1226.

Schmidt WA, Kraft HE, Vorpahl K, et al. Color duplex ultrasonography om the diagnosis of temporal arteritis. *N Engl J Med* 1997;337(19):1336–1342.

Schwedt TJ, Dodick DW. Patent foramen ovale and migraine: bringing closure to the subject. Headache 2006;46(4):663–671.

Schwedt TJ, Dodick DW. Thunderclap emboli: Embolic cerebellar infarcts presenting as thunderclap headache. Headache 2006;46(3):520–522.

Selim M. Perioperative stroke. *N Engl J Med* 2007;356:706–713.

Serfaty-Lacrosniere C, Civeira F, Lanzberg A, et al. Homozygous Tangier disease and cardiovascular disease. *Atherosclerosis* 1994;107(1):85–98.

Shaaban AM, Duerinckx AJ. Wall shear stress and early atherosclerosis. *AJR* 2000;174:1657–1665.

Sharshar T, Lamy C, Mas JL. Incidence and causes of strokes associated with pregnancy and puerperium: A study in public hospitals of Ile de France. *Stroke* 1995;26:930–936.

Sherman DG, Atkinson RP, Chippendale T, et al. Intravenous Ancrod for treatment of acute ischemic stroke. *JAMA* 2000;283;2395–2403.

Sievert H, Lesh MD, Trepels T, et al. Percutaneous left atrial appendage transcatheter occlusion to prevent stroke in high-risk patients with atrial fibrillation. *Circulation* 2002;105:1887–1889.

Silverman IE, Liu GT, Volpe NJ, Galetta SL. The crossed paralyses: The original brain-stem syndromes of Millard-Gubler, Foville, Weber, and Raymond-Cestan. *Arch Neurology* 1995;52(6);635–638.

Smith EE, Greenberg SM. Clinical diagnosis of cerebral amyloid angiopathy: Validation of the Boston Criteria. *Curr Athero Rep* 2003;5:260–266.

Smith RA. Risk factors, prevention and treatment of hypertension during pregnancy. *Minerva Gynecol* 2005;126:23.

Smith WS, Johnston SC, Skalabrin EJ, et al. Spinal manipulative therapy is an independent risk factor for vertebral artery dissection. *Neurology* 2003;60:1424.

Smith WS, Sung G, Starkman S, et al. Safety and efficacy of mechanical embolectomy in acute ischemic stroke: Results of the MERCI trial. *Stroke* 2005;36:1432–1438.

Spence JD, Bang H, Chambless LE, Stampfer MJ. Vitamin intervention for stroke prevention trial: An efficacy analysis. *Stroke* 2005;36:2404–2409.

Stam J. Thrombosis of the cerebral veins and sinuses. *N Engl J Med* 2005;352:1791–1798.

Stapf C, Mohr JP, Choi JH, Hartmann A, et al. Invasive treatment of unruptured brain arteriovenous malformations is experimental therapy. *Curr Opin Neurol* 2006;19:63–68.

Stapf C, Mast H, Sciacca RR, et al. Predictors of hemorrhage in patients with untreated brain arteriovenous malformation. *Neurology* 2006;66:1350–1355.

Stoll G, Bendszus M. Inflammation and atherosclerosis: Novel insights into plaque formation and destabilization. *Stroke* 2006;37:1923–1932.

Strandness ED, Ascher E, Haimovici H, Calligaro K, eds. Haimovici's Vascular Surgery, 5th ed. Oxford: Blackwell, 2004.

Strouse JJ, Hulbert ML, DeBaun MR, et al. Primary hemorrhagic stroke in children with sickle cell disease is associated with recent transfusion and use of corticosteroids. *Pediatrics* 2006;118:1916–1924.

Suarez JI, Tarr RW, Selman WR. Aneurysmal subarachnoid hemorrhage. *N Engl J Med* 2006;354: 387–396.

Subai BM. Chronic hypertension in pregnancy. *Obstet Gynecol* 2002;2:369.

Susac J, Murtagh FR, Egan RA, et al. MRI findings in Susac's syndrome. *Neurology* 2003;61:1783–1787.

Szkup P, Stoneham G. Spontaneous spinal and epidural haematoma during pregnancy: Case report and review of the literature. *Br J Rad* 2004:77;881–884.

Tang-Wai R, Webster RI, Shevell MI. A clinic and etiologic profile of spastic diplegia. *Pediatr Neurol* 2006;34:212–218.

Thom T, Haase N, Rosamond W, et al. Heart disease and stroke statistics—2006 update: A report from the American Heart Association statistics committee and stroke statistics subcommittee. *Circulation* 2006;113:85–151.

Tieleman RG, Gosselink AT. Efficacy, safety, and determinants of conversion of atrial fibrillation and flutter with oral amiodarone. *Am J Cardiol* 1997;79: 53–57.

Toole JF, Malinow MR, Chambless LE, et al. Lowering homocysteine in patients with ischemic stroke to prevent recurrent stroke, myocardial infarction, and death: The Vitamin Intervention for Stroke Prevention (VISP) randomized controlled trial. *JAMA* 2004;291:565–575.

Tormene D, Gavasso S, Rossetto V, Simioni P. Thrombosis and thrombophilia in children: A systematic review. *Semin Thromb Hemost* 2006;32:724–728.

Tumialan LM, Dhail SS, Tomak PR, Barrow DL. Alagille syndrome and aneurysmal subarachnoid hemorrhage: Case report and review of the literature. *Pediatric Neurosurg* 2006;42:57–61.

Ullrich NJ, Robertson R, Kinnamon DD, et al. Moyamoya following cranial irradiation for primary brain tumors in children. *Neurology* 2007;68:932–938.

Umphred DA. *Neurologic Rehabilitation*, 4th ed. Chicago: Mosby, 2001.

Van Gijn J, Kerr RS, Rinkel GJ. Subarachnoid hemorrhage. *Lancet* 2007;369:306–318.

von Kummer R. Early major ischemic changes on computed tomography should preclude use of tissue plasminogen activator. *Stroke* 2003;34:820–821.

Wannamethee SG, Shaper AG, Lennon L, Morris RW. Metabolic syndrome vs Framingham Risk Score for prediction of coronary heart disease, stroke, and type 2 diabetes mellitus. *Arch Int Med* 2005:165:2644–2650.

Weinberger J. Adverse effects and drug interactions of antithrombotic agents used in prevention of ischaemic stroke. *Drugs* 2005;66(4):461–471.

Weitz JI, Bates SM. New anticoagulants. *J Thromb Haemost* 2005;3:1843–1853.

West SG. Central nervous system vasculitis. *Curr Rheum Rep* 2003;5:116–127.

Westhout F, Hasso A, Jalili M, et al. Lemierre syndrome complicated by cavernous sinus thrombosis, the development of subdural empyemas, and internal carotid artery narrowing without cerebral infarction. Case report. *J Neurosurg* 2007;106(1 Suppl):53–56.

Wiebers DO. Unruptured intracranial aneurysms: Natural history and clinical management. Update on the International Study of Unruptured Intracranial Aneurysms. *Neuroimag Clin N Am* 2006;16:383–390.

Wiegman A, Hutten BA, de Groot E, et al. Efficacy and safety of statin therapy in children with familial hypercholesterolemia: A randomized controlled trial. *JAMA* 2004;292:331–337.

Wijdicks E, Hijdra A, Young GB, et al. Practice parameter: Prediction of outcome in comatose survivors after cardiopulmonary resuscitation. *Neurology* 2006;67:203–210.

Wolf SL, Winstein CJ, Miller JP, et al. Effect of constraint-induced movement therapy on upper extremity function 3 to 9 months after stroke: The EXCITE randomized clinical trial. *JAMA* 2006;296:2095–2104.

Wong R, Bequelin GZ, de Lima M, et al. Tacrolimus-associated posterior reversible encephalopathy syndrome after allogenic hematopoietic stem cell transplantation. *Br J Haemat* 2003;122:128–134.

Woo D, Kissela BM, Khoury JC, et al. Hypercholesterolemia, HMG-CoA reductase inhibitors, and risk of intracerebral hemorrhage: A case-control study. *Stroke* 2004;6;1360–1364.

Wu O, Robertson L, Langhorne P, et al. Oral contraceptives, hormone replacement therapy, thrombophilias and risk of venous thromboembolism: A systematic review. The Thrombosis: Risk and Economic Assessment of Thrombophilia Screening (TREATS) Study. *Thromb Haemost* 2005;94(1):17–25.

Yadav JS, Roubin GS, King P, Iyer S, et al. Angioplasty and stenting for restenosis after carotid endarterectomy. *Stroke* 1996;27:2075–2079.

Yaggi HK, Concato J, Kernan WN, et al. Obstructive sleep apnea as a risk factor for stroke and death. *N Engl J Med* 2005;353:2034–2041.

ABBREVIATIONS

ACA	anterior cerebral artery
ACE	angiotensin-converting enzyme
ADC	apparent diffusion coefficient
AED	antiepileptic drug
AF	atrial fibrillation
AGS	Alagille syndrome
AIF	apoptosis-inducing factor
ANA	antinuclear antibody
ANCA	antineutrophilic cytoplasmic antibodies
APMPPE	acute posterior multifocal placoid pigment epitheliopathy
apoA-1	apolipoprotein A-1
APS	antiphospholipid syndrome
aPTT	activated partial thromboplastin time
ARB	angiotensin receptor blocker
ASD	atrial septal defect
ATP	adenosine triphosphate
AV	atrioventricular
AVM	arteriovenous malformation
BI	Barthel Index
BMI	body mass index
CAA	cerebral amyloid angiopathy
CADASIL	cerebral autosomal dominant arteriopathy with subcortical infarcts and leukoencephalopathy

CBF	cerebral blood flow
CBV	cerebral blood volume
CCF	carotid cavernous fistula
CEA	carotid endarterectomy
CIMT	constraint-induced movement therapy
CK	creatine kinase
CMRO2	cerebral metabolic rate of oxygen
CMV	cytomegalovirus
CNS	central nervous system
C-RP	C-reactive protein
CSF	cerebrospinal fluid
CT	computed tomography
CTA	computed tomography angiography
CVT	cerebral venous thrombosis
DBP	diastolic blood pressure
DHE	dihydroergotamine
DIC	disseminated intravascular coagulopathy
dRVVT	dilute Russell's viper venom time
DVA	developmental venous anomaly
DVT	deep vein thrombosis
DWI	diffusion-weighted imaging
ECA	external carotid artery
ECG	electrocardiogram
EC-IC	extracranial-intracranial
EDS	Ehlers-Danlos syndrome
EEG	electroencephalogram
EMG	electromyogram
ESR	erythrocyte sedimentation rate
FDA	Food and Drug Administration
FDF	fibroblast-derived growth factor
FFP	fresh frozen plasma
FHM	familial hemiplegic migraine
FIM	Functional Independence Measure

FLAIR	fluid-attenuation inversion recovery
FMD	fibromuscular dysplasia
GABA	γ-aminobutyric acid
GI	gastrointestinal
GOS	Glasgow Outcome Scale
GRE	gradient echo
HCV	hepatitis C virus
HDL	high-density lipoprotein
HHT	hereditary hemorrhagic telangiectasia
HIF	hypoxia Inducible factor
HIT	heparin-induced thrombocytopenia
HIV	human immunodeficiency virus
HMGCoA	3-hydroxy-3-methylglutaryl coenzyme A
HRT	hormone replacement therapy
HTN	hypertension
ICA	internal carotid artery
ICD	intracardiac defibrillator
ICH	intracerebral hemorrhage
ICP	intracranial pressure
Ig	immunoglobulin
INO	internuclear ophthalmoplegia
INR	international normalized ratio
ITP	idiopathic thrombocytopenic purpura
IVIG	intravenous immunoglobulin
LA	lupus anticoagulant
LDL	low-density lipoprotein
LMWH	low-molecular-weight heparin
Lp-PL	A2 lipoprotein-associated phospholipase A2
LTP	long-term potentiation
MAP	mean arterial pressure
MCA	middle cerebral artery
MELAS	mitochondrial encephalomyopathy lactic acidosis and stroke-like symptoms

MMP	matrix metalloproteinases
MRA	magnetic resonance angiography
MRI	magnetic resonance imaging
mRS	modified Rankin Scale
MTHFR	methylenetetrahydrofolate reductase
MTT	mean transit time
NG	nasogastric
NIHSS	National Institutes of Health Stroke Scale
NINDS	National Institutes of Neurologic Disorders
NMDA	*N*-methyl-D-aspartate
NO	nitric oxide
NOS	nitric oxide synthase
NSE	neuron-specific enolase
OA	ophthalmic artery
OEF	oxygen extraction fraction
OPG	oculoplethysmography
OSA	obstructive sleep apnea
PACNS	primary angiitis of the central nervous system
PCA	posterior cerebral artery
PCC	prothrombin complex concentrate
PDGF	platelet-derived growth factor
PEG	percutaneous endoscopic gastrostomy
PFO	patent foramen ovale
PHACE	posterior fossa malformations, hemangiomas, arterial anomalies, coarctation of the aorta and other cardiac defects, and eye abnormalities
PRES	posterior reversible encephalopathy syndrome
PSV	peak systolic velocities
PT	prothrombin time
PTT	partial thromboplastin time
PWI	perfusion-weighted imaging
RCVS	reversible cerebral vasoconstriction syndrome
RRR	relative risk reduction

SAH	subarachnoid hemorrhage
SBP	systolic blood pressure
SCA	superior cerebellar artery
SCD	sickle cell disease
SDAVF	spinal dural arteriovenous fistula
SIS	Stroke Impact Scale
SLE	systemic lupus erythematosus
SMART	stroke-like migraine attacks after radiation therapy
SMT	spinal manipulative therapy
SPECT	single-photon emission tomography
TCD	transcranial Doppler
TEE	transesophageal echocardiograph
TGA	transient global amnesia
TIA	transient ischemic attack
t-PA	tissue plasminogen
TSH	thyroid-stimulating hormone
TTE	transthoracic echocardiograph
TTP	thrombotic thrombocytopenic purpura
VEGF	vascular endothelial growth factor
VLDL	very-low-density lipoprotein
VZV	Varicella zoster virus
WPW	Wolff-Parkinson-White